Hoyle Leigh

Genes, Memes, Culture, and Mental Illness

Toward an Integrative Model

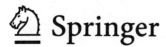 Springer

Hoyle Leigh
University of California
San Francisco
California
USA
hoyle.leigh@ucsf.edu

ISBN 978-1-4419-5670-5 (hardcover)   e-ISBN 978-1-4419-5671-2
ISBN 978-1-4614-0239-8 (softcover)
DOI 10.1007/978-1-4419-5671-2
Springer New York Dordrecht Heidelberg London

Library of Congress Control Number: 2010921915

Printed on acid-free paper

Springer is part of Springer Science+Business Media (www.springer.com)

For Vinnie,
My Partner in this Epigenetic Journey
Of Genes, Memes, Culture, and much more....

Preface

How do genes interact with the environment? How does the environment actually enter the body to affect the genes? When we perceive the environment, bits of information are encoded within the brain as memory, which consists of a series of neural connections, a brain code (see Chapter 9). When perception occurs, the new sensory input interacts with existing memory and creates new memory.

Primitive memory formed by trial and error died with the organism. With the evolution of complex brains, however, memory in the form of brain codes acquired the ability to skip from one brain to another, first by imitation as a shortcut to trial and error, and later, with language, as knowledge and information. When memory achieved portability, it became *memes*, bits of replicating information (see Chapters 8 and 9). Memes, like genes, undergo Darwinian evolution in a complex relationship with genes. In our time, it is the gene × meme × environment interaction that is fundamental in understanding mental health and illness.

This book integrates the concepts of genes and memes in understanding mental illness as a final common pathway brain dysfunction. The brain dysfunction is manifested by the symptoms and signs of mental illness that are determined by both genes and memes.

In Part I. What is Mental Illness? An Epigenetic Model, we consider the current model of mental illness based on gene × environment interaction and stress. The concept of epigenesis – how genes are switched on or off by the environment – is discussed. I introduce the concept of memes as perception and memory, neural entities introduced from the environment and interacting with genes and existing memes, and build a case for gene × meme × environment interaction model of mental illness.

In Part II. Evolution and Mental Health: Genes, Memes, Culture, and the Individual, we discuss and integrate the basic concepts of genetics, evolution, and memes and how learning led to the emergence of memes. We then examine how memes are actually stored in the brain, and how they evolve within the brain as well as outside the brain as elements of culture. We discuss beneficial, symbiotic, and pathogenic memes and how the latter may enter the brain "under the radar." I discuss mental health and mental illness in the light of gene × meme × environment interaction and propose that mental health is achieved when a democracy of memes representing the self (selfplexes) is achieved in the brain.

In Part III. Principles of Diagnosis and Treatment of Mental Illness, I propose a new psychiatric diagnostic scheme based on gene × meme interaction, epigenesis, and the concept of final common pathway brain dysfunction with replication of pathologic memes. I propose that the diagnostic scheme should be multiaxial, and that Axis I should be for phenomenological, neurophysiomemetic diagnosis based on a continuum of brain function while Axis II should be for genetic and neuroscience diagnosis. I then discuss existing and to-be-developed techniques for making a memetic diagnosis. I propose that effective treatment for mental illness should be geared toward both genes and memes, and discuss memetic therapeutic approaches.

Memetic therapy may be broad-spectrum or specific. I discuss existing psychotherapies from a memetic perspective as well as the need for novel meme-oriented therapies. Virtual reality therapy utilizing avatars (virtual image of oneself with desirable attributes) is a promising novel technique.

Prevention is of utmost importance as vulnerable individuals could be identified in early childhood and immunization against toxic memes may prevent an epigenetic cascade toward mental illness. Education plays a crucial role in strengthening the meme-filtering, meme-sorting, and other meme-processing skills.

In Part IV. Specific Psychiatric Syndromes, I discuss specific proposed Axis I (neurophysiomemetic) psychiatric syndromes under the categories of (1) attention-cognition spectrum syndromes (delirium, dementia, attention deficit and impulse control syndromes, obsessions, compulsions), (2) anxiety-mood spectrum syndromes (anxiety, panic, phobias, acute stress disorder (ASD), PTSD, borderline, mania, dependent traits and personality, avoidant traits and personality, depression-neurotic and major depressive syndrome, adjustment disorders), (3) reality perception spectrum syndromes (imagination, dissociation, conversion, somatoform, misattribution somatization, psychosis), (4) pleasure spectrum syndromes (substance use/abuse, addictions to substances, beliefs, fanaticism), (5) primary memetic syndromes (eating disorders, factitious disorders, malingering, meme-directed destructive behaviors). We focus on the memetic diagnosis, gene–meme interaction in development, and genetic–memetic treatment for each category. In the last chapter, Future Challenges, I briefly discuss the testable hypotheses derivable from our model of gene × meme × environment interaction, and the need to develop new techniques in memetic diagnosis and treatment as well as their ethical considerations.

The seemingly perennial dichotomy of mind and body becomes irrelevant with the concept of memes – there is no single mind but a sea of memes in the brain. What is perceived as my mind at a particular time is but a large wave crashing on the shore of my consciousness.

This work is intended to integrate the seemingly disparate languages and methods of biological and social sciences around the indivisible organism, the patient. It is intended to stimulate thinking and hopefully innovations among psychiatrists, physicians of other specialties, health-care professionals, psychologists, sociologists, anthropologists, and others who are interested in human behavior and emotions.

I am grateful to my colleagues and students who have stimulated my thinking through discussions and arguments. I thank Janice Stern of Springer for her support and help in all phases of this work, and Vinnie for putting up with my late and early hours of writing and exchanging genes, memes, culture, and much more.

Fresno and San Francisco, CA   Hoyle Leigh, MD
October, 2009

Contents

Part I
What Is Mental Illness? An Epigenetic Model

Chapter 1
Genes and Mental Illness

Contents

1.1 The Evolution of the Concept of Mental Illness

Alienists used to treat mental illness and those afflicted were considered "alienated" or strange. There have been essentially two lines of thought concerning the causes of mental illness: alien and endogenous. The alien causes may be a possession of the gods or the devil, or, more recently, microorganisms such as bacteria and virus. The endogenous causes may be an imbalance of the body fluids – the Hippocratic blood, phlegm, yellow bile, and black bile (thence the term, *melancholia*) or the modern version of an imbalance among serotonin, norepinephrine, and dopamine. It is also generally accepted that severe environmental factors such as extreme heat or cold can cause mental aberrations such as delirium.

Certain types of mental dysfunction, such as maladaptive patterns of behavior and neurosis, have been also attributed to faulty learning or bad modeling. Experimental "neuroses" and "learned helplessness" have been produced in animals by confusing rewards or inescapable punishment (Saunders et al., 1995; Seligman, 1972).

Mental illness is known to run in families. With the advent of biological psychiatry, it was hoped, in the latter part of the twentieth century, that the etiologic genes of mental illness would be discovered. In fact, the diagnostic and statistical manual for mental illness adopted by the American Psychiatric Association in 1980 (DSM III) was based on the research diagnostic criteria (Feighner et al., 1972) that were designed to isolate "pure cultures" of psychiatric illness for biological research.

H. Leigh, *Genes, Memes, Culture, and Mental Illness*,
DOI 10.1007/978-1-4419-5671-2_1, © Hoyle Leigh, 2010

At the time DSM III was introduced, the catecholamine theory of affective disorders (Schildkraut, 1965) was the prevailing theory of mood disorders, chlorpromazine the most commonly used antipsychotic, and the Human Genome Project was yet not even a gleam in anyone's eyes. Exciting developments have since occurred in molecular biology and genetics and the Human Genome Project has been completed ahead of schedule (2003). Psychiatric research, at least in part fostered by the rigorous diagnostic criteria of DSM III and its slight modification, DSM IV (1994), has made breathtaking advances, taking full advantage of these and other developments during the *Decade of the Brain*, including neuroimaging techniques. On the strength of these developments, a new theoretical model of psychiatric illness has emerged that is open and evidence based.

Many putative genes that code for vulnerability for psychiatric syndromes are evolutionarily conserved. This explains why schizophrenia which is associated with low fertility rates in the afflicted has not become extinct. Crow (1997a, b, 2000, 2007) and Mitchell and Crow (2005) postulate that vulnerability to schizophrenia may be the price that *Homo sapiens* had to pay for the development of language, i.e., the speciation of humans from their ancestral apes involves the same genes that caused the left hemispheric dominance and language. Crow proposes that there are gradations in the genetic predisposition to psychosis, across diagnostic categories of schizophrenia and bipolar disorder.

Certain genes that endow vulnerability to anxiety, for example, the short allele of the serotonin transporter promoter gene (more of this below), may confer sensitivity to the "smoke detector" of anxiety activation (Nesse, 2001) and be evolutionarily adaptive when humans dwelled in caves in fear of predator animals. In the modern world, however, such sensitivity to anxiety would be dysfunctional for the individual and thus be considered a psychiatric syndrome.

1.2 Gene-Environment Interaction and Brain Morphology and Function

The genes coding for predisposition to various psychiatric syndromes are currently being defined using various techniques including linkage studies and genome scan. As far as psychiatric diagnosis goes, current state of affairs can be summarized as follows: For each diagnostic category, there are many susceptibility genes, and a single gene or a few genes may code for the susceptibility for many different disorders. On the basis of genetic studies, Kendler et al. (1998) proposed that psychosis be reclassified as: (1) classic schizophrenia, (2) major depression, (3) schizophreniform disorder, (4) bipolar-schizomania, (5) schizodepression, and (6) hebephrenia.

What seems clear is that psychiatric disorders are syndromes, phenomenological convergence of a number of different genetic-pathophysiologic pathways. An analogy might be hypertension. Hypertension is a syndrome that has definable signs and complications that can be treated with "antihypertensive" drugs. Hypertension, however, is pathophysiologically heterogeneous – it may be nephrogenic, cardiogenic, neurogenic, endocrine, secondary to familial hyperlipidemia, stress-induced, etc.

1.3 Gene–Environment Interaction: Serotonin Transporter Gene as an Exemplar

A single gene that codes for the vulnerability to multiple psychiatric (and medical) conditions is the serotonin transporter gene (SERT) and its promoter region polymorphism (5-HTTLPR). SERT is highly evolutionarily conserved and regulates the entire serotoninergic system and its receptors via modulation of extracellular fluid serotonin concentrations. DNA screens of patients with autism, ADHD, bipolar disorder, and Tourette's syndrome have detected signals in the chromosome 17q region where SERT is located (Murphy et al., 2004). 5-HTTLPR polymorphism consists of short (s) and long (l) alleles, and the presence of the short allele tends to reduce the effectiveness and efficiency of SERT. The short allele has been identified as the underlying variation for the risk for the above disorders as well as anxiety, increased neuroticism scales, smoking oticism, smoking behavior, negative mood, social behavior, especially to reduce negative mood and feel stimulated, difficulty in quitting smoking, social phobia, major depression, and irritable bowel syndrome (Hu et al., 2000; Lerman et al., 2000; Lotrich and Pollock, 2004; Yeo et al., 2004).

Why does a single gene code for so many vulnerabilities? One simple answer may be that the gene codes for one or more basic evolutionarily adaptive predispositions that, in combination with other factors, may determine the development and severity of a psychiatric syndrome. When we look at the list of vulnerabilities above, it seems clear that there is a continuum, from anxiety to adaptive/maladaptive behavior to phobia to major depression, and/or to physical symptoms. The concept of endophenotype is useful in understanding traits associated with syndromes (e.g., eye-tracking abnormality in schizophrenics and relatives) (Gottesman and Gould, 2003) and might provide clues to a genotypic diagnosis.

Pezawas et al. (2005) showed that the short allele carriers show reduced gray matter in limbic regions critical for processing of negative emotion, particularly perigenual cingulate and amygdala. Functional MRI studies of fearful stimuli show a tightly coupled feedback circuit between the amygdala and the cingulate, implicated in the extinction of negative affect. Short allele carriers showed relative uncoupling of this circuit and the magnitude of coupling inversely predicted almost 30% of variation in temperamental anxiety. They also show increased amygdala activation to fearful stimuli (Bertolino et al., 2005; Hariri et al., 2002). Thus, this gene seems to increase the affected individual's brain's sensitivity to negative affect and anxiety (Gross and Hen, 2004). What other factors, then, may further predispose the individual for a major depression?

Caspi et al. (2002, 2003) have shown, in an elegant longitudinal study, that stress during the most recent 2 years in adulthood and maltreatment in childhood interacted with the 5-HTTLPR status. Individuals with two copies of the short allele who also had the stressors had greatest amount of depressive symptoms and suicidality than heterozygous individuals, and those with only the long alleles had the least amount of depression. The short allele carriers have been shown to have more neuroticism scores on Eysenck personality inventory, and those with both short allele

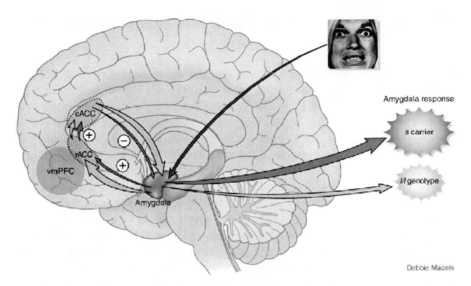

Differences in processing of emotional stimuli between *s* allele carriers (*darker arrows*) and homozygous *l* allele carriers (*lighter arrows*). Negative emotional stimuli are evaluated by the amygdale after preliminary analysis in the ventral visual pathway (not shown). Carriers of the *s* allele have markedly reduced positive functional coupling between the rostral anterior cingulate (rACC) and the amygdala, which results in a net decrease in inhibitory feedback from the caudal anterior cingulate (cACC), via connections between rACC and cACC (*short upward arrows*). Brain volume was also substantially reduced in *s* allele carriers in the rACC and, to a lesser extent, the cACC and amygdala. The consequence of these genotype-based alterations is an emotional hyperresponsivity to negative affective stimuli in *s* allele carriers (*large dark cloud*) compared with individuals lacking this allele (*small light cloud*), which may be related to an increased risk of developing depression. As found in a previous study, functional coupling between the vmPFC (*light circle on left*) and the amygdala was also increased in *s* allele carriers. (From Hamann, 2005, reprinted with permission)

and high neuroticism were at higher risk of developing lifetime depression (Munaro et al., 2005).

Studies in monkeys have shown that the anxiety-enhancing effect of the short allele is mitigated with good mothering in infancy (Barr et al., 2004; Suomi, 2003, 2005).

5-HTTLPR may also determine response to drugs. Depressed individuals with the short allele were found to respond better to antidepressants that are both serotonergic and noradrenergic (i.e., mirtazapine) rather than serotonin-specific reuptake blockers. On the other hand, individuals with the long allele may have more side effects with exactly those drugs that are more effective for those with the short allele (Murphy et al., 2004). Diet deficient in the serotonin precursor, tryptophan, has been shown to induce depression in healthy women with the 5-HTTLPR s/s regardless of family history of depression, while those l/l were resistant to depression regardless of family history of depression. Those with l/s without family history of depression were intermediate between l/l and s/s in depressive mood with tryptophan depletion, while l/s with family history of depression showed depressive response like the s/s (Neumeister, 2003; Neumeister et al., 2006, 2002, 2004a, b).

Thus, 5-HTTLPR short allele, in conjunction with childhood stress, confers an individual with the trait to respond to later stress with increased anxiety and neuroticism, which, in turn, predisposes the individual for later major depression, suicidality, and psychophysiologic disorders. Other gene–environment interactions predisposing to trait and disorder have been reported, including type 4 dopamine receptor gene (D4DR) and novelty seeking and ADHD (Ebstein et al., 1997; Keltikangas-Jarvinen et al., 2003), monoamine oxidase A (MAOA) and antisocial personality (Caspi et al., 2002; Craig, 2005), and dopamine transporter gene (DAT1) and ADHD (Brookes et al., 2006). The Val66Met allele of the brain-derived neurotrophic factor (BDNF) gene causes reduced dendritic branching in hippocampus, impaired contextual fear conditioning, and increased anxiety that is less sensitive to antidepressant treatment. There are alleles of the glucocorticoid receptor gene found in the normal population, which confer a higher sensitivity to glucocorticoids for both negative feedback and insulin reponsiveness or glucocorticoid resistance and an association with an increased likelihood of depression in several alleles and increased response to antidepressants in one of them (McEwen, 2007).

FKBP5 polymorphism (a glucocorticoid receptor-regulating gene) has also been shown to interact with childhood abuse in increasing the risk of PTSD in an urban general hospital population (Binder et al., 2008).

1.4 Emerging Model of Mental Illness: Gene × Meme Interaction

It seems clear, then, that modern model of psychiatric and medical illness must be based on *gene × environment interaction*. This model posits that the "vulnerability gene" has evolutionarily adaptive function as evidenced by its very conservation. It holds that there are critical interactions between the genotype and early environment in forming a personality trait which may in turn be adaptive or maladaptive at the individual level, e.g., anxiety-prone, exploratory, attention fluctuating, hypervigilant, etc. Kandel showed how environment (and learning) modifies gene expression (Kandel, 1979, 1998).

Recent and current stress may play the role of tipping the balance from a trait to a syndrome that has a course of its own.

How do environment and stress affect the genes exactly? To be precise, except in a few extreme cases of physical stress, environment and stress affect human beings only when they are perceived. As we have seen, the serotonin transporter promoter gene polymorphism may affect *how* the same stimulus may be perceived – as threatening or non-threatening – and may in turn result in activation or deactivation of genes. The fact that a recent meta-analysis failed to show a significant interaction between the serotonin transporter promoter polymorphism (5-HTTLPR) and stress in the risk of depression (Risch et al., 2009) highlights that the interaction is not a simple gene × stress, but rather mediated by the individual *traits and percepts*.

When a sensation from a sensory organ reaches the brain, it is processed against existing templates formed by both genetic predisposition and memory, the output of this process constitutes perception. The templates and the percept are memes as we will discuss in the next chapter. In sum, environment affects and interacts with genes through memes in the course of development, and mental health and mental illness are the outcomes of this interaction.

References

Barr, C. S., Newman, T. K., Lindell, S., et al. (2004) Interaction between serotonin transporter gene variation and rearing condition in alcohol preference and consumption in female primates. *Arch Gen Psychiatry*, **61**, 1146–1152.

Bertolino, A., Arciero, G., Rubino, V., et al. (2005) Variation of human amygdala response during threatening stimuli as a function of 5'HTTLPR genotype and personality style. *Biol Psychiatry*, **57**, 1517–1525.

Binder, E. B., Bradley, R. G., Liu, W., et al. (2008) Association of FKBP5 polymorphisms and childhood abuse with risk of posttraumatic stress disorder symptoms in adults. *JAMA*, **299**, 1291–1305.

Brookes, K. J., Mill, J., Guindalini, C., et al. (2006) A common haplotype of the dopamine transporter gene associated with attention-deficit/hyperactivity disorder and interacting with maternal use of alcohol during pregnancy. *Arch Gen Psychiatry*, **63**, 74–81.

Caspi, A., McClay, J., Moffitt, T. E., et al. (2002) Role of genotype in the cycle of violence in maltreated children. *Science*, **297**, 851–854.

Caspi, A., Sugden, K., Moffitt, T. E., et al. (2003) Influence of life stress on depression: Moderation by a polymorphism in the 5-HTT gene. *Science*, **301**, 386–389.

Craig, I. W. (2005) The role of monoamine oxidase A, MAOA, in the aetiology of antisocial behaviour: The importance of gene-environment interactions. *Novartis Found Symposium*, **268**, 227–237; discussion 237–241, 242–253.

Crow, T. J. (1997a) Is schizophrenia the price that Homo sapiens pays for language? *Schizophr Res*, **28**, 127–141.

Crow, T. J. (1997b) Temporolimbic or transcallosal connections: Where is the primary lesion in schizophrenia and what is its nature? *Schizophr Bull*, **23**, 521–523.

Crow, T. J. (2000) Schizophrenia as the price that homo sapiens pays for language: A resolution of the central paradox in the origin of the species. *Brain Res Brain Res Rev*, **31**, 118–129.

Crow, T. J. (2007) How and why genetic linkage has not solved the problem of psychosis: Review and hypothesis. *Am J Psychiatry*, **164**, 13–21.

Ebstein, R. P., Nemanov, L., Klotz, I., et al. (1997) Additional evidence for an association between the dopamine D4 receptor (D4DR) exon III repeat polymorphism and the human personality trait of Novelty Seeking. *Mol Psychiatry*, **2**, 472–477.

Feighner, J. P., Robins, E., Guze, S. B., et al. (1972) Diagnostic criteria for use in psychiatric research. *Arch Gen Psychiatry*, **26**, 57–63.

Gottesman, I. I., Gould, T. D. (2003) The endophenotype concept in psychiatry: Etymology and strategic intentions. *Am J Psychiatry*, **160**, 636–645.

Gross, C., Hen, R. (2004) The developmental origins of anxiety. *Nat Rev Neurosci*, **5**, 545–552.

Hamann, S. (2005) Blue genes: wiring the brain for depression. *Nat Neurosci*, **8**, 701–703.

Hariri, A. R., Mattay, V. S., Tessitore, A., et al. (2002) Serotonin transporter genetic variation and the response of the human amygdala. *Science*, **297**, 400–403.

Hu, S., Brody, C. L., Fisher, C., et al. (2000) Interaction between the serotonin transporter gene and neuroticism in cigarette smoking behavior. *Mol Psychiatry*, **5**, 181–188.

Kandel, E. R. (1979) Psychotherapy and the single synapse. The impact of psychiatric thought on neurobiologic research. *N Engl J Med*, **301**, 1028–1037.

Kandel, E. R. (1998) A new intellectual framework for psychiatry. *Am J Psychiatry*, **155**, 457–469.

Keltikangas-Jarvinen, L., Elovainio, M., Kivimaki, M., et al. (2003) Association between the type 4 dopamine receptor gene polymorphism and novelty seeking. *Psychosom Med*, **65**, 471–476.

Kendler, K. S., Karkowski, L. M., Walsh, D. (1998) The structure of psychosis: Latent class analysis of probands from the Roscommon Family Study. *Arch Gen Psychiatry*, **55**, 492–499.

Lerman, C., Caporaso, N. E., Audrain, J., et al. (2000) Interacting effects of the serotonin transporter gene and neuroticism in smoking practices and nicotine dependence. *Mol Psychiatry*, **5**, 189–192.

Lotrich, F. E., Pollock, B. G. (2004) Meta-analysis of serotonin transporter polymorphisms and affective disorders. *Psychiatr Genet*, **14**, 121–129.

McEwen, B. S. (2007) Physiology and neurobiology of stress and adaptation: Central role of the brain. *Physiol Rev*, **87**, 873–904.

Mitchell, R. L., Crow, T. J. (2005) Right hemisphere language functions and schizophrenia: The forgotten hemisphere? *Brain*, **128**, 963–978.

Munaro, M., Clark, T., Roberts, K., et al. (2005) Neuroticism mediates the association of the serotonin transporter gene with lifetime major depression. *Neuropsychobiology*, **24**, 1–8.

Murphy, G. M., Jr., Hollander, S. B., Rodrigues, H. E., et al. (2004) Effects of the serotonin transporter gene promoter polymorphism on mirtazapine and paroxetine efficacy and adverse events in geriatric major depression. *Arch Gen Psychiatry*, **61**, 1163–1169.

Murphy, D. L., Lerner, A., Rudnick, G., et al. (2004) Serotonin transporter: Gene, genetic disorders, and pharmacogenetics. *Mol Interv*, **4**, 109–123.

Nesse, R. M. (2001) The smoke detector principle. Natural selection and the regulation of defensive responses. *Ann NY Acad Sci*, **935**, 75–85.

Neumeister, A. (2003) Tryptophan depletion, serotonin, and depression: Where do we stand? *Psychopharmacol Bull*, **37**, 99–115.

Neumeister, A., Hu, X. Z., Luckenbaugh, D. A., et al. (2006) Differential effects of 5-HTTLPR genotypes on the behavioral and neural responses to tryptophan depletion in patients with major depression and controls. *Arch Gen Psychiatry*, **63**, 978–986.

Neumeister, A., Konstantinidis, A., Stastny, J., et al. (2002) Association between serotonin transporter gene promoter polymorphism (5HTTLPR) and behavioral responses to tryptophan depletion in healthy women with and without family history of depression. *Arch Gen Psychiatry*, **59**, 613–620.

Neumeister, A., Nugent, A. C., Waldeck, T., et al. (2004a) Neural and behavioral responses to tryptophan depletion in unmedicated patients with remitted major depressive disorder and controls. *Arch Gen Psychiatry*, **61**, 765–773.

Neumeister, A., Young, T., Stastny, J. (2004b) Implications of genetic research on the role of the serotonin in depression: Emphasis on the serotonin type 1A receptor and the serotonin transporter. *Psychopharmacology (Berl)*, **174**, 512–524.

Pezawas, L., Meyer-Lindenberg, A., Drabant, E. M., et al. (2005) 5-HTTLPR polymorphism impacts human cingulate-amygdala interactions: A genetic susceptibility mechanism for depression. *Nat Neurosci*, **8**, 828–834.

Risch, N., Herrell, R., Lehner, T., et al. (2009) Interaction between the serotonin transporter gene (5-HTTLPR), stressful life events, and risk of depression: A meta-analysis. *JAMA*, **301**, 2462–2471.

Saunders, B., Wilkinson, C., Phillips, M. (1995) The impact of a brief motivational intervention with opiate users attending a methadone programme. *Addiction*, **90**, 415–424.

Schildkraut, J. J. (1965) The catecholamine hypothesis of affective disorders: A review of supporting evidence. *Am J Psychiatry*, **122**, 509–522.

Seligman, M. E. (1972) Learned helplessness. *Annu Rev Med*, **23**, 407–412.

Suomi, S. J. (2003) Gene-environment interactions and the neurobiology of social conflict. *Ann NY Acad Sci*, **1008**, 132–139.

Suomi, S. J. (2005) Aggression and social behaviour in rhesus monkeys. *Novartis Found Symposium*, **268**, 216–222; discussion 222–216, 242–253.

Yeo, A., Boyd, P., Lumsden, S., et al. (2004) Association between a functional polymorphism in the serotonin transporter gene and diarrhoea predominant irritable bowel syndrome in women. *Gut*, **53**, 1452–1458.

Chapter 2
How Does Stress Work? The Role of Memes in Epigenesis

Contents

Since Selye's work on the role of stress on the activation of the adrenal cortex and the *general adaptation syndrome* (Selye, 1956), there has been an explosion of knowledge concerning the effects of stress on the organism in such fields as neuropsychoendocrinology and neuropsychoimmunology.

2.1 Stress, Aging, and Disease

Classically, stress response is the "fight–flight" reaction to a threatening stimulus such as a dangerous animal, mugger, or approaching fire. It is accompanied with the activation of the autonomic nervous system and hypothalamo-pituitary-adrenal (HPA) axis. The organism needs the normal stress response to survive such danger situations, and inadequate or excessive adrenocortical and autonomic response is deleterious for health and survival. The active process by which the body responds to stresses and maintains homeostasis has been termed allostasis (achieving stability through change) (Sterling and Eyer, 1988). The term *allostatic load or overload* has been introduced by McEwen to denote the wear and tear and resulting pathophysiology from insufficient management of allostasis either due to too much stress or inappropriate stress response (McEwen, 1998).

When the stress is of short duration, and the behavioral, endocrine, and autonomic responses have been successful in warding off the danger situation, the organism may be strengthened by the stress experience. On the other hand, if the

H. Leigh, *Genes, Memes, Culture, and Mental Illness*,
DOI 10.1007/978-1-4419-5671-2_2, © Hoyle Leigh, 2010

stress is prolonged and/or the organism is unable to master it (allostatic overload), there may be serious health consequences.

Sapolsky et al. proposed the *glucocorticoid cascade hypothesis* of stress and aging (Sapolsky et al., 1986). Aging animals have impaired ability to terminate the secretion of adrenocortical stress hormones at the end of stress, which may be due to the degeneration of negative feedback neurons. These neurons may further degenerate due to the toxic effects of excessive glucocorticoids, resulting in a feed-forward cascade with potentially serious pathophysiological consequences in the aged subject.

Epel and her colleagues found that perceived stress and chronicity of stress in healthy premenopausal women were significantly associated with higher oxidative stress, lower telomerase activity and shorter telomere length, which are known determinants of cell senescence and longevity in peripheral blood mononuclear cells. They found that women with the highest levels of perceived stress had shorter telomeres on average by the equivalent of at least one decade of additional aging (Epel et al., 2004).

The role of stress in various disease conditions from cancer to cardiac disease has been elucidated in numerous publications – as of this writing, there were more than 18,000 PubMed publications for stress and cancer, and more than 32,000 publications on stress and heart disease. As for the stress and the brain, there were more than 30,000 PubMed publications.

Posttraumatic stress disorder and *acute stress disorder* are results of massive identifiable stress and are manifested by emotional and behavioral symptoms. As we have seen, however, stress plays a prominent role in depression and anxiety, and, in fact, most psychiatric conditions are either precipitated by or contributed by stress. Even exacerbations of schizophrenia, often thought to be primarily biological, are induced by emotional stress (Marom et al., 2005).

2.2 Stress, Memes, and the Brain

Stress has been shown to change both the structure and function of the brain.

When a stimulus arrives at a sensory cortical area such as the visual cortex, auditory cortex (Wernicke's area), and/or the somatosensory postcentral gyrus and the thalamus, the neural impulses are projected to the association cortices resulting in a perception. Perception is determined by both genetically determined circuitry and neural projections determined by learning and memory formation, i.e., memes (see Section 2.5 and Chapter 8).

Then the cortical impulses constituting the percepts are projected to the amygdala, the hippocampus, and other limbic structures, all of which are interconnected with each other. Amygdala has a very tight feedback loop with the anterior cingulate gyrus which is connected with the thalamus, neocortex, and the entorhinal cortex. The negative feedback from the anterior cingulate reduces amygdalar activation. Stressful perceptions stimulate amygdala and result in the autonomic and

HPA activation. In memetic terms, the perceived human face (meme) arising in the primary visual cortex and arriving at amygdala may be elaborated into a *smiling* human face, the attribute meme of "smiling" coming from the anterior cingulate gyrus after processing of the original stimulus.

Hippocampus plays an important role in shutting off the HPA activation – any damage or atrophy of the hippocampus attenuates this resulting in a prolonged HPA activation to stress (McEwen, 2007). Longitudinal studies on aging in human subjects revealed that progressive increases in salivary cortisol during a yearly exam over a 5-year period predicted reduced hippocampal volume and reduced performance on hippocampal-dependent memory tasks (Lupien et al., 1998). Initially, it was thought that aging in hippocampus was associated with a loss of neurons, but subsequent studies on animal models of aging confer greater importance to a loss of synaptic connectivity or impairment of synaptic function (McEwen, 2007).

Neural regeneration is now known to occur in the brain, particularly in hippocampus. Certain types of acute stress and many chronic stressors suppress neurogenesis or cell survival in the dentate gyrus of the hippocampus. Glucocorticoids, excitatory amino acids acting on NMDA receptors, and endogenous opioids mediate the suppression (Gould et al., 1997). Stress also affects the shape and abundance of dendrites in the hippocampus, amygdala, and prefrontal cortex. Generally, stress results in retraction and simplification of dendrites. In memetic terms, stress memes tend to disconnect incoming memes from existing memes (memories).

Puberty seems to be a particularly vulnerable period for the effect of stress on the brain. Stress in peripubertal rats resulted in a stunting of growth in parts of the hippocampus and a sustained down-regulation of the hippocampal glucocorticoid receptor (GR) gene expression, resulting in deficits in the shut-off of the HPA activation. Daily infusions of corticosterone during puberty resulted in a reduction of both hippocampal volume and the number of neurons in parts of the hippocampus, while it produced only reduction in volume but not in the number of neurons in adults (McEwen, 2007).

Corticosteroids released by HPA activation interact with many chemicals and neurotransmitters in the hippocampus, including serotonin, endorphins, GABA-benzodiazepine receptors, and glutamate and other excitatory amino acids. Chronic stress in rats releases glutamate and affects the neural cell adhesion molecule (NCAM, PSA-NCAM). Chronic stress also releases the tissue plasminogen activator (tPA), an extracellular protease and signaling molecule, that is involved in the loss of spines and NMDA receptor subunits in the hippocampus (McEwen, 2007).

Neurotrophic factors such as brain-derived neurotrophic factor (BDNF) play a role in dendritic proliferation. BDNF knockout mice exhibit a paucity in dendrites and no further reduction in hippocampal dendritic length with chronic stress, while wild-type mice show reduced dendritic length with chronic stress. On the other hand, overexpression of BDNF prevents stress-induced dendritic reductions and an antidepressant-like action on forced swimming test in mice (Govindarajan et al.,

2006). Both stress-induced increases and decreases of BDNF expression have been reported, which may reflect that BDNF synthesis may be triggered by stress to off-set the depletion of BDNF caused by stress. BDNF and corticosteroids may oppose each other, with BDNF reversing the corticosteroid-induced reduction in hippocampal neuronal sensitivity. BDNF may facilitate meme introduction, replication, and synthesis.

Corticotropin-releasing factor (CRF) plays an important role in mediating stress in the brain. It regulates the ACTH release in the pituitary and also acts on the amygdala that controls the behavioral and autonomic responses to stress including the release of tPA that plays an important part in anxiety. When CRF is injected into the brain, it produces arousal and increased responsiveness to stressful stimuli that seem to be independent of the pituitary adrenal axis and can be reversed by specific and selective CRF antagonists. Such antagonists also reverse behavioral responses to stressors. An interaction between the norepinephrine and the CRF systems seems to occur both at the locus ceruleus and the amygdala. Noradrenergic neurons arising from the locus ceruleus are concerned with behavioral arousal and anxiety. CRF neurons seem to activate locus ceruleus. Norepinephrine, in turn, may stimulate CRF release in the paraventricular nucleus of the hypothalamus, the bed nucleus of the stria terminalis, and the central nucleus of the amygdala. Such a feed-forward system was hypothesized to be particularly important in stress situations where an organism must mobilize not only the HPA but also the central nervous system. Such a positive feedback system that accelerates anxiety response, however, might be particularly vulnerable to dysfunction (Koob, 1999).

Prefrontal cortex and amygdala are also affected by stress. Chronic stress in rats causes dendritic shortening in the medial prefrontal cortex but dendritic growth in the neurons in amygdala and in the orbitofrontal cortex. Glucocorticoids have been shown to produce retraction of dendrites in medial prefrontal cortex. Behaviorally, chronic stress remodeling of the prefrontal cortex impairs attention set shifting (McEwen, 2007). Chronic stress enhances amygdala-dependent unlearned fear and fear conditioning (Conrad et al., 1999). Chronic stress also increases aggression through hyperactivity of amygdala.

The amygdala exerts a regulatory influence on the stress response and is itself affected by stress. The serine protease tissue plasminogen activator (tPA), a key mediator of dendritic spine plasticity, is required for stress-induced facilitation of anxiety-like behavior. In the tPA knockout mice, repeated stress did not cause a reduction in the spine density (Bennur et al., 2007). BDNF may also play a role in amygdala in enhancing anxiety and increasing dendritic density.

All the brain structures mentioned, the prefrontal cortex, amygdala, and hippocampus, are closely interconnected and influence each other. Inactivation of amygdala blocks stress-induced impairment of hippocampal memory long-term potentiation (LTP) and spatial memory (Kim et al., 2005). Stimulation of medial prefrontal cortex reduces responsiveness of central amygdala output neurons and thus the prefrontal cortex plays an important role in fear extinction. Amygdala–hippocampus connections are required for the processing of emotional memories with contextual information (McEwen, 2007).

2.3 Role of Stress and Nurturing in Development: Epigenesis

Development is considered to be *epigenetic*, i.e., it occurs as an interaction between genes and environment. The phenotypic expression of a gene, i.e., whether it will be turned on or off in the life of an organism, depends on the organism's interaction with the environment. Stress figures in prominently in this epigenetic model of development. As I discussed in the previous chapter, the effect of childhood stress on the serotonin transporter promoter gene (5-HTTLPR) has been demonstrated and that noxious effects may be mitigated by good mothering in childhood at least in monkeys. But how exactly does stress affect the genes?

In a series of experiments, Szyf et al. (2007), Unterberger et al. (2006), Weaver (2007), and Weaver et al. (2007) studied the effects of different maternal behavior in rats. Maternal behavior in rats affects the neural systems that tonically inhibit corticotrophin-releasing factor (CRF) synthesis and release in the hypothalamus and amygdala, which in turn activate central norepinephrine in response to stress. Glucocorticoids initiate tonic negative feedback inhibition over CRF synthesis and release and thus dampen HPA responses to stress. This glucocorticoid negative feedback is, in part, mediated by glucocorticoid receptors (GR) which are found in many brain areas including hippocampus.

As adults, the offspring of high licking and grooming (LG) mothers show increased hippocampal GR expression and enhanced glucocorticoid feedback sensitivity by comparison to adult animals reared by low-LG mothers. Thus, adult offspring of high-LG mothers show decreased hypothalamic CRF expression and more modest HPA responses to stress. Eliminating the difference in hippocampal GR levels abolishes the effects of early-life experience on HPA.

In essence, the experience of high licking by the rat pup is a meme that forms neural connections as perception that in turn activates existing memes and the ensemble of memes increases hippocampal GR expression.

In addition to alterations in hippocampal GR expression, enhanced maternal LG behavior over the first week of life is associated with increased hippocampal neuronal survival, synaptogenesis, and improved cognitive performance under stressful conditions. Behaviorally, such pups become "neophilic" rats that are more exploratory in novel environments and less emotionally reactive. On the other hand, the pups with lower LG during their first week of life develop a "neophobic" phenotype with increased emotional and HPA reactivity and less exploration of a novel situation (McEwen, 2007).

When the pups of high-LG mothers were bred by low-LG mothers, and pups of low-LG mothers were bred by high-LG mothers (cross-breeding), the gene expression and stress response patterns followed what was expected of the early experience, i.e., the fostering mother's care, not the biological mother, determined the degree of gene expression and stress response.

How could the behavior of the caregiver cause a stable change in gene expression in the offspring long after the caregiver is gone? Szyf et al. propose an epigenetic mechanism in which the maternal behavior of the caregiver triggered an epigenetic change in the brain of the offspring.

2.4 Environment Changes Epigenome

The epigenome consists of the chromatin and its modifications and a covalent DNA modification through methylation. The DNA is wrapped around a protein-based structure termed chromatin. The basic building block of chromatin is the nucleosome, which is formed of an octamer of histone proteins. There are five basic forms of histone proteins. The histones are extensively modified by methylation, phosphorylation, acetylation, and ubiquitination, and such modifications play an important role in defining the accessibility of the DNA wrapped around the nucleosome core. The specific pattern of histone modifications forms a "histone code," that determines the parts of the genome to be expressed at a given point in time in a given cell type (Jenuwein and Allis, 2001; Taverna et al., 2007). Thus a change in histone configurations around a gene will change its level of expression and could switch a gene between functionality and "silence."

In addition to chromatin, the DNA molecule itself is modified by methylation of the cytosine rings in the dinucleotide sequence CG in vertebrates (Razin, 1998; Razin and Kantor, 2005) (Fig. 2.1). In the vertebrate genome, DNA methylation occurs in different patterns in different cell types. Since DNA methylation is part of the chemical structure of the DNA itself, it is more stable than other epigenetic markers. It is generally accepted that DNA methylation plays an important role in regulating gene expression. The methylation of DNA in distinct regulatory regions is believed to mark silent genes. Epigenomic screening of human chromosomes suggests that a third of the genes analyzed shows inverse correlation between the state of DNA methylation at the $5'$ regulatory regions and the gene expression (Eckhardt et al., 2004, 2006; Lesche and Eckhardt, 2007). Aberrant silencing of tumor suppressor genes by DNA methylation seems to be a common mechanism in cancer (Baylin, 2001; Rountree et al., 2001).

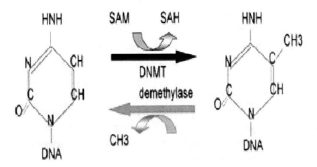

Fig. 2.1 The reversible DNA methylation reaction. DNA methyltransferases (DNMT) catalyze the transfer of methyl groups from the methyl donor S-adenosylmethionine to DNA releasing S-adenosylhomocysteine. Demethylases release the methyl group from methylated DNA as either methanol or formaldehyde. (From Szyf et al., 2007, reprinted with permission)

The DNA methylation pattern is established during early development and is maintained faithfully through life. It was long believed that DNA methylation pattern could be altered only during cell division when new unmethylated DNA is synthesized and serves as a substrate for maintenance DNA methyltransferase (DNMT). There is evidence, however, that DNMT exists in post-mitotic cells and that DNMT levels in neurons change in certain pathological conditions such as psychosis (Veldic et al., 2005). DNA methylation pattern probably represents a balance of methylation and demethylation in response to physiological and environmental signals.

The epigenome consisting of both histone configurations and DNA methylation status determines the accessibility of the transcription machinery (Szyf et al., 2007) and thus determines which genes are accessible for transcription (see Figs. 2.1, 2.2,

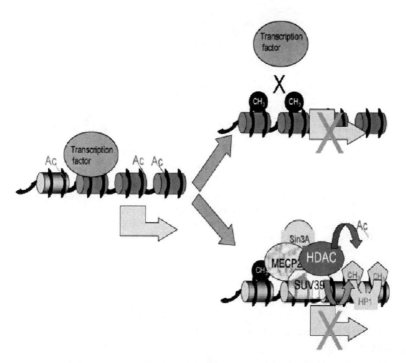

Fig. 2.2 Two mechanisms of silencing gene expression by DNA methylation. An expressed gene (transcription indicated by *horizontal arrow*) is usually associated with acetylated histones and is unmethylated. An event of methylation would lead to methylation by two different mechanisms. The methyl group (CH₃) interferes with the binding of a transcription factor which is required for gene expression resulting in blocking of transcription. The second mechanism shown in the *bottom right* is indirect. Methylated DNA attracts methylated DNA binding proteins such as Me CP2, which in turn recruits co-repressors such as SIN3A, histone methyltransferases such as SUV39 that methylates histones and histone deacetylases (HDAC), which remove the acetyl group from histone tails. Methylated histones (K9 residue of histone tails) recruit heterochromatin proteins such as HP1, which contribute to a closed chromatin configuration and silencing of the gene. (From Szyf et al., 2007, reprinted with permission)

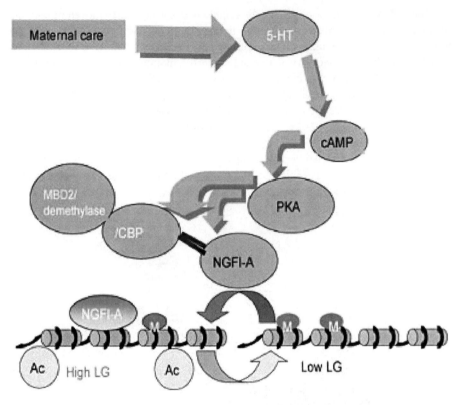

Fig. 2.3 Behavioral gene programming by maternal care. The sequence of events leading from maternal licking and grooming behavior to epigenetic programming of the GR exon 1, promoter CBP, a HAT (cAMP recognition element-binding protein, CREB), M, methylated CG, Ac, acetylated H3-Histone. (From Szyf et al., 2007, reprinted with permission)

and 2.3). Inaccessible genes are, therefore, silent whereas accessible genes are transcribed. In addition, another level of epigenetic regulation by small, non-coding RNAs (microRNAs) has recently been described (Bergmann and Lane, 2003).

Returning to the mechanisms of early experience affecting stress responsivity, maternal programming of individual differences in gene expression and stress responses in the rat seems to involve modifications of epigenetic mechanisms, including DNA methylation and histone modification of a nerve growth factor inducible protein A (NGFI-A) transcription factor binding site on a brain-specific GR promoter. Increased maternal LG behavior during the first week of life causes DNA demethylation, increased histone acetylation and NGFI-A binding, and increased hippocampal GR expression (Weaver et al., 2006). Thus, the NGFI-A binding site on the hippocampal GR promoter is methylated and hypoacetylated in offspring of low-LG mothers and demethylated and hyperacetylated in offspring of high-LG mothers.

Weaver et al. also report that the central infusion of the histone deacetylase inhibitor trichostatin A (TSA) eliminated the maternal effect on histone acetylation, DNA methylation, hippocampal GR expression, and HPA responses to stress in the adult offspring of low-LG mothers (Weaver et al., 2004). On the other hand, central infusion of the adult offspring of high-LG mothers with a methyl donor, L-methionine, a precursor to S-adenosylmethionine, resulted in increased methylation of the NGFI-A binding site on the hippocampal GR promoter, decreased GR expression, and increased HPA responses to stress (Weaver et al., 2005).

The difference in the methylation status between the offspring of high- and low-LG mothers emerged over the first week of life, was reversed with cross-fostering, and persisted into adulthood. Weaver et al. have also shown that maternal care early in life affected the expression of hundreds of genes in the adult hippocampus (Weaver et al., 2006).

Physical environment, including environmental chemicals and toxins which interact with the epigenetic machinery during this critical period might also have a profound impact on behavior later in life by interfering with the maternal care-driven epigenetic programming.

The epigenetic gene expression determined by the quality of maternal care during the first week of life seems to be potentially reversible as there is a dynamic equilibrium in methylation–demethylation reactions (Szyf et al., 2007).

The epigenetic reversal caused by TSA infusion discussed above was reported to be accompanied with a behavioral change so that the stress response of the TSA-treated adult offspring of low LG was indistinguishable from the offspring of high LG.

Such reversal of methylation could be achieved also by neurotransmitter activation that eventually stimulates histone acetyltransferases. Szyf et al. hypothesize that maternal care (LG) in early life elicits a thyroid hormone-dependent increase in serotonin (5-HT) activity at 5-HT_7 receptors, and the subsequent activation of cyclic adenosine $3'$, $5'$ monophosphate (cAMP) and cAMP-dependent protein kinase A (PKA), which is accompanied by increased hippocampal expression of NGFI-A transcription factor which, in turn, binds to the GR exon 1_7 promoter region. NGFI-A interacts with the transcriptional coactivator and histone acetyl transferase CREB binding protein (CBP). Signaling pathways that result in increased cAMP also activate CBP. Recruitment of CBP to the GR exon 1_7 promoter in response to maternal care could explain the increased acetylation and demethylation observed in offspring of high-LG (Szyf et al., 2007).

How does licking by mother or foster-mother affect the pup's neurotransmitter levels and gene methylation status in many parts of the brain? The perception of licking by the pup results in memes, i.e., new neural connections and potentiation of existing ones that may represent, in *homo sapiens* terms, "I am loved." It is these patterns of neural connections (memes) that affect other neural connections to result in neurotransmitter release and affect genes. The affected genes, in turn, affect the individual's perceptual bias and interpretation of life experiences in the future, and thus stress vulnerability or resilience.

Behavioral interventions which lead to firing of neurons and consistent and repetitive activation of signaling pathways might also lead to a change in DNA methylation of specific genes in the adult brain. In addition, drugs, both recreational and therapeutic, may alter DNA methylation patterns of genes in the brain. Vaproic acid, a mood stabilizer and anticonvulsant, is a histone deacetylase (HDAC) inhibitor and triggered replication-independent DNA demethylation in tissue culture, and inhibited DNA methylation in animal brain (Detich et al., 2003; Milutinovic et al., 2007; Tremolizzo et al., 2002).

2.5 Memes and Epigenesis

How does stress actually work? What is the *allo* in *allostasis?* We often talk about stress as though it is an obviously definable condition. In cases of physical stress, such as extreme heat or cold, or physical trauma, the physiologic demand may be direct and obvious, although these are also accompanied by meanings that may not be so obvious. In cases of psychological stress, however, the exact mechanism by which stress enters the body has not been well explained.

Perception obviously underlies all stress but why are certain percepts stressful to some but not others? Why do some neutral percepts, such as advertising jingles, sometimes recur in one's mind and cause annoyance?

Perceiving involves an integration of sensory impulses with an existing information base (memories) in the brain (see Chapter 9 for further discussion on this topic). Such an integration creates a percept, a bit of information that interacts with other information in the brain. Often such percepts are replicas of information from other brains or sources of information such as books, DVDs, etc.

Richard Dawkins coined the term, *memes,* to denote such bits of information that replicate themselves (Dawkins, 1976). Memes are created, stored, and replicated not only in human brains but also in computers, and replicated by copiers, fax machines, printers, and stored in books, DVDs, and other media (see Chapter 8, Chapter 9, and Chapter 10 for how memes rose, how they evolved, and exactly where they reside).

Perceiving may then be considered to be an act of meme infusion into the brain or meme creation making use of sensory input. Memes enter the brain through the *vehicle* of sensations. The perception of a stressful situation is the introduction of stress-response inducing memes. For this to occur, there has to be an interaction between the newly introduced meme and the preexisting memes, and the interaction must lead to an activation of the limbic system (resulting in emotional memes).

Is maternal behavior a meme when all she is doing is what comes instinctually? It is a meme generated by the mother either pre-programmed by genes or learned by observation of others or both. It is, however, the meme of being cared for, or licked, experienced by the pup that has long-term consequences – it is introduced into the pup through maternal behavior, and now resides in the pup as a meme, having caused gene modification and modification in the brain to interpret new experiences against the new template.

2.6 Stress Awakens Dormant Memes Resulting in Mental Illness

How does the concept of the meme clarify stress? The environment consists of memes and potential memes like a culture medium in a petri dish. The culture medium consists of molecules, some of them nutrients, some of them toxins, and others inert. Some enter the organism and become part of it or give it energy. Others may simply enter and stay without much effect. Under certain conditions, such as an increase in the concentration of the toxic molecules, some such molecules will penetrate the protective barrier of the organism and cause a reaction in the host – perhaps an immune reaction that gets rid of the toxic molecule, or the organism may succumb to the toxin. The shape and nature of the toxic molecule play important roles in whether it enters the host, and what happens afterwards. So with memes. The shapes and other characteristics of the vehicles of memes are physical in nature such as printed words, spoken words, melodies, rhythm, scenes, movements, facial expressions, touch, etc.

Memes contain various specific sensory components that can be identified and analyzed. For example, the news of the death of a loved one may be introduced into the brain in different memetic vehicles, e.g., as a phone call, a letter, a news item on TV, etc, which cause different patterns and sequence of brain activation and thus affective arousal. Thus, the sound of a phone call may reverberate (replicate) repeatedly in the brain while a visit by a friend bearing the news may be soon forgotten. Stress thus may be definable through an analysis of the types and quantities of memes and their vehicles that invade the brain.

While memes enter the brain through physical sensations, memes are bits of information, and like all information, a meme can be transcribed and translated into different languages and physical sensations. In the brain, memes are functional neuronal clusters (*neural cliques*) with specific long-term potentiation. Meme replication occurs in the brain when a meme-containing neuronal cluster is reinforced by stimulation, which may in turn infect other clusters to change configuration (see Chapter 9).

I noted in the previous section that stress changes the structure and function of the brain in various ways. The stress response in the brain may be seen to be a result of replications of stress memes triggered by the introduction of new stress memes. Memes are above all replicators. The invader in the culture medium analogy is a replicating virus. The stress memes interact with resident stress memes in the brain, which will tend to cause a cascade of stress meme replication. Counterbalancing this tendency is the host immune response, the negative feedback loop to amygdala from the cortex that may be effective in shutting off the stress response – if the protective memes are prepared and abundant. Chronic stress diminishes the number of hippocampal neurons and causes an attenuation of the hippocampal dendritic connections resulting in a disconnection between long-term memory (resident memetic store that may attenuate the stress response) and current stress meme infusion, a favorable circumstance for invasion of new memes.

The arousal and activation associated with acute stress may create a condition for heightened receptivity for meme infusion from the outside, while the deleterious effects of chronic stress on the brain serve to protect the stress memes from resident protective memes. Dormant stress memes, however, may be activated by the incoming stress memes, especially as the protective memes are attenuated.

Recognizing memes as independent replicators whose only concern is replication of themselves regardless of consequences to the host organism can explain why allostatic overload occurs so easily in human beings, whose brains are particularly favored by memes (see Chapter 9 for a discussion of the mechanisms of meme replication in the brain).

To summarize so far, we may conceptualize mental illness as a final common pathway dysregulation syndrome of normal brain function. In the course of development, particularly in critical periods in early life, genes are turned on or off depending on stress or nurturance, giving rise to vulnerability to stress in later life. Stress is introduced into the brain as memes that interact with resident memes resulting in acute arousal that serves the adaptive fight/flight reaction and receptivity to introduction of memes. Chronic stress attenuates memory function causing a disconnection between new memes and resident protective memes that are normally dominant. The new memes may then interact with dormant or suppressed resident memes to stimulate their replication. Thus, pathogenic, hitherto suppressed memes may become dominant. In such an allostatic overload situations, dysregulation of brain function may result in a psychiatric syndrome, in which there may be an unchecked replication of pathologic memes. But how do we acquire the resident memes in the first place? From the culture medium, which will be the topic of discussion in the next chapter.

References

Baylin, S. (2001) DNA methylation and epigenetic mechanisms of carcinogenesis. *Dev Biol (Basel)*, **106**, 85–87, discussion 143–160.

Bennur, S., Shankaranarayana Rao, B. S., Pawlak, R., et al. (2007) Stress-induced spine loss in the medial amygdala is mediated by tissue-plasminogen activator. *Neuroscience*, **144**, 8–16.

Bergmann, A., Lane, M. E. (2003) Hidden targets of microRNAs for growth control. *Trends Biochem Sci*, **28**, 461–463.

Conrad, C. D., LeDoux, J. E., Magarinos, A. M., et al. (1999) Repeated restraint stress facilitates fear conditioning independently of causing hippocampal CA3 dendritic atrophy. *Behav Neurosci*, **113**, 902–913.

Dawkins, R. (1976) *The Selfish Gene*. Oxford University Press, New York.

Detich, N., Bovenzi, V., Szyf, M. (2003) Valproate induces replication-independent active DNA demethylation. *J Biol Chem*, **278**, 27586–27592.

Eckhardt, F., Beck, S., Gut, I. G., et al. (2004) Future potential of the human epigenome project. *Expert Rev Mol Diagn*, **4**, 609–618.

Eckhardt, F., Lewin, J., Cortese, R., et al. (2006) DNA methylation profiling of human chromosomes 6, 20 and 22. *Nat Genet*, **38**, 1378–1385.

Epel, E. S., Blackburn, E. H., Lin, J., et al. (2004) Accelerated telomere shortening in response to life stress. *Proc Natl Acad Sci USA*, **101**, 17312–17315.

Gould, E., McEwen, B. S., Tanapat, P., et al. (1997) Neurogenesis in the dentate gyrus of the adult tree shrew is regulated by psychosocial stress and NMDA receptor activation. *J Neurosci*, **17**, 2492–2498.

Govindarajan, A., Rao, B. S., Nair, D., et al. (2006) Transgenic brain-derived neurotrophic factor expression causes both anxiogenic and antidepressant effects. *Proc Natl Acad Sci USA*, **103**, 13208–13213.

Jenuwein, T., Allis, C. D. (2001) Translating the histone code. *Science*, **293**, 1074–1080.

Kim, J. J., Koo, J. W., Lee, H. J., et al. (2005) Amygdalar inactivation blocks stress-induced impairments in hippocampal long-term potentiation and spatial memory. *J Neurosci*, **25**, 1532–1539.

Koob, G. F. (1999) Corticotropin-releasing factor, norepinephrine, and stress. *Biol Psychiatry*, **46**, 1167–1180.

Lesche, R., Eckhardt, F. (2007) DNA methylation markers: A versatile diagnostic tool for routine clinical use. *Curr Opin Mol Ther*, **9**, 222–230.

Lupien, S. J., de Leon, M., de Santi, S., et al. (1998) Cortisol levels during human aging predict hippocampal atrophy and memory deficits. *Nat Neurosci*, **1**, 69–73.

Marom, S., Munitz, H., Jones, P. B., et al. (2005) Expressed emotion: Relevance to rehospitalization in schizophrenia over 7 years. *Schizophr Bull*, **31**, 751–758.

McEwen, B. S. (1998) Stress, adaptation, and disease. Allostasis and allostatic load. *Ann NY Acad Sci*, **840**, 33–44.

McEwen, B. S. (2007) Physiology and neurobiology of stress and adaptation: Central role of the brain. *Physiol Rev*, **87**, 873–904.

Milutinovic, S., D'Alessio, A. C., Detich, N., et al. (2007) Valproate induces widespread epigenetic reprogramming which involves demethylation of specific genes. *Carcinogenesis*, **28**, 560–571.

Razin, A. (1998) CpG methylation, chromatin structure and gene silencing—a three-way connection. *EMBO J*, **17**, 4905–4908.

Razin, A., Kantor, B. (2005) DNA methylation in epigenetic control of gene expression. *Prog Mol Subcell Biol*, **38**, 151–167.

Rountree, M. R., Bachman, K. E., Herman, J. G., et al. (2001) DNA methylation, chromatin inheritance, and cancer. *Oncogene*, **20**, 3156–3165.

Sapolsky, R. M., Krey, L. C., McEwen, B. S. (1986) The neuroendocrinology of stress and aging: The glucocorticoid cascade hypothesis. *Endocr Rev*, **7**, 284–301.

Selye, H. (1956) *The Stress of Life*. McGraw Hill, New York.

Sterling, P., Eyer, J. (1988) Allostasis: A new paradigm to explain arousal pathology. In *Handbook of Life Stress, Cognition and Health* (J. Reason and S. Fisher eds.), pp. 629–649. Wiley, New York.

Szyf, M., Weaver, I., Meaney, M. (2007) Maternal care, the epigenome and phenotypic differences in behavior. *Reprod Toxicol*, **24**, 9–19.

Taverna, S. D., Li, H., Ruthenburg, A. J., et al. (2007) How chromatin-binding modules interpret histone modifications: Lessons from professional pocket pickers. *Nat Struct Mol Biol*, **14**, 1025–1040.

Tremolizzo, L., Carboni, G., Ruzicka, W. B., et al. (2002) An epigenetic mouse model for molecular and behavioral neuropathologies related to schizophrenia vulnerability. *Proc Natl Acad Sci USA*, **99**, 17095–17100.

Unterberger, A., Andrews, S. D., Weaver, I. C., et al. (2006) DNA methyltransferase 1 knockdown activates a replication stress checkpoint. *Mol Cell Biol*, **26**, 7575–7586.

Veldic, M., Guidotti, A., Maloku, E., et al. (2005) In psychosis, cortical interneurons overexpress DNA-methyltransferase 1. *Proc Natl Acad Sci USA*, **102**, 2152–2157.

Weaver, I. C. (2007) Epigenetic programming by maternal behavior and pharmacological intervention. Nature versus nurture: Let's call the whole thing off. *Epigenetics*, **2**, 22–28.

Weaver, I. C., Cervoni, N., Champagne, F. A., et al. (2004) Epigenetic programming by maternal behavior. *Nat Neurosci*, **7**, 847–854.

Weaver, I. C., Champagne, F. A., Brown, S. E., et al. (2005) Reversal of maternal programming of stress responses in adult offspring through methyl supplementation: Altering epigenetic marking later in life. *J Neurosci*, **25**, 11045–11054.

Weaver, I. C., D'Alessio, A. C., Brown, S. E., et al. (2007) The transcription factor nerve growth factor-inducible protein a mediates epigenetic programming: Altering epigenetic marks by immediate-early genes. *J Neurosci*, **27**, 1756–1768.
Weaver, I. C., Meaney, M. J., Szyf, M. (2006) Maternal care effects on the hippocampal transcriptome and anxiety-mediated behaviors in the offspring that are reversible in adulthood. *Proc Natl Acad Sci USA*, **103**, 3480–3485.

Chapter 3
Culture and Mental Illness

Contents

In the previous two chapters, we discussed a new model of mental illness based on gene × meme interaction. We visualized the individual organism as being in a petri dish surrounded by a medium of molecules representing memes. We examined how stress memes may awaken dormant memes resulting in mental illness. In this chapter, we will examine the petri dish as a container of cultural memes that affect mental health and illness.

3.1 Culture and Presenting Symptoms

It is well known that psychiatric syndromes are influenced by culture and cultural change, both in geographic and temporal senses. For example, waxy flexibility of catatonia and psychogenic fainting have diminished over time in Western cultures (van der Heijden et al., 2005) while previously rarely recognized conditions such as anorexia, fibromyalgia, and drug addiction have become commonplace.

For the same psychiatric condition, such as depression or schizophrenia, different symptomatic presentations depending on culture have been noted. For example, depressed Latinos presented with somatic symptoms much more than otherwise demographically matched Anglo-Americans whether they lived in North America or in their native lands (Escobar et al., 1983; Stoker et al., 1968). It has been reported that South American Indians who practice witchcraft often have hallucinations of "jungle spirits" and saints (Murphy, 1982). In fact, any clinician dealing with mental illness would note that religious delusions and hallucinations are common among the religious patients, while more persecutory delusions and hallucinations of non-religious objects, such as animals and space aliens, are more common among the nonreligious.

H. Leigh, *Genes, Memes, Culture, and Mental Illness*,
DOI 10.1007/978-1-4419-5671-2_3, © Hoyle Leigh, 2010

3.2 Culture-Specific Psychiatric Syndromes

There are culture-specific psychiatric syndromes that seem to be confined to geographic areas, such as koro, characterized by the patient's intense preoccupation of retraction of his penis and that he will die. This syndrome is endemic in Malaysia and Indonesia. Epidemics of koro have been reported affecting hundreds or thousands of people (Jilek and Jilek-Aall, 1977; Tseng and Streltzer, 1997). Latah, seen in Southeast Asian women, is characterized by a startle response in which they lose control, mimic others around them, and blindly obey commands. Ataques de nervios, a condition seen in Puerto Ricans, is characterized by anxiety, dissociation, and loss of control (Cintron et al., 2005; Guarnaccia, 1993; Oquendo et al., 1992).

Culture-specific syndromes seem to incorporate endemic memes and are readily accepted in the specific culture.

3.3 Enculturation and Memes

Culture is considered to consist of explicit and implicit patterns of behavior acquired and transmitted by symbols constituting distinctive achievement of human groups. The core of culture is considered to be traditional ideas and values (Tseng and Streltzer, 1997). Enculturation is a process through which the traditional ideas and values take up residence in the brain of the individual through repeated pattern formation in the neural networks, resulting in the formation and strengthening of certain synaptic and dendritic connections (see Chapter 9). Tseng and Streltzer note that the organization of culture has its psychobiological correlates in the organization of the brain, the microanatomy of individual neurons, and thus the organization of neural networks (Tseng and Streltzer, 1997).

In the previous chapter, I likened environment to a petri dish, and the nutrients and toxins that may enter the organism to memes. Culture, consisting of symbols – language, artifacts, rules, is then a pool of memes. Memes enter the brain and take up residence in the brain through long-term potentiation of neural network patterns. Endemic (cultural) memes introduced in childhood are strongly potentiated as they are repeatedly introduced during a period when the filtration system for meme introduction is immature. Eventually, existing memes contribute to the formation of the filtration system which filters out new memes that may conflict with or contradict the pre-existing potentiated memes.

3.4 Memes for Being Ill

Within the meme pool (culture) of most geographic areas, there are memes for being "crazy" or "insane" as well as memes for anxiety and dysphoria. This is no wonder as many memes started out as imitations (see Chapter 8). Imitating the crazy one is surely the best way to be crazy, and imitating the one recognized as not feeling well is a good way of communicating that you are not feeling well. In isolated cultures, certain unusual (for other cultures) memes denoting such states have evolved, such as koro, latah, and ataques de nervios.

New memes or ways of expressing an internal state do arise and may become fashionable, such as some cases of fibromyalgia, "burn-out," and multiple chemical sensitivity (Eriksen and Ursin, 2004).

As we saw in the previous chapter, sustained stress, by attenuating the connection to memory and thus dominant resident memes, provides the brain with favorable conditions for new meme infusion from the outside without normal filtration. Such unchecked infusion of new stress memes may interact with dormant pathogenic memes hidden in the brain, stimulating their replication. A contributing factor may be that chronic stress causes sensitization to bodily dysphoric sensations (Eriksen and Ursin, 2004), which may in turn stimulate the pathogenic memes.

An example of such pathogenic memes may be depressive memes. Memes such as "I am worthless," "I am a bad person," "Nobody loves me" exist in many individuals, but are not prominent (reinforced) in everyday life. Such memes are not uncommonly introduced in childhood by adults, peers, and by exposure to persons who are despised (empathy is a form of imitation, and thus leads to memes). Conversely, protective memes such as "I am loved (by parents, friends, spouse)," "I am competent," and "I am good" are introduced to varying degrees during a person's development.

We can now state that the resident memes, both protective and pathogenic, are memes the brain acquired from the meme pool that we call culture. The cultural environment in which the person grew up provided the individual with the memes that reside in the person's brain. Some of these memes were repeatedly introduced and were attached to positive emotions becoming dominant part of the personality, others may have been introduced repeatedly but consciously suppressed, become attached to negative emotions, and stayed in a dormant, repressed state within the brain. It is these repressed memes attached to unpleasant affect that chronic stress permits to multiply and reach consciousness.

References

Cintron, J. A., Carter, M. M., Sbrocco, T. (2005) Ataques de nervios in relation to anxiety sensitivity among island Puerto Ricans. *Cult Med Psychiatry*, **29**, 415–431.

Eriksen, H. R., Ursin, H. (2004) Subjective health complaints, sensitization, and sustained cognitive activation (stress). *J Psychosom Res*, **56**, 445–448.

Escobar, J. I., Gomez, J., Tuason, V. B. (1983) Depressive phenomenology in North and South American patients. *Am J Psychiatry*, **140**, 47–51.

Guarnaccia, P. J. (1993) Ataques de nervios in Puerto Rico: Culture-bound syndrome or popular illness? *Med Anthropol*, **15**, 157–170.

Jilek, W., Jilek-Aall, L. (1977) [Mass-hysteria with Koro-symptoms in Thailand]. *Schweiz Arch Neurol Neurochir Psychiatr*, **120**, 257–259.

Murphy, H. B. M. (1982) Culture and schizophrenia. In *Culture and Psychopathology* (I. Al-Issa ed.), pp. 49–82. University Park Press, Baltimore, MD.

Oquendo, M., Horwath, E., Martinez, A. (1992) Ataques de nervios: Proposed diagnostic criteria for a culture specific syndrome. *Cult Med Psychiatry*, **16**, 367–376.

Stoker, D. H., Zurcher, L. A., Fox, W. (1968) Women in psychotherapy: A cross-cultural comparison. *Int J Soc Psychiatry*, **15**, 5–22.

Tseng, W.-S., Streltzer, J. (1997) *Culture and Psychopathology*. Bruner/Mazel, New York.

van der Heijden, F. M., Tuinier, S., Arts, N. J., et al. (2005) Catatonia: Disappeared or under-diagnosed? *Psychopathology*, **38**, 3–8.

Chapter 4
Genetic–Memetic Model of Mental Illness – Migration and Natural Disasters as Illustrations

Contents

We have so far developed an epigenetic model of mental illness based on gene × meme interaction. Important in the equations are the nature of genes themselves (e.g., polymorphisms) and the culture that forms the meme pool in early life as well as childhood stress memes. Adult stress conditions result in an influx of new stress memes that may stimulate the replication of dormant pathogenic memes, as a carcinogen may trigger the uncontrolled growth of a cancer-prone (e.g., BRCA gene activated) cell. We will examine two stress conditions that affect large populations and consider the gene × meme interaction that may result in mental illness.

4.1 Migration

When an individual emigrates to another country, there is usually a change in culture (meme pool) to which the person has to adapt (stress).

In a classic 1932 study in Minnesota, Odegaard found a much higher incidence of state hospital admission for schizophrenia among the Norwegian immigrants as compared to native born, and even compared to Norwegians in Norway (Odegaard, 1932). More recent study in The Netherlands showed an increased risk of schizophrenia and other psychosis in immigrants from Morocco, Surinam, and Dutch Antilles but not in those from Turkey or western Europe (Schrier et al., 2001; Selten et al., 2001). There was an increased risk of psychosis among immigrants, especially in those from East Africa (Zolkowska et al., 2001). It is generally accepted that highest rates of psychosis occur in immigrants who are socially and economically disadvantaged and have poorer housing, less educational, and employment opportunities. A recent finding by Patino et al. indicates that there was a fourfold increase in the risk of psychotic symptoms in children who had a history of both immigration and family dysfunction (Patino et al., 2005).

Ndetei reviewed the phenomenology of mental illness of different cultural groups (Ndetei, 1988). The role of migration in West Indian immigrants to England has been studied extensively. West Indian patients admitted to a mental hospital in England and normal West Indians with no history of mental illness both shared a fundamentalist acceptance of the god and the devil having a personal control of one's health and disease as well as beliefs in the existence of ghosts and spirits of the dead. In the patients, religious delusions and persecutory delusions were common, i.e., an exaggeration of commonly held beliefs (memes). Some patients also had grandiose delusions of having special powers to help others, again congruent with the widely held belief in magic. West Indians in a mental hospital in London were found to have an excess of paranoia, somatic, and persecutory symptoms irrespective of actual diagnosis compared to English patients. The delusions found in West Indians were predominantly paranoid in nature (77%), and the hallucinations were predominantly auditory (92%) (Tewfik and Okasha, 1965).

Most of the West Indians who emigrated to England are descendents of slaves brought to the West Indies from West Africa. Thus, the West Indian culture contains a mixture of memes from traditional African culture and European cultures. There are also mutations such as the West Indian version of Pentecostal Christian beliefs to which some 25% of the Jamaican population subscribe. The traditional African beliefs include beliefs in witchcraft and evil spirits.

In Africans living in Africa, e.g., Sudan, Guinea Coast, and Congo, there is widespread belief in witchcraft that did not seem to be altered significantly by levels of education and Westernization (Ndetei, 1988). Even Christians returned to the traditional belief/behavior when under stress. This may indicate that the witchcraft and evil spirit memes may have lain dormant in the brains in which Western or Christian memes became dominant, but that the dormant memes awakened and multiplied under conditions of stress.

According to traditional African beliefs, health signifies peace with the spirits of ancestors and supernatural beings. When sick, they often go to the Western doctor for treatment of the illness, but also to the witch doctor to divine the cause of the disease. This practice may cut across educational and socioeconomic levels.

Ndetei states that any actions, beliefs, traditions, and cultural ways of thinking of many Africans are based on local laws of causality, i.e., every misfortune or disease is the doing of witches or evil people. Thus it makes sense to feel paranoid, i.e., an external agent is responsible, when one feels dysphoria. Since such external spirits exist, it is also natural to hear them in the form of auditory hallucinations. In memetic terms, brains infected with memes like witches and evil spirits are at a higher risk of paranoid forms of psychosis under stress.

The impact of migration on the individual would be different between voluntary migrants and involuntary ones. The voluntary immigrants who choose to migrate would have had increased and regular contact with the new culture (memes) to prepare for the migration, usually for economic or educational advancement, i.e., the infusion of the new memes would be gradual and in harmony with existing memes because of the positive affect attached to the new memes. Further, the voluntary immigrants are more likely to be either better educated, from a higher socioeconomic class, or novelty-seeking. Involuntary migration, as in refugees, exiles, and slaves, on the other hand, is often sudden and associated with negative affect. The exposure to the new culture and memes is unprepared and may result in a "culture shock." The loss of familiar culture (re-enforcing meme pool) and cultural identity (influx of memes contrary to dominant memes in the brain) may cause an acute grief reaction and has been called *cultural bereavement* (Bhugra and Becker, 2005; Eisenbruch, 1984).

Even among voluntary immigrants, the degree of acceptance by the new land and the degree of discrepancy between expectations and achievements play a role in the stress level and thence the risk of mental illness. High ethnic density (thus re-enforcing meme pool for familiar memes) may have a protective effect. Bhugra observed that there may be particular difficulties for individuals who migrate from a collectivistic or socio-centric societies, and who themselves are socio-centric, into individual or ego-centric societies (Bhugra and Becker, 2005). Obviously, there would be memetic conflict between the dominant socio-centric memes in the brain and the incoming ego-centric memes from the newly dominant meme pool.

While migration is generally stressful in the sense that there is an adaptational demand to a new location and culture, it is not universally pathogenic. For some groups of immigrants same or lower rate of psychiatric illness compared to indigenous people have been observed. For example, the East Asians (East Indians and Pakistanis) in England had similar or lower rates of psychosis compared to native-born English (Bhugra, 2000; Cochrane, 1977). This finding may be attributed to the increased social support in these groups. Social support in these groups may be in the form of frequent access to familiar meme pools from the original culture, and gradual and, therefore, filtered introduction of new memes.

People who emigrate might also be more sturdy individuals who are unafraid of change, and some such individuals may already harbor memes of the new culture through active exposure to books, films, etc. (Cochrane, 1979).

So far, we discussed the interaction of resident memes with stress that increases the risk of psychosis in some immigrants. What might be the role of genes in this interaction?

One hypothesis is that persons with genes associated with a higher risk for schizophrenia, i.e., eccentric, asocial, or unstable personalities, may be more predisposed to emigrate. The fact that many psychotic symptoms seen in immigrants do not seem to be "core symptoms" of schizophrenia but rather exaggerations of memes of culture of origin, tend to cast doubt to the completeness of this explanation. On the other hand, the so-called core symptoms, e.g., Schneiderian first-rank symptoms such as auditory hallucinations, have been reported to vary depending on culture (Ndetei, 1988). Therefore, given genetic vulnerability to psychosis, whether in native land or new land, the memes denoting psychosis (or memes that tell you how to be "crazy") may proliferate under stressful conditions.

An intriguing finding in monkeys may be relevant. Male rhesus monkeys leave their maternal group when they reach adolescence and roam in bands of male-only groups. The serotonin transporter promoter polymorphism discussed in Chapter 2 seems to determine the age of such departure. Those with the short alleles of 5-HTTLPR tended to leave the maternal troop earlier than those with the long alleles. Those with the short alleles tend to be antisocial, aggressive, and stress-sensitive, and also have lower levels of the serotonin metabolite, 5-hydroxyindoleacetic acid (5-HIAA), in the cerebrospinal fluid (Trefilov et al., 2000). Another study found that males with low central serotonin levels (and therefore low 5-HIAA) delay migration if they stayed until adolescence and show high levels of violence and premature death, but those that survive achieve higher dominance rank in the new troop (Howell et al., 2007). Perhaps, some humans who migrate might also be genetically more prone to be adventurous, more stress-sensitive, but can be more sturdy and achieve mastery if they survive the initial adjustment.

While there is clearly a higher rate of psychosis among immigrants, the rate of depression and anxiety seems lower, especially among the Asian immigrants to England. This might be due to resident memes that cause reluctance to express dysphoria or due to fatalistic memes or external locus or control that may be protective (Bhugra, 2004). Existing memes may also influence immigrants to express dysphoria as somatic symptoms rather than emotional suffering (Iwata et al., 2002; Ndetei, 1988). In other words, it is possible that there is a greater prevalence of memes denoting or describing depressive states in the Western culture so that the immigrants' expression of depressive memes may be smaller in comparison even in those whose brains may be experiencing a depressive state. On the other hand, there may be more memetic expression of somatic discomfort.

In summary, migration serves as an example of stress that may differentially affect different individuals depending on several factors. One is clearly the genetic composition of the individual and the early memetic environment that may have predisposed the individual to be stress-sensitive or stress resistant. Another factor is the memes that the individual has absorbed in early life, memes for expressing dysphoria and memes for being "crazy," and overarching memes that explain nature and misfortune. Then the degree of conflict or congruence between the pre-existing memes and the new meme pool of the new land would play a role, as well as the degree of support or filtering available from the sub-meme pool in the immigrant community playing a protective role.

4.2 Natural Disasters

Natural disasters such as tsunamis, floods, and hurricanes are well known to cause depression and posttraumatic stress disorders. However, not everyone who has been exposed to such disasters develops psychiatric syndromes. Kilpatrick and colleagues recently reported an association among the serotonin transporter promoter gene polymorphism (5-HTTLPR), the amount of exposure to disaster, and social support in the risk of development of depression and PTSD (Kilpatrick et al., 2007). They studied 589 victims of the 2004 Florida hurricane through interviews and DNA analysis to determine the extent of stressful exposure to the disaster, symptoms of depression and PTSD, and social support. Social support during the 6 months before the hurricanes was assessed, consisting of emotional (e.g., "someone available to love you and make you feel wanted"), instrumental (e.g., "someone available to help you if you were confined to bed"), and appraisal (e.g., "someone available to give you good advice in a crisis") aspects. In this study, the prevalence of post-hurricane PTSD was 3.2% and the prevalence of post-hurricane major depression was 5.6%. Low social support was associated with both PTSD and major depression and high hurricane exposure was associated with PTSD but not major depression. The serotonin transporter genotype by itself was not associated with the risk of PTSD or depression, but the short allele of 5-HTTLPR in interaction with the degree of exposure to stress and lack of social support increased the risk of depression and PTSD. This genotype-by-environment effect was found in both males and females.

Though no specific memetic data are available, this study shows the power of social support whose effect is largely memetic (someone to love you, make you feel wanted, give good advice, etc.) that may attenuate or exacerbate the stress of natural disasters.

References

Bhugra, D. (2000) Migration and schizophrenia. *Acta Psychiatr Scand Suppl*, **407**, 68–73.

Bhugra, D. (2004) Migration and mental health. *Acta Psychiatr Scand*, **109**, 243–258.

Bhugra, D., Becker, M. A. (2005) Migration, cultural bereavement and cultural identity. *World Psychiatry*, **4**, 18–24.

Binder, E. B., Bradley, R. G., Liu, W., et al. (2008) Association of FKBP5 polymorphisms and childhood abuse with risk of posttraumatic stress disorder symptoms in adults. *JAMA*, **299**, 1291–1305

Cochrane, R. (1977) Mental illness in immigrants to England and Wales. *Soc Psychiatry*, **12**, 25–35.

Cochrane, R. (1979) Psychological and behavioural disturbance in West Indians, Indians and Pakistanis in Britain: A comparison of rates among children and adults. *Br J Psychiatry*, **134**, 201–210.

Eisenbruch, M. (1984) Cross-cultural aspects of bereavement. I: A conceptual framework for comparative analysis. *Cult Med Psychiatry*, **8**, 283–309.

Howell, S., Westergaard, G., Hoos, B., et al. (2007) Serotonergic influences on life-history outcomes in free-ranging male rhesus macaques. *Am J Primatol*, **69**, 851–865.

Iwata, N., Turner, R. J., Lloyd, D. A. (2002) Race/ethnicity and depressive symptoms in community-dwelling young adults: A differential item functioning analysis. *Psychiatry Res*, **110**, 281–289.

Kilpatrick, D. G., Koenen, K. C., Ruggiero, K. J., et al. (2007) The serotonin transporter genotype and social support and moderation of posttraumatic stress disorder and depression in hurricane-exposed adults. *Am J Psychiatry*, **164**, 1693–1699.

Ndetei, D. M. (1988) Psychiatric phenomenology across countries: Constitutional, cultural, or environmental? *Acta Psychiatr Scand Suppl*, **344**, 33–44.

Odegaard, O. (1932) Emigration and insanity: A study of mental disease among the Norwegian-born population of Minnesota. *Acta Psychiatr Scand*, **7**, 1–206.

Patino, L. R., Selten, J. P., Van Engeland, H., et al. (2005) Migration, family dysfunction and psychotic symptoms in children and adolescents. *Br J Psychiatry*, **186**, 442–443.

Schrier, A. C., van de Wetering, B. J., Mulder, P. G., et al. (2001) Point prevalence of schizophrenia in immigrant groups in Rotterdam: Data from outpatient facilities. *Eur Psychiatry*, **16**, 162–166.

Selten, J. P., Veen, N., Feller, W., et al. (2001) Incidence of psychotic disorders in immigrant groups to The Netherlands. *Br J Psychiatry*, **178**, 367–372.

Tewfik, G. I., Okasha, A. (1965) Psychosis and immigration. *Postgrad Med J*, **41**, 603–612.
Trefilov, A., Berard, J., Krawczak, M., et al. (2000) Natal dispersal in rhesus macaques is related
   to serotonin transporter gene promoter variation. *Behav Genet*, **30**, 295–301.
Zolkowska, K., Cantor-Graae, E., McNeil, T. F. (2001) Increased rates of psychosis among
   immigrants to Sweden: Is migration a risk factor for psychosis? *Psychol Med*, **31**, 669–678.

Part II
Evolution and Mental Health: Genes, Memes, Culture, and the Individual

In Part I, we focused on mental illness and how genes, memes, stress, and culture interact in the development of vulnerability or resistance to mental illness. In Part II, we will examine in some detail how memes arose in the course of evolution, how they are stored in the brain and externally, and how they are evolving. Here, I redefine the meme as a brain code, which is replicated both inside and outside of the brain. I then describe an integrated model of mental health and illness based on gene x meme x environment interaction.

Chapter 5
What Do We Inherit from Our Parents and Ancestors?

Contents

We are composed of genes and memes. We inherit genes from our parents, and by extension, our ancestors, human and pre-human. Memes are mostly information from our cultural environment that are also inherited from our parents, and ancestors. Some memes are introduced into the environment from other cultures or de novo by creative persons. Memes are dispersed in the environment around us, like chemicals in a petri dish. Some of the memes forcibly penetrate our brains, others are passively absorbed by our brains. This chapter discusses the broad concepts of cultural inheritance and meme's role in it.

5.1 Like Parent, Like Child

What do we inherit from our parents, other than money for those who are lucky? Like father, like son is a commonly accepted idea as is the saying, "the baby has her mother's eyes and her father's mouth." Physical characteristics are obviously passed on to the next generation, much of the time according to Mendelian genetics as discussed in the next chapter. But what about behavior and psychology?

"Like father, like son" may mean both physical characteristics *and* behavior, e.g., if the father is a drunkard, then the son might also be one, too. Does this mean that the father's habit of driving while intoxicated will pass on to the child as well? What are the cultural influences for such situations? Would the son be a drunkard and drive while intoxicated if he became a Muslim and forswore drinking alcohol? Would he *want to or be able to* stop drinking given his inherited genes from father?

H. Leigh, *Genes, Memes, Culture, and Mental Illness*,
DOI 10.1007/978-1-4419-5671-2_5, © Hoyle Leigh, 2010

Even for inheritance of property, the rules are not as simple as might be supposed. For example, males historically inherited larger portions of the parents' property in most Western and Eastern cultures, and they still do under Islamic law where the sons get exactly double of what the daughters get. Just how the property was to be divided among heirs was complex depending on culture, for example, the spouse vs. the eldest son vs. the male and female siblings. The net result of just which property (for example, the house and the car) will go to whom and how much of the money would go to whom is, therefore, a result of a complex set of rules that are specific to the situation and culture. And these rules are passed on from generation to generation unless a cultural change occurs.

5.2 How Does Culture Affect Behavior?

It is generally believed that individuals learn to absorb and adapt to the cultural norms through learning, mostly following the reward–punishment paradigm of operant conditioning and the development of representations of cultural values transmitted through parents – the superego.

Culture consists of not only values but also language, modes of dress, food, and recreational activities. Such cultural items are passed on from generation to generation mainly through imitation and identification. For example, longer hairdo for women, men wearing trousers and not skirts. Culture does change – either through exposure to other cultures, or through mutation. Thus sushi became a popular food in the West, and most Japanese wear Western attire. Through mutation, the Greek *era* became *eorthe* in old English, then *earth* today (Merriam-Webster). Our ancestors walked and ran, then rode horses, and now we ride automobiles, ships, and airplanes.

5.3 Memes and Cultural Change

How exactly does culture mutate? Certainly, horses did not mutate into automobiles, and kimonos did not mutate into Western suits. In fact, horses and kimonos still exist side by side with automobiles and Western suits. What changes is inside our brains – what is accepted as desirable or preferable. What changes is the brain's reaction to the cultural information, e.g., kimono and Western suit, what has been perceived. "Sushi is delicious, and eating it is good" defeats the once prevalent idea, "Eating raw fish is disgusting." Richard Dawkins coined the term *Meme* to denote the elements of cultural information that is largely transmitted through imitation (Dawkins, 1976, 2006). As discussed earlier, memes, like genes, are replicators, i.e., they are copied by brains and transmitted to others by means of behavior and language, and nowadays by electronic means and by computers, and reside in books, DVDs, and computer hard drives as well as in human brains. See Chapter 8 for further discussion on this topic.

5.4 Memeplexes

Individuals are immersed in the cultural environment consisting of memes. The culture medium in a petri dish affects the bacterial colony in it through the chemical molecules that may be nutrients or poisons. In the same way, the memes in our environment are introduced into our brains by absorption, diffusion, or forced penetration as by incessant TV advertisements or roadside billboards. The term, *memeplex*, denotes a complex of memes that tend to travel together and co-evolve. A memeplex conjures up often multimodal images and sounds, for example, national anthem, Mona Lisa, self, Christmas. Memeplexes have survival advantage just as multicellular organisms do. Consider the strength of the memeplex "National Anthem" to the meme "national." National anthem is copied (sung) each time there is a ceremony, including the opening of sporting events.

References

Dawkins, R. (1976) *The Selfish Gene*. Oxford University Press, New York.
Dawkins, R. (2006) *The Selfish Gene* (30th anniversary edn). Oxford University Press, Oxford; New York.
Merriam-Webster. *Merriam-Webster Dictionary*.

Chapter 6
Genes

Contents

This chapter is a review of basic genetics as a preliminary for discussion of evolution.

6.1 Human Genes

In the previous chapter, we discussed how we inherit cultural heritage through memes. In this chapter, we will examine how our physical characteristics are inherited. We know now that genes are the basis of hereditary transmission and that they are double-helix DNA strands consisting of four nucleotides, thymine, guanine, cytosine, and adenine. All of the some 30,000 human genes have now been mapped.

All our genes are in the 23 pairs of chromosomes that exist in every cell of our body (except for sperms and eggs that have half the number of chromosomes). The chromosomes consist of 22 pairs of autosomes and two sex chromosomes, XX or XY. The reproductive cells, eggs and sperms, have only one half of the chromosomes, and thus a sperm can have only one X or Y.

Genes have been discussed and argued over long before it was known that they consisted of DNA. Hippocrates, for example, believed in hereditary material accumulating throughout life and that strong impressions, i.e., acquired characteristics, could be transmitted to the offspring. An illustration is his famous defense of a woman who gave birth to a black child as, he believed, she was very impressed with

H. Leigh, *Genes, Memes, Culture, and Mental Illness*,
DOI 10.1007/978-1-4419-5671-2_6, © Hoyle Leigh, 2010

an African man (Hippocrates). The idea that acquired characteristics are genetically transmitted was considered to be a well-established fact until the nineteenth century.

6.2 Mendelian Genetics

Gregor Johann Mendel (1822–1884) was an Austrian Augustinian monk who is considered to be the father of modern genetics (Bardoe, 2006). He studied the inheritance patterns of specific aspects of the pea plant and discovered that they followed simple mathematical rules. Mendel came to the conclusion that the hereditary determinants were particulate in nature called genes. He believed that each gene consists of a pair of alleles that may be dominant or recessive. Only the dominant allele is expressed as the phenotype unless there are two recessive alleles. Mendel published his work in 1866 as *Experiments on Plant Hybridization* in the *Proceedings of the Natural History Society of Brünn*. His discoveries, however, remained unrecognized until after his death, when in 1900 they were "rediscovered" by Hugo De Vries, Carl Correns, and Erich Von Tschermak.

Now it is known that a heterozygote carrying a copy of both a dominant and a recessive trait may result in a phenotype that contains both traits to a greater or lesser extent.

6.3 Genes and Mutation

The function of genes is to tell the cells of the offspring how to build a body that resembles the parents. As an offspring requires the contribution of genes from two parents, there is inevitably a recombination of the genes, and the offspring is never an exact copy of the parent. In addition to such recombinations, mutations occur that may change the offspring drastically.

The *genetic code* is the set of rules by which information encoded in genetic material (DNA or RNA sequences) is translated into proteins. The code maps trinucleotide sequences called *codons* that specify a single amino acid to be produced.

Mutation is a change in the genetic code, which may occur simply by accident or by influences such as chemicals and radiation (see Figs. 6.1 and 6.2). Extra nucleotides may be inserted into a DNA sequence (*Insertion*) or segments of DNA may be *deleted*. There may be a *frame shift*, i.e., the sequence of the codon may be altered by insertion or deletion so that the resulting protein, if it exists, would be incorrect. *Substitution* is a mutation in which there is a substitution of one base for another, e.g., A for G, CTGGAG for CTGGGG. Substitution may result in a codon that produces a different amino acid resulting in a small change in the protein produced. An example is the sickle cell anemia caused by a substitution in the beta hemoglobin gene that alters a single amino acid (valine for glutamic acid) resulting in Hemoglobin S. Substitution may change a codon that encodes the same amino acid, resulting in no change in the protein produced (*silent or synonymous*

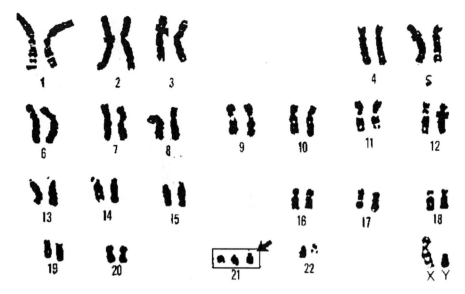

Fig. 6.1 Human chromosomes in Down's syndrome, which results from trisomy of chromosome 21. (Figure from http://ornl.gov/sci/techresources/Human_Genome/publicat/primer/fig6.html)

mutation). At times, an amino acid-coding codon may change to a single "stop" codon, causing an incomplete protein which may not function correctly.

A *single nucleotide polymorphism, or SNP* (pronounced *snip*), is a DNA sequence variation occurring when a single nucleotide (A, T, C, or G) in the genome differs between members of a species or between paired chromosomes in an individual. For example, two DNA fragments from different individuals, AAGCCTA and AAGCTTA, contain a difference in a single nucleotide, i.e., there are two alleles, C and T, for this gene. Almost all common SNPs have two alleles. SNPs may occur within coding sequences of genes, noncoding regions of genes, or between genes.

Missence mutation refers to a substitution of a single nucleotide that results in the production of a different amino acid and, therefore, a different protein (or in some cases, no protein). When an amino acid is replaced by another of very similar chemical properties, the protein may still function normally (*neutral or quiet mutation*). Some amino acids may be encoded by more than one codon (*degenerate coding*), in which case a mutation in one codon would not result in any change in the protein, which would be a synonymous mutation. Some missence mutations cause serious diseases, e.g., epidermolysis bullosa, sickle cell disease, and some forms of amyotrophic lateral sclerosis.

An illustration of Mendelian genetic transmission of a human disease caused by a single nucleotide mutation is sickle cell anemia. Sickle cell anemia is caused by a mutation in the beta hemoglobin gene (HBB) located on the short arm of chromosome 11. The 17th nucleotide of this gene is changed from codon GAG that codes for glutamic acid to GTG, which codes for valine, so the amino acid in position 6 is incorrectly substituted (see Fig. 6.3).

Mutation

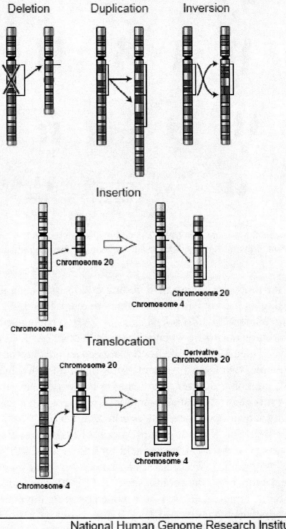

Fig. 6.2 Gene mutations

This mutation results in production of abnormal Hemoglobin S, which tends to stick together and form long, rigid molecules. The rigid HbS molecules bend red blood cells into a sickle (crescent) shape. These abnormal cells die prematurely, which may lead to anemia. The sickle-shaped cells can also occlude small

Fig. 6.3 Chromosome 11
and HBB. (From
http://ghr.nlm.nih.gov/gene=hbb)

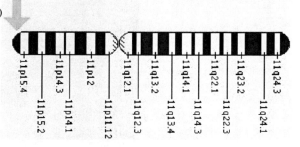

Fig. 6.4 Genetics of sickle
cell disease

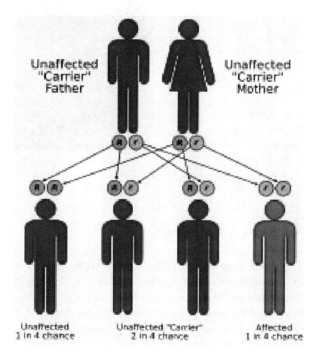

blood vessels, causing pain and tissue damage (http://ghr.nlm.nih.gov/gene=hbb)
(Figs. 6.4 and 6.5).

Sickle cell anemia is a Mendelian autosomal recessive disease, and one quarter
of the offsprings of carrier parents are expected to be affected. Sickle cell trait is
a heterozygous form of this illness with variable severity of symptomatology. The
sickle cell gene is quite common in sub-Saharan Africa where malaria is prevalent
(Makani et al., 2007). This is no wonder as sickle cells are resistant to malarial
infection, and thus confers protection against it (Timmann et al., 2007).

Fig. 6.5 Sickle cells

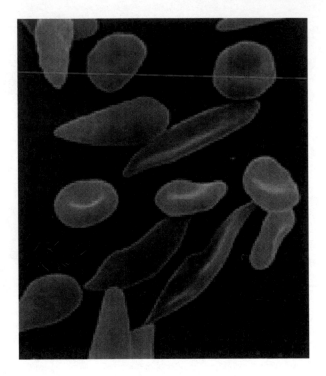

6.4 Sex-Linked Genes

The genes that reside in the sex chromosomes, X and Y, not only cause sexual differentiation but also may be associated with disease. The genes in the Y chromosomes can only be manifested in males – only a few genes in the Y chromosomes have been identified, one of them the testis-determining factor that causes the male phenotype to develop. Even one X-linked recessive trait will be expressed in a male (lacking another X chromosome that might carry the dominant trait) but in a female only if she carries another X chromosome with the same recessive trait.

An example of sex-linked condition is red-green color blindness, which is an X-linked recessive trait. Thus, the children of a color-blind father (X'Y) and a carrier mother (X'X) would result in X'X', X'X, YX', and YX, so that 50% of the male children and 50% of the female children would be color blind. On the other hand, if the father is not color blind (XY) and mother is a carrier (X'X), then the children would be XX', XX, YX', and YX, i.e., 50% of the male children and no female children would be phenotypically color blind (Wiggs, 2000).

If the father is color blind (X'Y) and mother is not a carrier (XX), then none of the sons would be color blind, while 50% of the daughters would be carriers.

6.5 Polygenic Inheritance

Many genetic traits and conditions such as size, intelligence, and behavioral dispositions in humans and animals are determined by the interaction of many different genes as well as with environment as discussed in Chapters 1 and 2. One gene makes one protein but the effects of the proteins usually interact. The term, epistasis, is used to denote the interference of one gene in the expression of another.

There are many genes that have more than two alleles, such as the ABO blood type in humans. Multiple alleles result from different mutations of the same gene. Human ABO blood types are determined by alleles, A, B, and O. Both A and B alleles are codominant over O. Thus, AA and AO types produce A antigen, BB and BO produce B antigen, AB produces both A and B antigens, and OO type produces neither antigen.

Polygenic traits are usually expressed as a gradation of small differences (continuous variation) rather than discrete characteristics as in simple Mendelian inheritance. Such variations usually result in a bell-shaped curve, as in height, weight, skin color, etc. Traits showing continuous variation may be controlled by two or more separate gene pairs. The inheritance of each gene in such polygenic inheritance does follow Mendelian rules (Farabee, 2001).

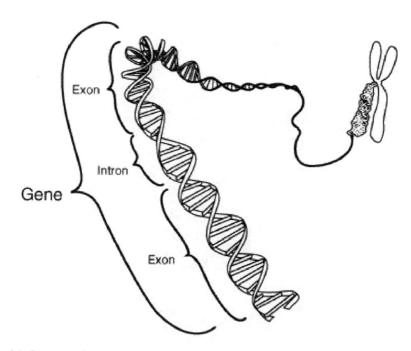

Fig. 6.6 Structure of a gene

6.6 How Do Genes Work?

Genes are segments of the chromosome that contain strands of DNA that make messenger RNAs (ribonucleic acid, mRNA). Genes are associated with a promoter, the DNA region that is usually upstream to the coding sequence. The promoter binds and directs RNA polymerase (RNAP, RNApol) to the correct transcriptional start site and thus permits the initiation of *transcription*. Through this process, a copy of RNA complementary to the DNA template is produced.

Of particular interest is polymorphism of gene promoters such as the serotonin transporter promoter gene (5-HTTLPR) mentioned in Chapters 1 and 2.

RNA polymerase can also elongate the mRNA chain by adding nucleotides to it. The mRNA leaves the nucleus of the cell and becomes ribosomal RNA (mRNA) that makes a protein using the amino acids presented to it by the transport RNA (tRNA). The only function of genes is to make proteins.

However, not all the DNAs that make up the chromosome are genes. There are large portions of the DNA that do not code for proteins, and even in a gene, there are

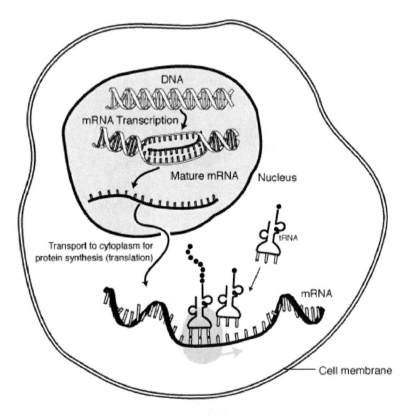

Fig. 6.7 DNA and RNA. (This image is in the *public domain* because it contains materials that originally came from the *National Institutes of Health*)

segments that do not make proteins. That segment of the gene that is expressed to make proteins is called an exon, and the silent portion is called an intron (Fig. 6.6). The DNA that does not produce proteins has been called collectively "junk DNA." Even when a DNA has made an RNA, some portions of the RNA may not get translated into protein (untranslated RNA, UTR) (Fig. 6.7).

It turns out that such "junk DNA" and UTR are not junk at all, but seem to have important functions in regulating the genes and, even at times, reverse engineering the genes (Andolfatto, 2005; Lolle et al., 2005).

Each cell has the entire DNA code, but cells in different tissues are different and serve different functions, i.e., only certain genes are activated and others are not. What activates the specific genes to make specific cells? It seems the DNA produces cell type-specific noncoding RNA that attracts molecules called *epigenetic activators*, which, in turn, bind to DNA elements in the target gene, activating or silencing it (Beisel et al., 2002; Brene et al., 2000; Sanchez-Elsner et al., 2006).

References

Andolfatto, P. (2005) Adaptive evolution of non-coding DNA in Drosophila. *Nature*, **437**, 1149–1152.

Bardoe, C. (2006) *Gregor Mendel: The Friar Who Grew Peas*. HN Abrans, New York.

Beisel, C., Imhof, A., Greene, J., et al. (2002) Histone methylation by the Drosophila epigenetic transcriptional regulator Ash1. *Nature*, **419**, 857–862.

Brene, S., Messer, C., Okado, H., et al. (2000) Regulation of GluR2 promoter activity by neurotrophic factors via a neuron-restrictive silencer element. *Eur J Neurosci*, **12**, 1525–1533.

Farabee, M. (2001) *Gene interactions*. http://www.emc.maricopa.edu/faculty/farabee/BIOBK/BioBookgeninteract.html#Interactions%20among%20genes

Hippocrates.   http://duke.usask.ca/~niallm/233/Hippocra.htm   http://ghr.nlm.nih.gov/gene=hbb HBB

Lolle, S. J., Victor, J. L., Young, J. M., et al. (2005) Genome-wide non-mendelian inheritance of extra-genomic information in Arabidopsis. *Nature*, **434**, 505–509.

Makani, J., Williams, T. N., Marsh, K. (2007) Sickle cell disease in Africa: Burden and research priorities. *Ann Trop Med Parasitol*, **101**, 3–14.

Sanchez-Elsner, T., Gou, D., Kremmer, E., et al. (2006) Noncoding RNAs of trithorax response elements recruit Drosophila Ash1 to Ultrabithorax. *Science*, **311**, 1118–1123.

Timmann, C., Evans, J. A., Konig, I. R., et al. (2007) Genome-wide linkage analysis of malaria infection intensity and mild disease. *PLoS Genet*, **3**, e48.

Wiggs, J. L. (2000) Color vision. In *Ophthalmology* (M. Yanoff and J. S. Duker eds.). St. Louis, Mosby.

Chapter 7
Evolution

Contents

7.1 In the Beginning . . .

In the beginning, there was the Big Bang. Then the universe inflated, after which there was only hot plasma of quarks and gluons and other relativistic particles. Particle and antiparticle pairs were continuously formed and destroyed in extreme heat. A small excess of quarks and leptons over antiquarks and antileptons resulted in the predominance of matter over antimatter. At about 10^{-6} s, quarks and gluons combined to form baryons such as protons and neutrons. As the temperature dropped with continuing expansion of universe, no new proton–antiproton or neutron–antineutron pairs could be formed, and a mass annihilation of particle and antiparticle occurred (Kolb and Turner, 1990). In 3 min, the universe was filled with light (photons), and with continued cooling of the universe in the span of 380,000 years, protons became hydrogen by acquiring an electron, photons were decoupled from matter to fly away eventually becoming the microwave background of today. Aggregates of molecules of hydrogen and helium became densely packed with gravity, finally igniting nuclear fusion, forming stars. In about a billion years after the Big Bang, quasars and galaxies began to form. Large populations of stars were born, aged, and died, in spectacular explosions as supernovae, or shrinking into a black hole. Heavier elements including carbon and metals were created in the nuclear furnace of stars and then scattered in space when the stars went supernova. From the debris of exploded stars, the cosmic dust, new stars were born and new galaxies were formed, continuing the process of cosmic evolution (Bertschinger, 1998).

According to Smolin, black holes may produce other universes, just as our universe seems to have started from a black hole through the Big Bang (Smolin, 1999). In this multiverse theory, there would be many universes, some of which may be adapted to multiply and eventually to produce life, and others would simply shrink back into a black hole and give rise to another universe.

In our universe, by around 9 billion years, or 4,500 million years ago (MA), a small, insignificant planet was formed of cosmic dust in the gravitational system of a medium-sized star called the sun in an outer spiral of the milky way galaxy, an ordinary galaxy among billions (Wikipedia, 2008; Wright, 2004). Early earth was very hot and the atmosphere was composed of hydrogen and helium, much of which flew away escaping earth's gravity. Volcanic activity spewed out gasses that formed the bulk of atmosphere, including H_2O, CO_2, SO_2, CO, S_2, Cl_2, N_2, H_2, NH_3 (ammonia), and CH_4 (methane). As the earth cooled in the Archean period some 3,800 million years ago (MA) to 2,500 MA, H_2O congealed into water; oceans, continental plates, and rocks were formed. Some of the H_2O on the surface of the planet was broken up by ultraviolet rays to form oxygen in the atmosphere.

The atmosphere of the primitive earth was a strongly reducing one, in which glycine was synthesized from formaldehyde and hydrogen cyanide. Adenine was synthesized through hydrogen cyanide polymerization. Various nucleotides may have been formed catalyzed by metals and clay in various parts of the earth including volcanic vents, and some might have also been formed outside earth but arrived in meteorites and comets. So there were places on earth teeming with molecules ready for the next phase of earth's evolution – life (Fig. 7.1).

Perhaps, on a dark and stormy night about 3.5 billion years ago, in the pools of hot soup consisting of water, ammonia, and other organic molecules that were all colliding with each other, copies of some molecules were formed in the mix. Such molecules may have been lowly clay or simple linear polymers (Cairns-Smith, 1982). Some such molecules, particularly those consisting of RNA, found themselves inside spontaneously formed vesicles whose walls consisted of phospholipids (Hanczyc and Szostak, 2004). Such vesicles may spontaneously bud and divide, and those replicating molecules that were kept together in such vesicles and divided had a survival advantage, eventually resulting in stable cells (Fig. 7.2). The RNA in some such vesicles may have attracted the right chemicals to build a cell wall. Some RNA probably formed DNA, a reverse process of modern RNA being copied from DNA. Even a single DNA-containing replicating cell so formed could be the origin of all cells as it gave rise to more cells, most of them identical, but some not, due to copying errors. Copying errors gave rise to *variation* in the offspring cells that in turn had variation.

Some such cells happened to incorporate chemicals within the cell that were able to capture the photons to store energy – photosynthesis by cyanobacteria, which contributed to a change in the composition of the earth's environment by adding more oxygen to it.

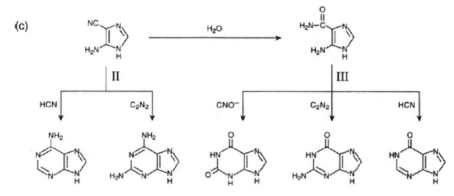

Fig. 7.1   Steps in possible prebiotic syntheses of adenine from HCN. (**a**) The formation of the HCN tetrane. (**b**) The conversion of HCN tetramer to AICN. (**c**) The formation of purines from AICN or from its hydrolysis product 4-amino-imidazole-5-carboxamide (III). From (Orgel, 2004)

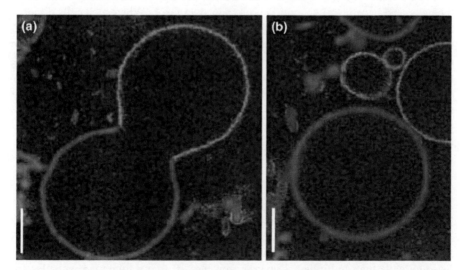

Fig. 7.2   Giant phospholipid vesicles were labeled with two different domain-specific dyes. A fission sequence triggered by heating the vesicles was captured by two-photon microscopy. (From Baumgart et al., 2003, reproduced with permission from Nature)

7.2 In a Changing, Hostile World

As we have seen, the atmosphere of early earth was frankly toxic, but perhaps such a hot atmosphere bombarded by meteorites and infused with gasses and debris from constant volcanic activity might have produced just the kind of mixing and shaking and turmoil to produce the beginnings of life. But life must have been hard for the self-replicating cells, and above all unpredictable. Many replicating molecules and protocells must have been formed, had a brief existence, and then perished in the changing, toxic environment. This constant churning of emergence and destruction of replicating entities resulted in the survival of those that could adapt to the constantly changing environment. Thus arose an algorithm that is evolution (Dennett, 1995), i.e., replicate with errors (variation), and those that can adapt (survive and replicate) in a changed environment will prevail. Evolution is based on *survival of the most stable*, in which survival of the fittest is a special case (Dawkins, 1976) (See Tables 7.1 and 7.2).

As Dennet states, algorithms are *blind* – there is no meaning or direction, just a procedure – in this case, the procedure by which variants that can best replicate in changed environment will survive and replicate again. At this point, it is important to recognize that what is survived is not the cell itself, but the replicators, the information that makes the cell the way it is, i.e., the gene. When we speak of variation, we are really referring to variations in the genetic information. DNA arose from RNA; cells from protocells. Multicellular organisms arose through this algorithm as replication with variation. Replication is more efficient when cells cooperate and effectuate a division of labor – obtaining and storing energy on one hand and replication on the other. Ancient bacteria invaded some cell lines, became incorporated into the cells, and became mitochondria with their own DNA. When such cells divided, they carried the genes (information) for both the original cell (in the nucleus) and the mitochondria (in the cytoplasm where mitochondria reside). Cells and bodies are survival machines for the genes, Dawkins calls evolution a means of perpetuating the *selfish gene* (Dawkins, 1976). This blind procedure, evolution, may lead to many different directions, some fertile, others blind alleys. This procedure, over eons of time, can produce exquisite intricacies in structure as well as complexities that are, in retrospect, functional but stupid, such as the human eye. But we are getting ahead of our story.

7.3 The Selfish Gene

Richard Dawkins clarified the fundamental principle of inheritance of living things in his 1976 landmark book, *The Selfish Gene*. Life as we know it began with naked RNAs that obtained clothes (cell walls), then DNAs arose with instructions for building cells that multiplied. Dawkins saw that all living things are vehicles for strands of DNA with instructions to preserve themselves through the copying process called reproduction. We are all vehicles of genes, and the genes' only interest is their own survival and replication.

It should be clearly stated here that the teleologic figure of speech commonly adopted in discussions of evolution is just that – figure of speech for convenience. Genes do not have any "desire" to replicate or "intention" to survive. It is just that in the course of time, natural laws have it that replicating genes and organisms (or packets of tissue containing genes) that happen to be sturdy (better containers) tend to survive and multiply with the result that "genes that build better vehicles survive and multiply."

For genes to be successful, they require three characteristics: longevity, fecundity, and copying fidelity. In other words, the organism (vehicle) must live long enough to reproduce, and reproduce in large quantities, and the copies must resemble the original.

A severe constraint is placed on the replicating genes by the environment. The environment surrounding the genes (and the vehicles for them, the organisms) consists of other genes and their vehicles, nutrients, toxins, and other hazards. When the resources (e.g., food) are scarce, which was the state of affairs much of the time, then there is naturally competition among the organisms to obtain the resources for survival. From the selfish gene's point of view, then, all other genes that are not like themselves are rivals.

Another resource that is an object of severe competition is a mate for reproduction, as without it, the genes would perish. Organisms better built to find a mate will make more of their own.

From the selfish gene's point of view, altruism is not a problem at all. When particular genes are widely distributed in a group of organisms (vehicles), the act of one vehicle signaling others of danger, even if it risks sacrifice of that particular individual, results in the preservation of large numbers of others that contain the same selfish genes (Fig. 7.3).

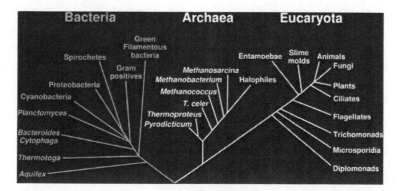

Fig. 7.3 A phylogenetic tree of living things, based on RNA data and proposed by Carl Woese, showing the separation of bacteria, archaea, and eukaryotes. Trees constructed with other genes are generally similar, although they may place some early-branching groups very differently, thanks to long-branch attraction. The exact relationships of the three domains are still being debated, as is the position of the root of the tree. It has also been suggested that due to lateral gene transfer, a tree may not be the best representation of the genetic relationships of all organisms. For instance some genetic evidence suggests that eukaryotes evolved from the union of some bacteria and archaea (one becoming the nucleus and the other the main cell). [Image from Wikimedia, public domain]

7.4 Wonderful Random Errors

Fidelity of copying, a requisite of successful genes, results in the same gene with the same instructions for building the organism. If this fidelity were perfect, then there would be only single-celled organisms inhabiting the earth!

Fortunately for us, nature provided errors for gene replication. Errors in copying resulted in variation and diversity. These errors arose from several factors: pure random statistical errors that occur in any copying process, due to bombardment by waves and particles such as photons, electromagnetic, thermal, and cosmic rays, and other molecules and atoms. Many organisms thus formed by inexact copying were incompatible with life or replication, but some survived, perhaps by dumb luck. And then, the environment changed!

As we know, the earth's crust and atmosphere changed rather drastically over the eons of earth's existence (see Table 7.1). Cells that emerged and replicated in the Archean eon could hardly survive in the oxygen-rich atmosphere of the Proterozoic eon. But the few cells with the errors in DNA so that they could survive in the toxic oxygen atmosphere did survive, and some formed aggregates (e.g., green algae) that resulted in better protection and efficiency in metabolism. Thanks to the random errors, there was variation in the offspring, and the process of evolution of life had begun.

Evolution is, then, the survival of the genes through mutation that are adapting to the demands of changing environment. See Tables 7.1 and 7.2 for an overview of evolution through time on planet earth.

7.5 Wonderful Invention of Sex

A wonderful but puzzling invention relatively early in the course of evolution is sex. From a purely multiplication point of view, sexual reproduction is inefficient, i.e., takes up more energy, slow, and yields less numbers of offsprings compared to asexual reproduction. For example, half of the population (males) does not reproduce directly. Then, why is sex?

The most primitive organisms known to undergo meiosis and to reproduce sexually are protists, the primitive unicellular eukaryotes that arose early in Proterozoic eon (1800 MA). Protists still exist, including those that cause malaria. Perhaps sex originated when some parasites exchanged their genes with the host for transmission and propagation with the host's offspring (Hickey, 1982).

In prokaryotes such as bacteria and archaea that lack a nucleus, genes are typically stored in a single large, circular chromosome, sometimes supplemented by additional small circles of DNA called plasmids, which usually consist of only a few genes. Plasmids are easily transferable between individuals. For example, the plasmids may contain genes that encode for antibiotic resistance. They can be passed between individual cells, even those of different species, via horizontal or lateral gene transfer. Some organisms may have ingested another whose genes may have been incorporated into the host genome.

What is the advantage of such lateral gene transfer? Such newly incorporated genes may have provided survival advantage, i.e., sturdiness, resistance to other parasites. Sex seems to have been optional for most protists with asexual reproduction as needed.

Sex may have arisen as a form of vaccination. Eukaryan fusion sex may have arisen from prokaryan unilateral sex-as-infection (Sterrer, 2002). In prokaryotes, the single circular chromosome is haploid. Their "sex" is unilateral, a donor such as plasmids and bacteriophages penetrates the organism and becomes a genetic symbiont (Snyder and Champness, 1997). It has been reported that in some gram positive bacteria, those lacking a certain plasmid secrete pheromone-like chemicals that attract donors that contain the plasmid and induce conjugation (Dunny et al., 1995). The relationship between the bacteria and their genetic symbionts ranges from antagonistic to mutualistic. Such a symbiont may kill its bacterial host and infect new bacteria laterally, or become integrated into the host's chromosome and be passed on vertically by the replicating host while providing immunity to superinfection by another symbiont of the same type (Sterrer, 2002).

In fact, the emergence of eukaryotes may be due to an infection of bacteria by archae, the prokaryote single cell organism whose genome resembles that of the cellular nucleus. Archae survives even in the present in extreme environments (such as in geysers above 100°C) like those of ancient times (Lopez-Garcia and Moreira, 2006). Alternate theories concerning the origin of cell nucleus include viral infection theory, and exomembrane theory postulates that the nucleus developed when the intracellular elements developed a second membrane enclosing it (de Roos, 2006).

When a symbiont genome became integrated with the host genome in the nucleus, "safe sex" emerged as "reciprocal vaccination." If a mating resulted in additive resistance, then there would have been selective advantage to such diploid heterozygotes (Sterrer, 2002).

With the emergence of multicellular eukaryotic organisms, sex served as reciprocal vaccination of two conspecific genomes. Meiosis and recombination developed as a mechanism of keeping the symbionts in check by breaking them up into fragments and preventing their assembly into large pieces that may return to their original virulence. In order to benefit from the vaccination, the offsprings had to go through the "bottleneck" of having single-celled parents (Maynard Smith and Szathmary, 1995).

The "safe sex" between two complete genomes in eukaryotes marks the distinction between self, mate, and foreign; self being an identical genome. "Mates" are nonidentical but compatible genomes that carry complementary resistance genes, considered to be the origin of mate selection for heterozygosity (Reusch et al., 2001).

Once sex has been invented, there are other reasons why sex is maintained in spite of its costs. One is that sex provides the means for efficient removal of deleterious genes through meiosis and recombination. Diploid organisms can repair a mutated section of the DNA through homologous recombination as there are two copies of the gene in the cell and one copy is presumably not damaged. Sex also mixes up genes and facilitates the creation and propagation of genes for advantageous traits. The "Red Queen" hypothesis (Bell, 1988) proposes that sex creates unique genotypes that may be better adapted to changing environment, i.e., like the red queen in *Through the Looking Glass* by Lewis Carroll, you have to keep on running (adapting) to remain in the same place (maintain the organism's niche vis-a-vis coevolving organisms such as parasites in the changing environment).

Infection of organisms by others resulting in the infusion and incorporation of new information in the form of genetic instructions seems to have given rise to the wonderful complexity of sex, whose function is to constantly mix up and create new information. This process led to the evolution of most extant living things including ourselves.

7.6 Darwin and Natural Selection

Charles Darwin (1809–1882) proposed the theory of evolution based on careful observation of geologic and biologic evidence in his book, *The Origin of Species* (1859).[1] Darwin was an English naturalist who first studied medicine at Edinburgh University, then theology at Cambridge.

The captain of the expedition ship, HMS Beagle, committed suicide during her first voyage and Captain Robert FitzRoy took over. For the second voyage, FitzRoy decided he needed a "gentleman companion" and hired young Darwin in that capacity. The second voyage of HMS Beagle lasted 5 years though originally planned for two and carried out detailed surveys sailing across the Atlantic Ocean and around the coasts of southern South America, Tahiti, and Australia, circumnavigating the earth. Darwin collected and studied fossils, plants, and animals during the voyage that formed the basis of his theory of evolution and natural selection. Darwin published his journal written during the voyage, *The Voyage of the Beagle*, which earned him a name as a naturalist.

In *The Origin of Species*, he proposed on the basis of his careful observations and other scientific evidences that all species of life evolved over time from common ancestors through the process of natural selection. Alfred Russel Wallace, a naturalist working in Borneo, had similar ideas and communicated them with Darwin, which resulted in a joint publication of Wallace's paper and an abstract of Darwin's forthcoming book. It was Darwin's book, however, that eventually revolutionized science and formed the foundation of biology by providing a unifying principle. Darwin explored human evolution and sexual selection in *The Descent of Man, and Selection In Relation to Sex* (Darwin, 2002–2008; van Wyhe, 2008).

---

[1] The original 1859 full book title was *On the Origin of Species by Means of Natural Selection* or the *Preservation of Favoured Races in the Struggle for Life*, which was changed to *The Origin of Species* in the 1872 edition.

Natural selection is the mechanism Darwin proposed in 1859 through which there was a gradual change in the phenotype of some members of the species that was better adapted to a changing environment. Eventually, the gradual change was enough that interbreeding between the changed and unchanged phenotype did not occur, and thus a new species would emerge. Darwin described natural selection as an analogy to artificial selection, in which humans systematically and selectively breed animals with traits desirable to humans until such traits became defining traits of the brood. At the time of Darwin's writing, there was no general theory of inheritance and genetics. It was not until the twentieth century that the works of Gregor Mendel, who was a contemporary of Darwin but whose works lay in obscurity, would be rediscovered (1900 by Hugo de Vries and Carl Correns), and molecular genetics would emerge with the discovery of DNA as genes (1943 by Oswald Avery) and the structure of DNA as double helix (1953 by James Watson and Francis Crick). The discovery and elucidation of the DNA-based molecular mechanisms of genetic inheritance gave rise to modern evolutionary theory. See Figures 7.5 and 7.6.

Darwin's illustrations of beak variation in the finches of the Galápagos Islands hold 13 closely related species that differ most markedly in the shape of their beaks. The beak of each species is suited to its preferred food, suggesting that beak shapes evolved by natural selection (Fig. 7.4).

Fitness is a central concept of natural selection. Though Darwin's term, *survival of the fittest*, implies individual survival, natural selection is in fact based on reproductive success. The phenotypes that lead to most number of offsprings will prevail. In addition to natural selection, Darwin described *sexual selection* as a means of gradual accentuation of traits that do not have survival advantage, for example, peacock's tail. Sexual selection is based on advantages in competing for a mate for reproduction.

Fig. 7.4 Darwin's Finches. Journal of researches into the natural history and geology of the countries visited during the voyage of HMS Beagle round the world, under the command of Captain Fitz Roy, R.N. 2nd edition. From Darwin's 1845 book, "Voyage of the Beagle" this image is in the public domain because its copyright has expired in those countries with a copyright term of life of the author plus 100 years or less [from Wikimedia]

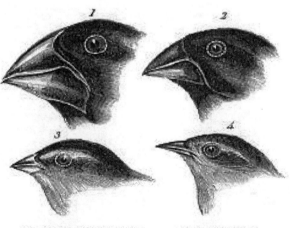

1. Geospiza magnirostris   2. Geospiza fortis
3. Geospiza parvula   4. Certhidea olivacea

Finches from Galapagos Archipelago

Fig. 7.5 An overview of the
structure of DNA

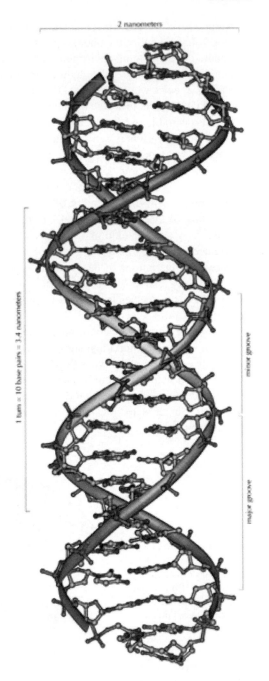

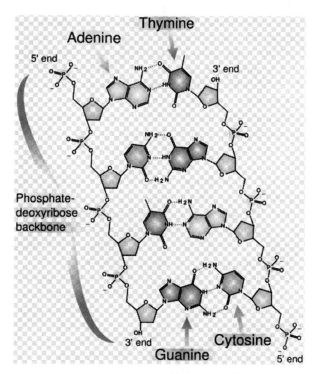

Fig. 7.6 Chemical structure of DNA. The backbone of the DNA strand is made from alternating phosphate and sugar residues. The sugars are joined together by phosphate groups that form phosphodiester bonds between the third and fifth carbon atoms of adjacent sugar rings. These asymmetric bonds mean a strand of DNA has a direction. In a double helix the direction of the nucleotides in one strand is opposite to their direction in the other strand. The asymmetric ends of DNA strands are referred to as the 5′ (*five prime*) and 3′ (*three prime*) ends. One of the major differences between DNA and RNA is the sugar, with 2-deoxyribose being replaced by the alternative pentose sugar ribose in RNA. The DNA double helix is stabilized by hydrogen bonds between the bases attached to the two strands. The four bases found in DNA are adenine (A), cytosine (C), guanine (G), and thymine (T). These bases are classified into two types; adenine and guanine are fused five- and six-membered heterocyclic compounds called purines, while cytosine and thymine are six-membered rings called pyrimidines. A fifth pyrimidine base, called uracil (U), usually takes the place of thymine in RNA and differs from thymine by lacking a methyl group on its ring. Uracil is not usually found in DNA, occurring only as a breakdown product of cytosine [From Wikipedia]. *Permission is granted to copy, distribute and/or modify this document under the terms of the* "GNU Free Documentation License," Version 1.2 or any later version published by the Free Software Foundation; with no Invariant Sections, no Front-Cover Texts, and no Back-Cover Texts. A copy of the license is included in the section entitled "GNU Free Documentation License" [From Wikimedia]

George C. Williams first explicitly advocated the gene-centric view of evolution in his 1966 book *Adaptation and Natural Selection*. He proposed an evolutionary concept of gene in which natural selection favored some genes over others.

Richard Dawkins argued in *The Selfish Gene* (Dawkins, 1976) and *The Extended Phenotype* (Dawkins, 1982) that the gene is the only replicator in living systems.

He argued that only genes transmit their structure largely intact and are potentially immortal through the copying process. Therefore, genes are the units of selection. Dawkins redefines the word "gene" to mean "an inheritable unit" instead of the generally accepted definition of "a section of DNA coding for a particular protein." Dawkins describes the idea of gene-centric selection in *River Out of Eden* by describing life as a river of compatible genes flowing through geological time. Scoop up a pail of genes from the river of genes, and we have an organism serving as temporary survival machines for the genes. A river of genes may fork into two or more branches representing noninterbreeding species as a result of geographical separation.

In gene-centric view of evolution, a gene need not have a function in the construction of the phenotype as long as the organism will keep on reproducing the vessels for the gene. The so-called junk DNA may be an example. "Junk" DNA does not contain instructions for protein coding, but they may be critically important to an organism's evolutionary survival by affecting others that do or by affecting the stability of the chromosome itself. In one study with the fruit fly (*Drosophila melanogaster*), the "junk DNA" regions, which account for about 80% of the fly's total genome, were found to be evolving more slowly than expected due to natural selection pressures on the nonprotein-coding DNA to remain the same over time. The "junk" regions also exhibit an unusually large amount of functional genetic divergence between different species of *Drosophila*. This implies that, like evolutionary changes to proteins, changes to these "junk" parts of the genome also play an important role in the evolution of new species. The largest differences between major species groups including fruit flies, reptiles, and mammals seem to be the amount of "junk" DNA rather than the number of genes (Andolfatto, 2005).

7.7 Somatic Evolution

We have seen that our bodies may be conceptualized as temporary containers for genes that attain immortality through replication. To be precise, however, it is the cells in our bodies that contain the genes. It is natural, then, to expect evolutionary processes occurring at the cellular level. Indeed, such somatic evolution plays an important role in both disease and health.

Somatic evolution of neurons is an extremely important topic for our purposes and will be discussed in Chapter 8.

Somatic evolution has been extensively studied in cancer. Some cells undergo mutation that increases cell growth and others may have already mutated oncogenes in them. For example, the human colonic epithelium is renewed every 3–5 days. For such a high rate of turnover, there are large numbers of cells undergoing mitoses and, therefore, large number of mutations. Cancers develop through genomic instability, which generates diversity, from which clonal evolution may occur. In colorectal cancers, three identifiable processes involved in generating diversity at the genetic or epigenetic level have been reported (Boland and Goel, 2005). Colorectal cancers may have chromosomal instability (CIN), microsatellite instability (MSI), or the

CpG island methylator phenotype (CIMP). Each of these processes is reported to be associated with a unique mutational or epigenetic "signature" identifiable in the tumor cells.

After acquiring somatic mutations for cell growth, some of the cancer cells may evolve to escape from the control of the microenvironment that is designed to keep them in place through various messenger systems. Not all mutated cells can do this, some may undergo enhanced proliferation without escaping environmental control. For example, the prevalence of small thyroid tumors in postmortem examination of people between the ages of 50–70 was 36%, while the incidence of clinically apparent thyroid cancer in age-matched population was 0.1% (Harach et al., 1985).

Most cancer cells are aneuploid (abnormal number of chromosomes), which is often manifested by the gain or loss of a whole of parts of chromosomes. Tumor cells often have excess chromosomes, often 60–90 per cell. There may be other chromosomal abnormalities such as deletions, inversions, duplications, and translocations. Such chromosomal abnormalities often result in loss of heterozygosity of particular genes. In an average tumor, about 25–30% of the normal alleles are lost, in some cases as high as 75% (Lengauer et al., 1998). The loss of these alleles, especially those of tumor suppressor and cell–cell adhesion control genes, may benefit the rapidly replicating clonal populations of tumor cells as they allow cells to rapidly adapt to the changing microenvironment (Smalley et al., 2005).

The effects of environmental evolutionary pressure on tumor cells have been demonstrated in experimental models. The sequential passage of melanoma cells through a reconstituted basement membrane (which mimics invasion into the dermal microenvironment) or in serum-free media selects for clones that are tenfold more invasive, metastatic and grow more rapidly in both serum-free and growth factor-depleted media (Kath et al., 1991). The selected invasive melanoma cells required continuous evolutionary pressure to maintain their phenotype and reverted to the parental phenotype when the environmental stimuli were removed. Although the effects of environmental selection pressure pushed the parent cells toward a more aggressive phenotype, it seems that these changes were not fixed.

It appears that the tumor cell clones that manage to escape their local environment have lost strong cell to cell contact with their neighbors and are no longer dependent on exogenous environmental cues to regulate their behavior (Smalley et al., 2005). In most cancers, a critical first step in this local escape seems to be a downregulation of E-cadherin expression or function. In melanoma, the first step in the transformation is the escape from keratinocyte control. As keratinocytes regulate melanocyte growth very tightly, loss of keratinocyte–melanocyte interaction at an early stage permits the earliest rounds of clonal expansion. E-cadherin inactivation or loss is required for escape of the earliest tumor cells from the primary focus (Hirohashi, 1998). Melanoma cells also undergo a cadherin switch and upregulate expression of N-cadherin (Hsu et al., 1996). There is evidence that the upregulation of N-cadherin rather than loss of E-cadherin is more important for the invasive and metastatic behavior of cancer cells. Upregulation of N-cadherin results in a number of survival advantages, such as reducing the rate of apoptosis, and less strong cell–cell adhesion thereby permitting greater mobility.

Immunocytes that are important in resistance to invading organisms through the production of antibodies have been demonstrated to evolve through clonal selection. The enormous diversity in antibody-producing cells is achieved by a variety of mechanisms including somatic recombination and mutation (Edelman, 1994).

7.8 Universal Darwinism

The process of evolution by natural selection is not unique to living things, though Darwin first proposed it as an explanation of how species evolved from common ancestors over time. To the extent that environment changes and entities (organic or nonorganic) arise and disintegrate, natural selection takes place so that entities that are better adapted to the changing environment will tend to become more numerous. This principle has been applied to quantum physics to explain the emergence of classical reality from quantum reality (Ollivier et al., 2004; Zurek, 2007). In quantum wave function, decoherence resulting from interference from outside (e.g., observation) gives rise to existence of individual particles, the location of which is statistical, i.e., many possible realities. Among all such possible realities, only those that can interact with the environment and decohere (i.e., become real) can produce information progeny.

Darwinian natural selection has been proposed as the mechanism by which the current universe evolved from many possible universes that evolved from a series of bouncing black holes that gave rise to daughter universes (Smolin, 1999, 2004, 2006). Smolin states that the physical processes that strongly influence the number of black holes produced are nucleosynthesis, galaxy formation, star formation, stellar dynamics, supernova explosions, and the formation and stability of neutron stars. Through the process of such cosmic evolution, our universe may have developed complexity enough to produce civilizations like ours.

Appendix

Table 7.1 Geologic timescale (From Wikipedia, the free encyclopedia)

Graphical timelines

The second and third timelines are each subsections of their preceding timeline as indicated by asterisks.

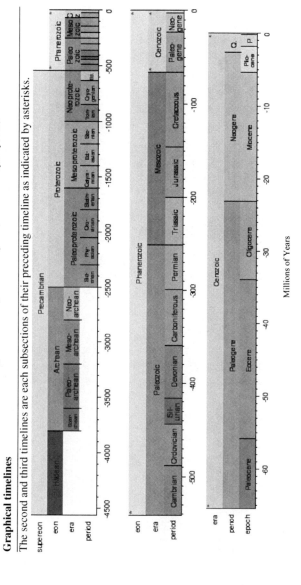

The Holocene (the latest epoch) is too small to be shown clearly on this timeline.

Table 7.2 Table of geologic time (From Wikipedia. All text I saw available under the terms of the GNU-Free Documentation License). The table summarizes the major events and characteristics of the periods of time making up the geologic timescale. As above, this timescale is based on the International Commission on Stratigraphy. (See *lunar geologic timescale* for a discussion of the geologic subdivisions of Earth's moon.) The height of each table entry does not correspond to the duration of each subdivision of time. As this table is a subsection of the Wikipedia article, the citations do not begin with 1 and a.

$v \cdot d \cdot e$ Geologic timescale template

Supereon	Eon	Era	Period[6]	Series/epoch	Faunal stage/geologic age	Major events	Start, million years ago[7]
	Phanerozoic	Cenozoic	Neogene[8]	Holocene	Quaternary	The last glacial period ends and rise of human civilization	0.011430 ±0.00013[9]
				Pleistocene	Late/Tyrrhenian Stage	Flourishing and then extinction of many large mammals (*Pleistocene megafauna*)	0.126 ±0.005*
						Evolution of anatomically modern humans	
					Middle		0.500?
					Early		1.806 ±0.005*
					Gelasian		2.588 ±0.005*
				Pliocene	Piacenzian/ Blancan	Intensification of present ice age; cool and dry climate.	3.600 ±0.005*
						Australopithecines, many of the existing genera of mammals, and recent mollusks appear.	
						Homo habilis appears. Present ice age begins	
					Zanclean		5.332 ±0.005*

Table 7.2 (continued)

v · d · e Geologic timescale template

Supereon	Eon	Era	Period[6]	Series/epoch	Faunal stage/geologic age	Major events	Start, million years ago[7]
				Miocene	Messinian	Moderate climate; Orogeny in northern hemisphere. Modern mammal and bird families became recognizable. Horses and mastodons diverse Grasses become ubiquitous. First apes appear (for reference see the article: "Sahelanthropus tchadensis")	7.246 ± 0.05*
					Tortonian		11.608 ± 0.05*
					Burdigalian		13.65 ± 0.05*
					Serravallian		15.97 ± 0.05*
					Langhian		20.43 ± 0.05*
					Aquitanian		23.03 ± 0.05*
			Paleogene[8]	Oligocene	Chattian	Warm climate; rapid evolution and diversification of fauna, especially mammals. Major evolution and dispersal of modern types of flowering plants	28.4 ± 0.1*
					Rupelian		33.9 ± 0.1*

Table 7.2 (continued)

v · d · e Geologic timescale template

Supereon	Eon	Era	Period[6]	Series/epoch	Faunal stage/geologic age	Major events	Start, million years ago[7]
				Eocene	Priabonian	Archaic mammals (e.g., Creodonts, Condylarths, Uintatheres) flourish and continue to develop during the epoch. Appearance of several "modern" mammal families. Primitive whales diversify. First grasses. Reglaciation of Antarctica and formation of its ice cap; current ice age begins	37.2 ± 0.1*
					Bartonian		40.4 ± 0.2*
					Lutetian		48.6 ± 0.2*
					Ypresian		55.8 ± 0.2*
				Paleocene	Thanetian	Climate tropical. Modern plants appear; Mammals diversify into a number of primitive lineages following the extinction of the dinosaurs. First large mammals (up to bear or small hippo size)	58.7 ± 0.2*
					Selandian		61.7 ± 0.3*
					Danian		65.5 ± 0.3*

Table 7.2 (continued)

v · d · e Geologic timescale template

Supereon	Eon	Era	Period[6]	Series/epoch	Faunal stage/geologic age	Major events	Start, million years ago[7]
		Mesozoic	Cretaceous	Upper/late	Maastrichtian	Flowering plants proliferate, along with new types of insects. More modern teleost fish begin to appear Ammonites, belemnites, rudist bivalves, echinoids and sponges all common. Many new types of dinosaurs (e.g., Tyrannosaurs, Titanosaurs, duck bills, and horned dinosaurs) evolve on land, as do Eusuchia (modern crocodilians); and mosasaurs and modern sharks appear in the sea Primitive birds gradually replace pterosaurs Monotremes, marsupials, and placental mammals appear. Break up of Gondwana	70.6 ± 0.6*
					Campanian		83.5 ± 0.7*
					Santonian		85.8 ± 0.7*
					Coniacian		89.3 ± 1.0*
					Turonian		93.5 ± 0.8*
					Cenomanian		99.6 ± 0.9*
				Lower/early	Albian		112.0 ± 1.0*
					Aptian		125.0 ± 1.0*
					Barremian		130.0 ± 1.5*
					Hauterivian		136.4 ± 2.0*

Table 7.2 (continued)

v · d · e Geologic timescale template

Supereon	Eon	Era	Period[6]	Series/epoch	Faunal stage/geologic age	Major events	Start, million years ago[7]
			Jurassic	Upper/late	Valanginian		140.2 ± 3.0*
					Berriasian		145.5 ± 4.0*
					Tithonian	Gymnosperms (especially conifers, Bennettitales, and cycads) and ferns common. Many types of dinosaurs, such as sauropods, carnosaurs, and stegosaurs Mammals common but small. First birds and lizards. Ichthyosaurs and plesiosaurs diverse. Bivalves. Ammonites, and belemnites abundant. Sea urchins very common, along with crinoids, starfish, sponges, and terebratulid and rhynchonellid brachiopods Breakup of Pangaea into Gondwana and Laurasia	150.8 ± 4.0*
					Kimmeridgian		155.7 ± 4.0*
					Oxfordian		161.2 ± 4.0*
				Middle	Callovian		164.7 ± 4.0
					Bathonian		167.7 ± 3.5*
					Bajocian		171.6 ± 3.0*
					Aalenian		175.6 ± 2.0*
				Lower/early	Toarcian		183.0 ± 1.5*

Table 7.2 (continued)

$v \cdot d \cdot e$ Geologic timescale template

Supereon	Eon	Era	Period[6]	Series/ epoch	Faunal stage/geologic age	Major events	Start, million years ago[7]
					Pliensbachian		$189.6 \pm 1.5^{*}$
					Sinemurian		$196.5 \pm 1.0^{*}$
					Hettangian		$199.6 \pm 0.6^{*}$
			Triassic	Upper/late	Rhaetian	Archosaurs dominant on land as dinosaurs, in the oceans as Ichthyosaurs and nothosaurs, and in the air as pterosaurs. Cynodonts become smaller and more mammal like, while first mammals and crocodilia appear. *Dicrodium* flora common on land. Many large aquatic temnospondyl amphibians Ceratitic ammonoids extremely common. Modern corals and teleost fish appear, as do many modern insect clades	$203.6 \pm 1.5^{*}$
					Norian		$216.5 \pm 2.0^{*}$
					Carnian		$228.0 \pm 2.0^{*}$
				Middle	Ladinian		$237.0 \pm 2.0^{*}$
					Anisian		$245.0 \pm 1.5^{*}$
				Lower/early ("Scythian")	Olenekian		$249.7 \pm 1.5^{*}$
					Induan		$251.0 \pm 0.7^{*}$

Table 7.2 (continued)

$v \cdot d \cdot e$ Geologic timescale template

Supereon	Eon	Era	Period[6]	Series/epoch	Faunal stage/geologic age	Major events	Start, million years ago[7]
		Paleozoic	Permian	Lopingian	Changhsingian	Landmasses unite into supercontinent Pangaea, creating the Appalachians. End of Permo-Carboniferous glaciation. Synapsid reptiles (pelycosaurs and therapsids) become plentiful, while pararreptiles and temnospondyl amphibians remain common. In the mid-Permian, coal-age flora are replaced by cone-bearing gymnosperms (the first true seed plants) and by the first true mosses. Beetles and flies evolve. Marine life flourishes in warm shallow reefs; productid and spiriferid brachiopods, bivalves, forams, and ammonoids all abundant. Permian-Triassic extinction event occurs 251 mya: 95% of life on Earth becomes extinct, including all trilobites, graptolites, and blastoids	253.8 ± 0.7*
				Guadalupian	Wuchiapingian		260.4 ± 0.7*
					Capitanian		265.8 ± 0.7*

Table 7.2 (continued)

v · d · e Geologic timescale template

Supereon	Eon	Era	Period[6]	Series/ epoch	Faunal stage/geologic age	Major events	Start, million years ago[7]
				Cisuralian	Wordian/Kazanian		268.4 ± 0.7*
					Roadian/Ufimian		270.6 ± 0.7*
					Kungurian		275.6 ± 0.7*
					Artinskian		284.4 ± 0.7*
					Sakmarian		294.6 ± 0.8*
					Asselian		299.0 ± 0.8*
			Carbon- iferous[10]/ Pennsylvanian	Upper/Late	Gzhelian	Winged insects radiate suddenly; some (esp. Protodonata and Palaeodictyoptera) are quite large. Amphibians common and diverse. First reptiles and coal forests (scale trees, ferns, club trees, giant horsetails, *Cordaites*, etc.). Highest-ever atmospheric oxygen levels. Goniatites, brachiopods, bryozoa, bivalves, and corals plentiful in the seas and oceans. Testate forams proliferate	303.9 ± 0.9*
				Middle	Kasimovian		306.5 ± 1.0*
					Moscovian		311.7 ± 1.1*
				Lower/Early	Bashkirian		318.1 ± 1.3*

Table 7.2 (continued)

$v \cdot d \cdot e$ Geologic timescale template

Supereon	Eon	Era	Period[6]	Series/epoch	Faunal stage/geologic age	Major events	Start, million years ago[7]
			Carboniferous[10]/Mississippian	Upper/late	Serpukhovian	Large primitive trees, first land vertebrates, and amphibious sea-scorpions live amid coal-forming coastal swamps Lobe-finned rhizodonts are dominant big fresh-water predators. In the oceans, early sharks are common and quite diverse; echinoderms (especially crinoids and blastoids) abundant. Corals, bryozoa, goniatites, and brachiopods (Productida, Spiriferida, etc.) very common. But trilobites and nautiloids decline. Glaciation in East Gondwana	$326.4 \pm 1.6^*$
				Middle	Viséan		$345.3 \pm 2 1^*$
				Lower/early	Tournaisian		$359.2 \pm 2.5^*$

Table 7.2 (continued)

v · d · e Geologic timescale template

Supereon	Eon	Era	Period[6]	Series/epoch	Faunal stage/geologic age	Major events	Start, million years ago[7]
			Devonian	Upper/late	Famennian	First clubmosses, horsetails, and ferns appear, as do the first seed-bearing plants (progymnosperms), first trees (the progymnosperm *Archaeopteris*), and first (wingless) insects Strophomenid and atrypid brachiopods, rugose and tabulate corals, and crinoids are all abundant in the oceans. Goniatite ammonoids are plentiful, while squid-like coleoids arise. Trilobites and armored agnaths decline, while jawed fishes (placoderms, lobe-finned and ray-finned fish, and early sharks) rule the seas. First amphibians still aquatic. "Old Red Continent" of Euramerica	374.5 ± 2.6*
					Frasnian		385.3 ± 2.6*
				Middle	Givetian		391.8 ± 2.7*
					Eifelian		397.5 ± 2.7*
					Emsian		407.0 ± 2.8*
				Lower/early	Pragian		407.0 ± 2.8*
					Lochkovian		416.0 ± 2.8*

Table 7.2 (continued)

v · d · e Geologic timescale template

Supereon	Eon	Era	Period[6]	Series/epoch	Faunal stage/geologic age	Major events	Start, million years ago[7]
			Silurian	Pridoli	No faunal stages defined	First vascular plants (the rhyniophytes and their relatives), first millipedes, and arthropleurids on land. First jawed fishes, as well as many armored jawless fish, populate the seas. Sea-scorpions reach large size. Tabulate and rugose corals, brachiopods (*Pentamerida*, Rhynchonellida, etc.), and crinoids all abundant. Trilobites and mollusks diverse; graptolites not as varied	418.7 ± 2.7*
				Ludlow/Cayugan	Ludfordian		421.3 ± 2.6*
					Gorstian		422.9 ± 2.5*
				Wenlock	Homerian/Lockportian		426.2 ± 2.4*
					Sheinwoodian/Tonawandan		428.2 ± 2.3*
				Llandovery/Alexandrian	Telychian/Ontarian		436.0 ± 1.9*
					Aeronian		439.0 ± 1.8*
					Rhuddanian		443.7 ± 1.5*

Table 7.2 (continued)

v · d · e Geologic timescale template

Supereon	Eon	Era	Period[6]	Series/epoch	Faunal stage/geologic age	Major events	Start, million years ago[7]
			Ordovician	Upper/late	Hirnantian	Invertebrates diversify into many new types (e.g., long straight-shelled cephalopods). Early corals, articulate brachiopods (*Orthida*, *Strophomenida*, etc.), bivalves, nautiloids, trilobites, ostracods, bryozoa, many types of echinoderms (crinoids, cystoids, starfish, etc.), branched graptolites, and other taxa all common. Conodonts (early planktonic vertebrates) appear. First green plants and fungi on land. Ice age at end of period	445.6 ± 1.5*
					Other faunal stages		460.9 ± 1.6*
				Middle	Darriwilian		468.1 ± 1.6*
					other faunal stages		471.8 ± 1.6*
				Lower/early	Arenig		471.8 ± 1.7*
					Tremadocian		488.3 ± 1.7*

Table 7.2 (continued)

v · d · e Geologic timescale template

Supereon	Eon	Era	Period[6]	Series/epoch	Faunal stage/geologic age	Major events	Start, million years ago[7]
			Cambrian	Furongian	Other faunal stages	Major diversification of life in the Cambrian Explosion. Many fossils; most modern animal phyla appear. First chordates appear, along with a number of extinct, problematic phyla. Reef-building Archaeocyatha abundant; then vanish. Trilobites, priapulid worms, sponges, inarticulate brachiopods (unhinged lampshells), and many other animals numerous. Anomalocarids are giant predators, while many Ediacaran fauna die out. Prokaryotes, protists (e.g., forams), fungi, and algae continue to present day. Gondwana emerges	496.0 ± 2.0[x]
					Paibian/Ibexian/ Ayusokkanian/ Sakian/Aksayan		501.0 ± 2.0*
				Middle	Other faunal stages		513.0 ± 2.0
				Lower/early	Other faunal stages		542.0 ± 1.0*

Table 7.2 (continued)

v · d · e Geologic timescale template

Supereon	Eon	Era	Period[6]	Series/epoch	Faunal stage/geologic age Major events	Start, million years ago[7]
Precambrian[11]	Proterozoic[12]	Neoproterozoic	Ediacaran		Good fossils of the first multi-celled animals. Ediacaran biota flourish worldwide in seas. Simple trace fossils of possible worm-like *Trichophycus*, etc. First sponges and trilobitomorphs. Enigmatic forms include many soft-jellied creatures shaped like bags, disks, or quilts (like *Dickinsonia*)	630 +5/−30*
			Cryogenian		Possible "Snowball Earth" period. Fossils still rare. Rodinia landmass begins to break up	850[13]
			Tonian		Rodinia supercontinent persists. Trace fossils of simple multi-celled eukaryotes. First radiation of dinoflagellate-like acritarchs	1000[13]
		Mesoproterozoic	Stenian		Narrow highly metamorphic belts due to orogeny as Rodinia formed	1200[13]
			Ectasian		Platform covers continue to expand. Green algae colonies in the seas	1400[13]
			Calynmian		Platform covers expand	1600[13]
		Paleoproterozoic	Statherian		First complex single-celled life: protists with nuclei. Columbia is the primordial supercontinent	1800[13]
			Orosirian		The atmosphere became oxygenic. Vredefort and Sudbury Basin asteroid impacts. Much orogeny	2050[13]
			Rhyacian		Bushveld formation formed. Huronian glaciation	2300[13]
			Siderian		Oxygen catastrophe: banded iron formations formed	2500[13]
	Archean[11]	Neoarchean			Stabilization of most modern cratons; possible mantle overturn event	2800[13]
		Mesoarchean			First stromatolites (probably colonial cyanobacteria). Oldest macrofossils	3200[13]
		Paleoarchean			First known oxygen-producing bacteria. Oldest definitive microfossils	3600[13]
		Eoarchean			Simple single-celled life (probably bacteria and perhaps archaea). Oldest probable microfossils	3800
	Hadean[11, 12, 14]	Lower Imbrian[12]			This era overlaps the end of the late heavy bombardment of the inner solar system	c.3850

Table 7.2 (continued)

v · d · e Geologic timescale template

Supereon	Eon	Era	Period[6]	Series/epoch	Faunal stage/geologic age Major events	Start, million years ago[7]
		Nectarian[12]			This era gets its name from the lunar geologic timescale when the Nectaris Basin and other major lunar basins were formed by large impact events	c.3920
		Basin Groups[12]			Oldest known rock (4,100 Ma). The first lifeforms self-replicating RNA molecules may have evolved on earth around 4 bya during this era	c.4150
		Cryptic[12]			Oldest known mineral (Zircon, 4,400 Ma). Formation of Earth (4,567.17–4,570 Ma)	c.4570

[6] Paleontologists often refer to faunal stages rather than geologic (geological) periods. The stage nomenclature is quite complex. See The Paleobiology Database. Retrieved on March 19, 2006 for an excellent time ordered list of faunal stages.

[7] Dates are slightly uncertain with differences of a few percent between various sources being common. This is largely due to uncertainties in radiometric dating and the problem that deposits suitable for radiometric dating seldom occur exactly at the places in the geologic column where they would be most useful. The dates and errors quoted above are according to the International Commission on Stratigraphy 2004 time scale. Dates labeled with a* indicate boundaries where a Global Boundary Stratotype Section and Point has been internationally agreed upon: see List of Global Boundary Stratotype Sections and Points for a complete list.

[8] *a* *b* Historically, the Cenozoic has been divided up into the Quaternary and Tertiary sub-eras, as well as the Neogene and Paleogene periods. However, the International Commission on Stratigraphy has recently decided to stop endorsing the terms Quaternary and Tertiary as part of the formal nomenclature.

[9] The start time for the Holocene epoch is here given as 11,430 years ago ± 130 years (that is, between 9610 BC–9560 BC and 9350 BC–9300 BC). For further discussion of the dating of this epoch, see Holocene.

[10] *a* *b* In North America, the Carboniferous is subdivided into Mississippian and Pennsylvanian Periods.

[11] *a* *b* *c* The Precambrian is also known as Cryptozoic.

[12] *a* *b* *c* *d* *e* *f* The Proterozoic, Archean, and Hadean are often collectively referred to as the Precambrian Time or sometimes, also the Cryptozoic.

[13] *a* *b* *c* *d* *e* *f* *g* *h* *i* *j* *k* *l* Defined by absolute age (Global Standard Stratigraphic Age).

[14] Though commonly used, the Hadean is not a formal eon and no lower bound for the Archean and Eoarchean have been agreed upon. The Hadean has also sometimes been called the Priscoan or the Azoic. Sometimes, the Hadean can be found to be subdivided according to the *lunar geologic time scale*. These eras include the Cryptic and Basin Groups (which are subdivisions of the pre-Nectarian era), Nectarian, and lower Imbrian eras.

References

Andolfatto, P. (2005) Adaptive evolution of non-coding DNA in Drosophila. *Nature*, **437**, 1149–1152.

Baumgart, T., Hess, S. T., Webb, W. W. (2003) Imaging coexisting fluid domains in biomembrane models coupling curvature and line tension. *Nature*, **425**, 821–824.

Bell, G. (1988) Uniformity and diversity in the evolution of sex. In *The Evolution of Sex* (R. Michod, B. Levin eds.), pp. 126–138. Sinauer, Sunderland, MA.

Bertschinger, E. (1998) Simulations of structure formation in the universe. *Annu Rev Astron Astrophys*, **36**, 599–654.

Boland, C. R., Goel, A. (2005) Somatic evolution of cancer cells. *Semin Cancer Biol*, **15**, 436–450.

Cairns-Smith, A. (1982) *Genetic Takeover and the Mineral Origin of Life*. Cambridge University Press, Cambridge.

Darwin, C. (2002–2008) *The Complete Work of Charles Darwin Online*. University of Cambridge, Cambridge.

Dawkins, R. (1976) *The Selfish Gene*. Oxford University Press, New York.

Dawkins, R. (1982) *The Extended Phenotype: The Gene as the Unit of Selection*. Freeman, Oxford [Oxfordshire]; San Francisco.

de Roos, A. D. (2006) The origin of the eukaryotic cell based on conservation of existing interfaces. *Artif Life*, **12**, 513–523.

Dennett, D. C. (1995) *Darwin's Dangerous Idea: Evolution and the Meanings of Life*. Simon, Schuster, New York.

Dunny, G. M., Leonard, B. A., Hedberg, P. J. (1995) Pheromone-inducible conjugation in Enterococcus faecalis: Interbacterial and host-parasite chemical communication. *J Bacteriol*, **177**, 871–876.

Edelman, G. M. (1994) The evolution of somatic selection: The antibody tale. *Genetics*, **138**, 975–981.

Hanczyc, M. M., Szostak, J. W. (2004) Replicating vesicles as models of primitive cell growth and division. *Curr Opin Chem Biol*, **8**, 660–664.

Harach, H. R., Franssila, K. O., Wasenius, V. M. (1985) Occult papillary carcinoma of the thyroid. A "normal" finding in Finland. A systematic autopsy study. *Cancer*, **56**, 531–538.

Hickey, D. (1982) Selfish DNA: A sexually-transmitted nuclear parasite. *Genetics*, **101**, 519–531.

Hirohashi, S. (1998) Inactivation of the E-cadherin-mediated cell adhesion system in human cancers. *Am J Pathol*, **153**, 333–339.

Hsu, M. Y., Wheelock, M. J., Johnson, K. R., et al. (1996) Shifts in cadherin profiles between human normal melanocytes and melanomas. *J Invest Dermatol Symp Proc*, **1**, 188–194.

Kath, R., Jambrosic, J. A., Holland, L., et al. (1991) Development of invasive and growth factor-independent cell variants from primary human melanomas. *Cancer Res*, **51**, 2205–2211.

Kolb, E., Turner, M. (1990) *The Early Universe*. Addison-Wesley, Redwood City.

Lengauer, C., Kinzler, K. W., Vogelstein, B. (1998) Genetic instabilities in human cancers. *Nature*, **396**, 643–649.

Lopez-Garcia, P., Moreira, D. (2006) Selective forces for the origin of the eukaryotic nucleus. *Bioessays*, **28**, 525–533.

Maynard Smith, J., Szathmary, E. (1995) *The Major Transitions in Evolution*. Oxford University Press, Oxford.

Ollivier, H., Poulin, D., Zurek, W. (2004) Objective properties from subjective quantum states: Environment as a witness. *Phys Rev Lett*, **93**, 220401.

Orgel, L. E. (2004) Prebiotic chemistry and the origin of the RNA world. *Crit Rev Biochem Mol Biol*, **39**, 99–123.

Reusch, T. B., Haberli, M. A., Aeschlimann, P. B., et al. (2001) Female sticklebacks count alleles in a strategy of sexual selection explaining MHC polymorphism. *Nature*, **414**, 300–302.

Smalley, K. S., Brafford, P. A., Herlyn, M. (2005) Selective evolutionary pressure from the tissue microenvironment drives tumor progression. *Semin Cancer Biol*, **15**, 451–459.

Smolin, L. (1999) *The Life of the Cosmos*. Oxford University Press, New York.

Smolin, L. (2004) Scientific alternatives to the anthropic principle. arXiv:hep-th/0407213, **3**.

Smolin, L. (2006) The status of cosmological natural selection. arXiv:hep-th/0612185v1.

Snyder, L., Champness, W. (1997) *Molecular Genetics of Bacteria*. ASM Press, Washington, DC.

Sterrer, W. (2002) On the origin of sex as vaccination. *J Theor Biol*, **216**, 387–396.

van Wyhe, J. (2008) Charles Darwin: Gentleman naturalist: a biographical sketch. Retrieved on 17/11/2008, from http://darwin-online.org.uk/darwin.html

Wikipedia (2008) Timeline of the Big Bang. In *Wikipedia*.

Wright, E. (2004) Big Bang Nucleosynthesis.

Zurek, W. (2007) Relative states and the environment: Einselection, envariance, quantum Darwinism, and the existential interpretation. http://arxiv.org/PS_cache/arxiv/pdf/0707/0707.2832v1.pdf

Chapter 8
Learning, Imitation, and Memes

Contents

8.1 Evolution of Complex Organisms

In the course of evolution, complex organisms arose as effective survival machines for genes. This is not to say that complex organisms replaced simple ones; rather the building of complex structures turned out to be another successful path of survival. Thus humans and bacteria coexist and are both successful, so far.

Once cells aggregated and formed cooperating complex structures, the genes for the structures coevolved to meet the demands of changing environment. Thus the structures changed with time, attaining greater complexity. The evolution of such complex organs as the mammalian eye is thus a result of eons of gradual modifi-cations of primitive light-sensitive collection of cells – and it turns out the eye is a result of design compromises because it started out from a transparent organism and thus the retina being inside out was not a problem in the beginning, but now is! (Nesse and Williams, 1994). The marvels of evolution have been achieved through laborious work of cranes rather than miraculous "sky hooks" (Dennett, 1995). Sometimes the cranes would put up pillars on the wrong side of the skyscraper, and the whole edifice would fall, the end of an evolutionary line. Evolution occurs through trial and error, with successful trials continuing the line.

H. Leigh, *Genes, Memes, Culture, and Mental Illness*,
DOI 10.1007/978-1-4419-5671-2_8, © Hoyle Leigh, 2010

8.2 Trial and Error

Trial and error is a basic process of evolution and occurs from the beginning in the sense that replication with variation is in fact trial and error. Trial and error became more organized, however, when cells acquired mobility. In plants, increased photosynthetic cell replication on the side facing the sun provided survival advantage. Eventually, movements of the multicellular organisms we call animals became directed and the incipient forms of sense organs and nervous systems appeared as it is more advantageous for the animal to move in the direction of food. In order to find food, it developed sensors that describe the state of the external environment in all directions (sense organs) and information channels for communication between these sensors and the motor apparatus, i.e., the nervous system.

Early nervous system was quite primitive. Sense organs simply distinguished a few situations to which the animal must respond differently. During the process of evolution the sense organs became more complex and transmitted an increasing amount of information about the external environment. The motor systems also made increasing demands on the nervous system for coordination. Special formations of nerves appeared – nerve centers which convert information received from the sense organs into information controlling the organs of movement, i.e., the brain.

8.3 Learn or Perish

As the primitive brain evolved, it developed the capacity to store prior experience as a shortcut to trial and error. If you have already done the trial and error, then you can cut down on the error rate by remembering what worked. This storage of past experience, memory, will be discussed in the next chapter; we will focus on learning itself for the present. It is important to remember, however, that learning and memory form an intrinsic whole.

At a very basic level, experience modifies organisms through habituation and sensitization. Repeated neutral stimulus results in habituation, i.e., a reduction in the animal's reaction to it. On the other hand, repeated noxious stimulus may cause sensitization, i.e., an exaggeration of response. Phenomena like learning has been demonstrated even in bacteria (Bruggeman et al., 2000). By studying the sea snail, *Aplysia californica* that has only 6 motor neurons and 24 sensory neurons, Kandel and colleagues demonstrated long-term habituation and sensitization at the level of a single synapse in response to repeated stimuli, mediated by functional changes in calcium channels and neurotransmitter release (Kandel, 1979).

Associative learning increasingly conferred serious survival advantage to those who were good at it. Both classical (Pavlovian) conditioning and operant (Skinnerian) conditioning are forms of associative learning. As with the Pavlovian dog who associated the ringing of the bell with food and salivated, animals increased the efficiency of finding food and avoiding danger through association of stimuli. In operant conditioning, animals who became ill with certain vegetation learned to avoid plants that had similar shapes and learned through experience what fruits were good to eat and what sorts of animals were easier to hunt. Such survival advantage selected for animals with better and better capacity for learning, i.e., better equipped brains.

As the brain became more complex with better capacity for association and memory storage, a new type of learning began to appear. Why go through the process of strenuous trial and painful error yourself if you can watch others? Why not just imitate the behavior of the successful one? Of course, the animals did not reason this out, it just happened that animals that happened to imitate the successful ones were able to survive better and reproduce better.

8.4 Imitation, Shortcut to Learning

Imitation occurs in nature at the gene level without necessarily involving the brain. Nonpoisonous mushrooms that resemble poisonous ones are not readily eaten by animals and thus have a survival advantage. So with nonpoisonous snakes that resemble poisonous ones.

Female fireflies of the Photuris species imitate the flash of other species of fireflies to lure the males and eat them. Furthermore, by eating them, they acquire chemicals from the victims that render them less attractive to their own predator spiders (Eisner et al., 1997).

Cephalopods such as octopuses and squids can imitate the coloring of their surroundings to blend in and avoid predators. Unlike the mushrooms and snakes that resemble the poisonous ones from the beginning, the cephalopods' imitation probably involves rather sophisticated brain activity (Wood and Jackson, 2004). Songbirds imitate their parents and "learn" to sing. Monkeys are of course well known for their imitations of humans. With songbirds and primates, the brain is clearly in charge in imitative learning. With the development of complex nervous systems, imitation became the basis of many repertoires of behavior that are added to those inherently encrypted in the genes.

Before imitation, the only way a new behavior could be passed on from one generation to another was purely by mutation, i.e., if the new behavior happened to be based on a mutation that passed on to the offspring. No learned behavior, such as those acquired by conditioning, could be passed on. With imitation, new generations can learn behaviors from their elders. Imitation, then, may be seen to be a new mode of cross-generational informational transmission that complements traditional genetic transmission.

Imitation replicates the behaviors and emotional expressions that are generated by another organism's experience, i.e., memory. Through imitation, memory is replicated in another brain. For example, monkey A happens to crack a nut with a stone, memory is formed, and remembers the action and uses a stone the next time he obtains a nut. Monkey A's son, monkey B, observes his father successfully cracking a nut with a stone, forms a memory of it, and when he (monkey B) obtains a nut, he copies his father's behavior that was stored in his own brain and cracks the nut with a stone.

Social learning is, of course, not based solely on imitation, though trying out what someone else does form its foundation. It is also not necessarily cross-generational – in fact, imitating peers is the norm both in humans and animals. For example, a young female Japanese macaque discovered that she could wash the sand grains off her sweet potatoes in water, and this behavior spread throughout the troop (Heyes and Galef, 1996). Chimpanzees learn from others how to insert stalks and twigs into an ant nest and harvest them to eat (Goodall, 1964; Sugiyama, 1995).

At a certain level of complexity of the brain, ideas or concepts arose. An idea is a brain code based on processed memories, i.e., an abstract meme. Ideas can be communicated to another either through imitation, emotional expression, or other means of communication. For example, an animal may cry out at the sight of a predator, and others who have not seen the predator may get the idea that there is danger and flee. Some ideas spread, i.e., ideas became infectious, i.e., they replicated themselves in other brains as memes. Some ideas are gene derived within an individual's brain, others are memes from outside that took up residence in the individual's brain.

Eventually, with the advent of language, memes could be propagated through words (which are themselves memes) instead of the action the words represent.

8.5 Coevolution of the Brain and Memes

It is well known that humans have the largest brains among all animals. The brain size of early hominids up to about 2.5 million ago was not much larger than present day chimpanzees, but it grew rapidly with the transition from *Australopithecus* to *Homo*. By about 100,000 years ago, human brain size achieved that of modern *Homo sapiens* (Blackmore, 1999).

The modern human brain volume is approximately 1,350 cm^3, about three times the size of existing apes of comparable body size (Jerison, 1973). With this large brain, humans have developed civilizations and technologies quite unlike any other animal. Clearly, from the point of view of pure genetic survival, such large amount of brain activity is quite unnecessary. Brain is an expensive organ to keep – it consumes 20% of the body's energy, weighing only 2% of the body's weight. To quote Steven Pinker, "Why would evolution ever have selected for sheer bigness of brain, that bulbous, metabolically greedy organ? Any selection on brain size itself would surely have favored the pinhead" (Pinker, 1994).

In addition to being expensive to maintain, the brain is an expensive organ to build, requiring much resource during early life for myelination and growth, more than tripling in size in the first few years. It is also a dangerous organ for reproduction as it is often too big for the birth canal. And it is getting bigger! What might be the evolutionary selection pressures that resulted in the large brain?

Susan Blackmore proposed that a turning point in evolution occurred with the advent of memes, i.e., memes changed the environment in which genes were selected, and that the direction of change was determined by the outcome of memetic selection (Blackmore, 1999). She argues that genes were selected for bigger and bigger brains in humans because of the selective advantage of imitation, i.e., memes.

Blackmore suggests that there are three skills needed for imitation – making decisions about what to imitate, complex transformation from one point of view to another, and the production of matching bodily actions. The skills needed in imitation, i.e., putting oneself in another's shoes and then imagining oneself doing it to achieve the same end, she argues, are exactly the skills needed in advanced social skills known as Machiavellian intelligence or theory of mind (TOM). Machiavellian intelligence involves the ability to manipulate and deceive others as well as to form and dissolve alliances to achieve social or political success, and involves exactly the skills of putting oneself in the other's shoes and taking the other's point of view, and imagining what it would be like to be the other. This intelligence is most prominent in humans, but has been demonstrated in other primates such as rhesus monkeys (Chicago, 2007).

Homo habilis, which means "handy man," some 2.5 million years ago first started using stone tools. Tool making probably spread through imitation, with further refinements and changes in styles, which also spread. With tool making, the better imitators of better tool makers obviously had better chance of success. And more successful imitators of more successful people had better chance of success in survival and mating (Blackmore, 1999). The escalation in skills for making better tools and the skills to imitate the successful ones who were skillful or had high Machiavellian intelligence led to an escalation in increase in brain size in humans. And with increased brain size came increased complexity both in tools and in social structure, i.e., memes that are the basis of culture and civilization. Memes and genes for brain size and complexity must have coevolved.

Another example of gene–meme coevolution is that of lactose absorption and dairy farming. There is a correlation between lactose tolerance and history of dairy farming in populations, i.e., over 90% of populations with history of dairy farming are lactose tolerant, while only about 20% of populations without the history of dairy farming have sufficient lactase activity (Leland and Odling-Smee, 2000). A population genetics analysis revealed that the allele for high lactase activity depends on the probability that the children of the milk users will adopt the meme for milk consumption (Feldman and Cavalli-Sforza, 1976). Furthermore, they found a broad range of conditions under which the lactase allele does not spread in spite of fitness advantage, demonstrating that memes complicate the genetic selection process.

The "Machiavellian intelligence" or the "social brain" hypothesis posits that large brains and distinctive cognitive abilities of humans have evolved through intense social competition in which the competitors developed increasingly sophisticated "Machiavellian" strategies as a means to achieve higher social and reproductive success. A mathematical model was constructed in which genes control brains which invent and learn strategies (memes) which are used by males to gain advantage in competition for mates. In that model, Gavrilets and Vose found that the dynamics of intelligence had three distinct phases (Gavrilets and Vose, 2006). During the dormant phase only newly invented memes were present in the population. During the cognitive explosion phase the population's meme count and the learning ability, cerebral capacity (controlling the number of different memes that the brain can learn and use), and Machiavellian fitness of individuals increased in a runaway fashion. During the saturation phase natural selection resulting from the costs of having large brains checked further increases in cognitive abilities. The results suggest that the mechanisms underlying the "Machiavellian intelligence" hypothesis can result in the evolution of significant cognitive abilities on the timescale of 10–20,000 generations. They showed that cerebral capacity evolves faster and to a larger degree than learning ability. Their model suggests that there may be a tendency toward a reduction in cognitive abilities driven by the costs of having a large brain as the reproductive advantage of having a large brain decreases and the exposure to memes increases.

Memes arose when genetic evolution reached a certain complexity of the brain and facilitated the brain's growth, which in turn helped the spread of memes. The relationship between genes and memes is not, however, always facilitative. Certain brains may be wired to reject memetic spread, and memes can interfere with the spread of genes through such practices as celibacy, birth control, and suicide.

From the gene's point of view, our bodies are just vehicles or containers for their perpetuation. From the meme's point of view, our brains are just vehicles or containers for their perpetuation. Genes have evolved to make better, sturdier, and more efficient containers for themselves, and so have the memes in producing better and bigger brains. Memes have, in addition, evolved a means of existing and replicating outside of brains, in electronic media, books, DVDs, and computers. Eventually, memes might not need brains at all to survive and replicate. Would this mean the end of genes? Not necessarily. Genes are packets of information encoded in DNA consisting of four nucleotides. Seen in this light, genes are nothing but memes encoded in nucleotides. Although the concept of memes as we currently use the term arose from imitative learning and storage and transmission of information at a fundamental level, memes invented genes, invented bodies, brains, and computers. The evolution of memetic containers will go on, relentlessly trying out different materials and forms.

8.6 Empathy and Mirror Neuron System

We saw in the previous section that what is required in imitation is an ability to put oneself in the other's shoes. When it comes to feelings, this is exactly what we call empathy; empathy is imitation of another's feeling. Empathy is usually achieved through a reading of the other's facial expression, body language, as well as verbal communication and an understanding of the person's situation. What is the neural substrate of empathy?

Mirror neurons were first described in the ventral premotor cortex of the rhesus macaque brain and later in the inferior parietal lobule. These neurons fire when a monkey performs a goal directed hand and mouth actions as well as when it observes the same action being performed by others (Ferrari et al., 2003; 2005a; b). This mirror neuron system (MNS) may form the neural substrate for understanding others' actions as well as intentions via a simulation mechanism whereby observing others' actions elicits neural activity in neurons that would be activated if the animals were actually engaging in the same activity. Thus, the mirror neuron system may form the basis of imitation in primates.

Mirror neuron system has been demonstrated in humans that encompasses the pars opercularis of the inferior frontal gyrus and adjacent ventral premotor cortex and the anterior inferior parietal lobule (Iacoboni and Dapretto, 2006; Rizzolatti and Craighero, 2004). The MNS, in concert with activity of the anterior insula and amygdala, is considered to be involved in the decoding of others' emotional states (Carr et al., 2003; Gazzola et al., 2006; Lenzi et al., 2008; Schulte-Ruther et al., 2007).

Observing facial muscles denoting a particular expression elicits firing of mirror neurons that are fired when one has similar expressions oneself. The frontal component of the MNS then modulates the activity of the amygdala and the limbic system to match the expression through connection to anterior insula. MNS activity in response to nonemotional stimuli has been associated with cognitive aspects of empathy, such as perspective-taking abilities (Gazzola et al., 2006), as well as with empathic concern (Molnar-Szakacs et al., 2006). As for emotionally laden stimuli, personal distress and, to a lesser extent, perspective taking have been associated with MNS activity in response to disgusted and pleased emotional expressions (Jabbi et al., 2007). Emotional empathy and empathic concern have also been linked to MNS activity in the right inferior frontal cortex while viewing angry and fearful facial expressions (Schulte-Ruther et al., 2007).

It seems thus that, with the development of mirror neuron system, imitation is built into the brain which reciprocally reinforces the theory of mind (TOM, Machiavellian intelligence), or the ability to think and feel like the other.

8.7   Meme Generation and Meme Infection

We discussed how our brains may have evolved to accommodate increasing memes. Are all memes in our brains then parasites? Not necessarily. Some memes obviously arose de novo in certain individuals, then, spread through imitation, and in humans, through symbolic communication, i.e., language. The mirror neuron system provides a direct example of how memes may arise in the form of motor expression before they have been fully assembled with emotion and meaning, i.e., before connections have been made with neurons in the limbic system and association cortices.

The activity of the mirror neuron system may later be connected with the cortex and the limbic system, especially if the activity is efficacious.

Some memes arose from plain trial and error – like the first monkey who happened to crack a nut with a stone. Then, "crack a nut with stone" meme spreads throughout the troop by observation (infection).

Memes are essentially memories that skip brains and infect other brains. When these memories are recalled and reassembled to meet current needs, we have *information*. Existing information is compared with incoming information leading to appropriate action.

Then, is all information memes? Yes to an extent. The "crack a nut with stone" idea would be a successful meme within the monkey as it would be replicated over and over again when he found a nut. If the "crack a nut with stone" idea stayed in one monkey's brain without being transmitted to other monkeys, it is not a successful meme in terms of longevity across generations. On the other hand, most likely, other monkeys would see the monkey cracking a nut and imitate it, and then the meme would spread successfully horizontally. Just as certain RNA's and DNA's are potential but not successful genes, memes may arise and fall without ever becoming successful, success being defined as the ability to infect and replicate.

Not only information about facts and behaviors but also emotions can be memes as long as they can be remembered and transmitted. A recent finding from the Framingham heart study social network is that happiness is contagious. In a 20-year follow-up of nearly 5,000 people, clusters of happy and unhappy people were found in the network. The clusters of happiness seem to result from the spread of happiness and not just a tendency of happy people to associate with each other. According to this study, a person's probability of being happy is increased by 25% if a friend who lives within a mile and becomes happy. Coresident spouses and siblings who live within a mile, and next door neighbors had similar increases in probability to be happy (by 8, 14, and 34%, respectively) (Fowler and Christakis, 2008). Happiness spread even to people who were separated by three degrees of separation and not even known to each other.

What exactly is meme contagion or infection? Does a meme physically enter the brain of the host?

In a sense, the answer is yes. A meme is a packet of information, i.e., an idea, emotion, or behavior, or a recipe to create the idea or emotion or behavior. Information content should not be confused with the carrier or vehicle through which it travels, which themselves are also memes. For example, the information content of the meme of "love" is not the assemblage of the letters l-o-v-e (which are themselves memes), but rather the *idea* that can be expressed as "amour," "Liebe," "名爱," or "hluv." Because we have in our brains the genetic and memetic apparatus to process memes that associate themselves with various forms of conveyance (languages, images, sounds), we have the capacity to understand, empathize, and influence other brains as they do ours.

Information changes the brain just as a virus (a packet of DNA or RNA, genetic code) changes a cell. The exact mechanism of meme-induced brain changes in the form of memory will be discussed in the next chapter.

When you throw a pebble in a lake, waves are formed that cause all the water in the lake to resonate without the pebble touching all the water molecules. Likewise, a new meme may affect all brains exposed to it. Of course, you can create a counter-wave in the lake to neutralize the pebble waves. The brains may also have counter-memes that may already be there, or newly introduced.

As memes have discovered new carriers outside of the brain such as books, computers, electromagnetic waves, DVDs, memes can now reside independently of human brains. In fact, some such memes have flown out of the planet Earth in space ships. Some such memes may infect nonhuman hosts in other planets and find a separate path of evolution (Fig. 8.1).

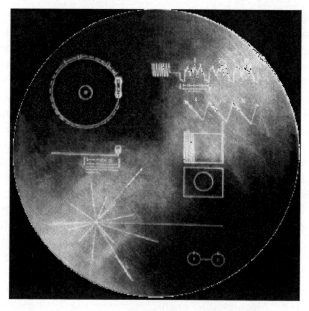

Fig. 8.1 The Voyager Interstellar Record with 2 h of images and sounds of earth. A 33 rpm grooved gold record 1977 (http://www.cedmagic.com/featured/voyager/voyager-record.html)

8.8   What Is a Meme?

A meme is memory that is transferred or has the potential to be transferred. The transfer of a meme may be from one brain to another, from a brain to a medium such as books, recordings, and digital media. Memes may be broadcasted, i.e., dispersed from the brain like seeds or spores. Memes are replicators. Replication occurs either within the brain or outside the brain. Replication occurs in two forms: direct replication as in being copied by a Xerox machine, or through transmission to other brains and then to other brains, etc. Within the brain, replication may occur through direct contact with other neurons and conferring the memory to them, or through reinforcement of the memory within the neuron which results in increased potential for the meme to reach consciousness and thus to be broadcasted or transmitted to other brains or media.

Memes need not be consciously transferred to be spread. Imitation is an example in which memes are created by simple observation. Such memes created through imitation may be either transmitted consciously in language or transmitted nonverbally through imitation by others. What is critical here is that the behavior that is imitated is remembered, i.e., memory has been formed that is potentially transferred.

Since Dawkins described memes as an analog of genes, there has been confusion concerning what the relationship between genes and memes is. Before the discovery of DNA, genes were defined purely by the phenotype, e.g., genes for blue eyes, color blindness. Now we know that strands of DNA make up the basis of protein synthesis that underlies the phenotypes. There are, however, many strands of DNA that do not produce protein ("junk DNA") but are faithfully replicated and may affect other DNA strands. DNA replication is dependent, however, on the phenotype's success in mate selection. Genes are a sequence of replicating nucleotides that carry *both* the information and the machinery for replication.

Memory is the precursor and foundation of memes. Memory served to reduce the error rate of trial and error. Out of memory arose *ideas*, interconnection among neuronal clusters containing memories that facilitated learning. As the complexity of the nervous system increased through evolution, imitation became a shortcut to trial and error. When ideas and actions acquired the means of replication through observation and imitation, they became memes, or replicating information. Memes are encoded in the neurons of the brain as "brain codes" as will be discussed in the last section of Chapter 9. As memory and ideas are interconnected, assemblies of memories and ideas formed, which were more convenient to store and retrieve. Some of these assemblies were particularly useful and thus tended to be imitated or learned together. Such assemblies are sometimes called memeplexes. However, it should be noted that when we talk of memes, much of the time we are talking about memeplexes.

The advent of mirror neurons facilitated imitation and a new means of meme manipulation – the Machiavellian intelligence. With the development of language (which is nothing but new containers of memes), memes acquired the means of spreading beyond the brain's immediate proximity of time and space.

Memes, consisting of only information, did not possess the means of replication, which has to be dependent on matter–energy-dependent processes (Crofts, 2007). Memes, as pure information or code, were stored as memory, constructed as thought, schema, knowledge, and emotion, emitted as sound, expression, and eventually in language, none of which carried the machinery for replication. Of necessity, meme replication was done by brains infecting other brains.

What, exactly, is meme replication? Karl Marx wrote *Das Kapital*, which gave rise to the meme, *communism*. It spread from brain to brain, eventually resulting in the meme taking over the governing structures of many countries during the twentieth century. It also evolved differently in different locations, so that the communisms practiced in different countries, e.g., Soviet Union, China, North Korea, Hungary, were very different. One can see that the complex memeplex that is communism consisted of many memes, including ideas concerning economics, equality, fairness, labor, profit, collectivism, ends justify means, authoritarianism, universalism, nationalism, etc. Many of the component ideas were also mutually contradictory while others were mutually reinforcing. Thus a meme complex can be replicated in many different ways through component memes and may mutate rapidly while maintaining the label and some vestiges of the original meme. Memeplexes often organize people or groups of people for their perpetuation and replication – such as political and religious organizations that reinforce the memes, and schools and institutions to replicate themselves in fresh brains.

Memes have been likened to a virus, which can replicate only when it finds a suitable cell. A meme, say an idea written in a book, does not enter the brain and make books in the brain. Memes are more like prions. Once a prion is in contact with a suitable protein, it changes the configuration of the existing protein, which, in turn, changes the configuration of an adjacent protein. So does an infected brain change adjacent brains through communication.

With the advent of computers and the information age, however, memes may have acquired the material means of self-replication, i.e., memes no longer need brains for actualization and replication. In fact, it may be that the achievement of a certain level of information-processing capacity inevitably means the ability to decode memes, regardless of their origin. This would be the hope if the Voyager disk were to be understood by an intelligent being in another part of the galaxy. It is also possible that memes may find that an efficient way of self-replication is encoding themselves with nucleotides in a new environment!

References

Blackmore, S. J. (1999) *The Meme Machine*. Oxford University Press, Oxford; New York.

Bruggeman, F. J., van Heeswijk, W. C., Boogerd, F. C., et al. (2000) Macromolecular intelligence in microorganisms. *Biol Chem*, **381**, 965–972.

Carr, L., Iacoboni, M., Dubeau, M. C., et al. (2003) Neural mechanisms of empathy in humans: A relay from neural systems for imitation to limbic areas. *Proc Natl Acad Sci USA*, **100**, 5497–5502.

University of Chicago. (2007) Humans and monkeys share Machiavellian intelligence. http://www.sciencedaily.com/releases/2007/10/071024144314.htm

Crofts, A. R. (2007) Life, information, entropy, and time: Vehicles for semantic inheritance. *Complexity*, **13**, 14–50.

Dennett, D. C. (1995) *Darwin's Dangerous Idea: Evolution and the Meanings of Life*. Simon and Schuster, New York.

Eisner, T., Goetz, M., Hill, D., et al. (1997) Firefly "femmes fatales" acquire defensive steroids (lucibufagins) from their firefly prey. *Proc Natl Acad Sci USA*, **94**, 9723–9728.

Feldman, M., Cavalli-Sforza, L. (1976) On the theory of evolution under genetic and cultural transmission with application to the lactose absorption problem. In *Mathematic Evolutionary Theory* (M. Feldman ed.), pp. 145–173. Princeton University Press, Princeton.

Ferrari, P. F., Gallese, V., Rizzolatti, G., et al. (2003) Mirror neurons responding to the observation of ingestive and communicative mouth actions in the monkey ventral premotor cortex. *Eur J Neurosci*, **17**, 1703–1714.

Ferrari, P. F., Maiolini, C., Addessi, E., et al. (2005a) The observation and hearing of eating actions activates motor programs related to eating in macaque monkeys. *Behav Brain Res*, **161**, 95–101.

Ferrari, P. F., Rozzi, S., Fogassi, L. (2005b) Mirror neurons responding to observation of actions made with tools in monkey ventral premotor cortex. *J Cogn Neurosci*, **17**, 212–226.

Fowler, J. H., Christakis, N. A. (2008) Dynamic spread of happiness in a large social network: Longitudinal analysis over 20 years in the Framingham Heart Study. *BMJ*, **337**, a2338.

Gavrilets, S., Vose, A. (2006) The dynamics of Machiavellian intelligence. *Proc Natl Acad Sci USA*, **103**, 16823–16828.

Gazzola, V., Aziz-Zadeh, L., Keysers, C. (2006) Empathy and the somatotopic auditory mirror system in humans. *Curr Biol*, **16**, 1824–1829.

Goodall, J. (1964) Tool using and aimed throwing in a community of free living chimpanzees. *Nature*, **201**, 1264–1266.

Heyes, C. M., Galef, B. G. J. (eds.) (1996) *Social Learning in Animals*. Academic Press, San Diego.

Iacoboni, M., Dapretto, M. (2006) The mirror neuron system and the consequences of its dysfunction. *Nat Rev Neurosci*, **7**, 942–951.

Jabbi, M., Swart, M., Keysers, C. (2007) Empathy for positive and negative emotions in the gustatory cortex. *Neuroimage*, **34**, 1744–1753.

Jerison, H. (1973) *Evolution of the Brain and Intelligence*. Academic Press, New York.

Kandel, E. R. (1979) Psychotherapy and the single synapse. The impact of psychiatric thought on neurobiologic research. *N Engl J Med*, **301**, 1028–1037.

Leland, K., Odling-Smee, J. (2000) The evolution of the meme. In *Darwinizing Culture: The Status of Memetics as a Science* (R. Aunger ed.), pp. 121–141. Oxford University Press, Oxford.

Lenzi, D., Trentini, C., Pantano, P., et al. (2009) Neural basis of maternal communication and emotional expression processing during infant preverbal stage. *Cereb Cortex*, **19**, 1124–1133.

Molnar-Szakacs, I., Kaplan, J., Greenfield, P. M., et al. (2006) Observing complex action sequences: The role of the fronto-parietal mirror neuron system. *Neuroimage*, **33**, 923–935.

Nesse, R. M., Williams, G. C. (1994) *Why We Get Sick*. Random House, New York.

Pinker, S. (1994) *The Language Instinct*. Morrow, New York.

Rizzolatti, G., Craighero, L. (2004) The mirror-neuron system. *Annu Rev Neurosci*, **27**, 169–192.

Schulte-Ruther, M., Markowitsch, H. J., Fink, G. R., et al. (2007) Mirror neuron and theory of mind mechanisms involved in face-to-face interactions: A functional magnetic resonance imaging approach to empathy. *J Cogn Neurosci*, **19**, 1354–1372.

Sugiyama, Y. (1995) Tool-use for catching ants by chimpanzees at Bossou and Monts Nimba, West Africa. *Primates*, **36**, 193–205.

Wood, J., Jackson, K. (2004) *Why cephalopods change color*. Bermuda Biological Station for Research.

Chapter 9
Storage and Evolution of Memes in the Brain

Contents

9.1 Storage of Memes as Memory

We have seen that genes have achieved immortality by developing perpetually replicating bodies. Through the algorithm of Darwinian evolution, bodies better suited for reproduction prevailed. A result of this evolution was the development of the brain.

Bigger brains mean more capacity for learning and memory. If you remember what was successful in your trial and error in a given situation, then you do not have to repeat the cumbersome and often dangerous trial and error to know what to do when a similar situation arises.

We discussed in the previous chapter that memory is the precursor and foundation of memes, i.e., memes are portable memory, and interconnected, assembled memories are memeplexes called ideas. Then, how is memory formed and stored in the brain?

The exact mechanism of the formation and storage of memory at the neuronal level has been elucidated recently through the works of Eric Kandel and others (Kandel, 2006) and will be discussed below.

Memory may be classified as implicit or explicit, and short term or long term. Implicit or procedural memory is the more fundamental form of memory, which is not necessarily conscious and does not necessarily involve language. It occurs in all animals. Explicit or declarative memory is subject to conscious recall and consists

H. Leigh, *Genes, Memes, Culture, and Mental Illness*,
DOI 10.1007/978-1-4419-5671-2_9, © Hoyle Leigh, 2010

of personal experiences (episodic memory) and what we call knowledge (semantic memory), e.g., what is your name, what is the capital of the United States. Both types of memory may be short or long term.

9.1.1 Implicit Memory

9.1.1.1 Short-Term Memory

Kandel showed that learning takes place even at the level of a single synapse in the sea slug, *Aplysia californica* (Kandel, 2001). Both habituation and sensitization occur at the level of the single synapse to repeated stimuli. In the synapse between a sensory neuron and a motor neuron, habituation causes the sensory neuron to release less and less amounts of the neurotransmitter, glutamate. In sensitization, it releases more glutamate.

In sensitization, Kandel et al. discovered that serotonin-releasing interneurons play a role, modulating the synaptic strength. The interneurons have synapses both at the cell body and the presynaptic terminal of the sensory neuron. When serotonin is released at the synaptic cleft, it enters a receptor and activates cyclic AMP, which in turn activates protein kinase A. Protein kinase A then enhances the release of glutamate.

9.1.1.2 Long-Term Memory

In long-term memory, there is, in addition to enhanced release of neurotransmitter, anatomical change in the presynaptic neuron, i.e., it grows more terminals and forms more synaptic connections. The mechanism of long-term memory formation involves genetic engineering.

Kandel and colleagues showed that genes encoding for protein synthesis at the synapse were turned on in *Aplysia* when new synaptic connections were made (Kandel, 2006).

Repeated stimuli activate serotonin release by interneurons which, in turn, activates cyclic AMP in the sensory neuron which, in turn, activates protein kinase A, which moves into the nucleus together with MAP kinase which it recruited (see Fig. 9.1). In the nucleus, the kinases activate a gene regulatory protein, CREB, which binds to a promoter gene. There are two forms of CREB protein, CREB-1 and CREB-2. CREB-1 activates gene expression and CREB-2 suppresses gene expression. Protein kinase A activates CREB-1 and MAP kinase inactivates CREB-2, thus, jointly, they enhance gene expression, making proteins for the new synaptic structure. The opposing action of CREB-1 and CREB-2 in enhancing and suppressing gene expression may serve to regulate long-term memory formation, i.e., which event will be stored and which will not.

When genes are activated by CREB proteins, they produce messenger RNAs (mRNAs) that are distributed throughout the cell (see Figs. 9.2 and 9.3). The mRNAs that reach synapses are in a dormant form and do not make proteins. When

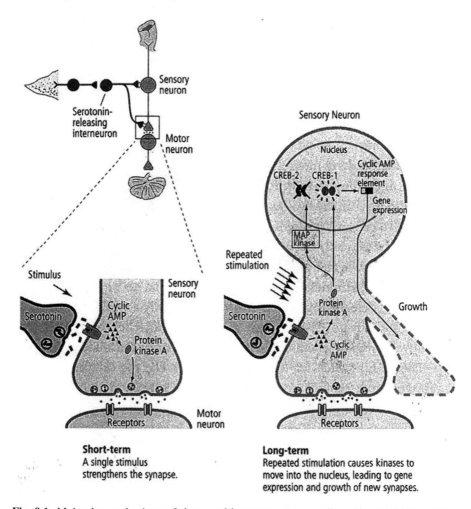

Fig. 9.1 Molecular mechanisms of short- and long-term memory. (From Kandel, 2006, p. 261, reprinted with permission)

a synapse has been repeatedly stimulated by serotonin released by an interneuron, the CPEB (cytoplasmic polyadenylation element-binding protein) that was present becomes activated, which in turn awakens the dormant mRNA, which now makes proteins and stabilizes the synapse. CPEB is a *prion-like* protein. Prions are proteins that cause the "mad cow" disease (bovine spongioform encephalopathy) and Creutzfeldt–Jakob disease. Prions can fold into two distinct shapes, an infectious (dominant) and a noninfectious (recessive) form. The noninfectious form is a normal protein found throughout the body. The infectious form is self-perpetuating and can transform the noninfectious form into the infectious form. There are normal genes that encode prions giving rise to the noninfectious form, but it can become infectious by contact with infectious prions, or sometimes spontaneously. Thus prion infection

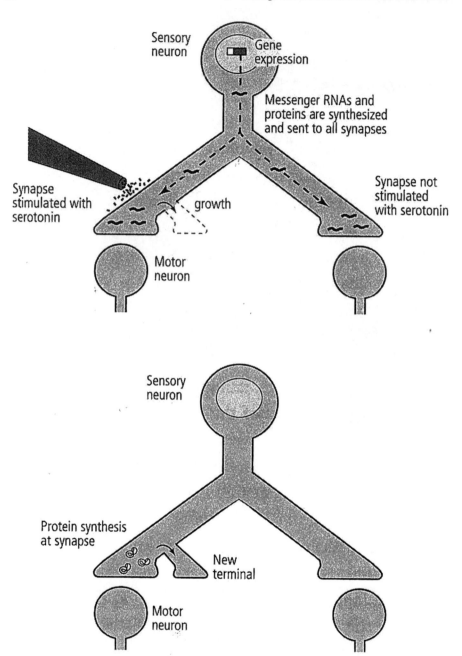

Fig. 9.2 Two mechanisms of long-term change. New proteins are sent to all of the synapses (*above*). Only synapses stimulated with serotonin use them to initiate the growth of new terminals. Proteins synthesized locally (*below*) are needed to sustain the growth initiated by gene expression. (From Kandel, 2006, p. 271, reprinted with permission)

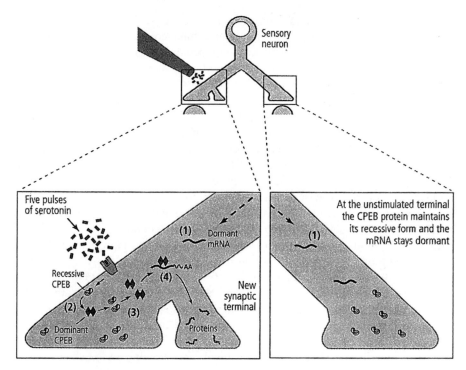

Fig. 9.3 Role of repeated stimulation in memory formation. (From Kandel, 2006, p. 274, reprinted with permission)

does not result in replication of the foreign prion, but rather it converts the existing noninfectious prion into the infectious conformation. In the case of CPEB, it becomes infectious when stimulated with serotonin. The infectious form of CPEB replicates itself and maintains local protein synthesis at the synapse. It perpetuates synaptic facilitation and thus long-term storage of memory.

Repetition is in general necessary for long-term memory. So-called flashbulb memory may occur if an event is highly emotionally charged and causes a massive influx of MAP kinase and protein kinase A into the nucleus to activate all CREB-1 protein and inactivate all CREB-2, thus directly creating a long-term memory.

While implicit memory can be stored in any synapse, basal ganglia and the cerebellum seem to be particularly involved in its storage in mammals.

9.1.2 Explicit Memory

Storage of explicit memory, unlike implicit memory that can be achieved at the level of a single synapse, involves the brain as consciousness and language involves the integrative function of the brain.

The sensory and association cortices, speech centers, the limbic system, especially hippocampus and amygdala, and the entorhinal cortex are intimately involved in explicit memory. Among the structures, hippocampus is considered to be the brain structure that is involved in consolidating short-term memory into long-term memory. Attention, mediated by the neurotransmitter dopamine, is necessary for explicit memory to occur. BDNF is considered to be essential in maintaining long-term explicit memory (Bekinschtein et al., 2008).

In animals, a *spatial map* develops when they enter a new environment, i.e., the hippocampus develops a multisensory representation of the new environment. The spatial map was destabilized and did not last long when protein kinase A was blocked, showing that it is memory dependent. Such a representation may be a form of explicit memory in animals (Kandel, 2006). The spatial map was destabilized when dopamine blockers were administered and enhanced when dopamine receptors were activated, indicating the necessity of attention.

Repeated rapid stimulation of neuronal pathway to the hippocampus leads to strengthening of the connection for hours and days. This type of synaptic facilitation is called long-term potentiation (LTP) (Bliss and Lomo, 1973). Glutamate is the principal excitatory neurotransmitter in the brain. Glutamate acts on both the AMPA and the NMDA receptors in the hippocampal neurons. The AMPA receptor mediates normal synaptic transmission, responding to potential from presynaptic neuron. When the postsynaptic neuron is stimulated repeatedly and rapidly, the AMPA receptor powerfully depolarizes the cell membrane allowing an ion channel in the NMDA receptor to open, allowing calcium ion influx (Kauer et al., 1988; Lynch et al., 1988). Calcium then acts as a second messenger akin to cyclic AMP discussed above, triggering activation of kinases which in turn activate CREB resulting in structural change of the neuron associated with LTP. Rhythmic bursting activity is highly effective in inducing LTP and the endogenous hippocampal theta rhythm may play a role in LTP induction in vivo (Lynch et al., 1990).

In LTP of rat hippocampal neurons, dopamine rather than serotonin (as in *Aplysia*) modulates the prion-like CPEB protein (CPEB-3) that results in perpetuation of the structural change at the synapse.

9.1.3 Learned Fear

Conditioned fear response is a basic learned response that involves long-term memory. The brain has to remember the stimulus associated with fear to elicit the response.

When a tone is paired with an electric shock in the rat, the tone travels through the auditory nerve to the medial geniculate body of the thalamus. The signal is then carried by two separate pathways: one goes directly to the lateral nucleus of amygdala, and another pathway goes to the auditory cortex first, then to the lateral nucleus of amygdala.

The electric shock activates pain fibers that terminate in the somatosensory thalamus. From the thalamus, there again emerge two separate pathways, one directly
to the lateral nucleus of amygdala, the other through the somatosensory cortex to
the same nucleus.

The existence of two separate pathways for sensory input to amygdala, one
through the cortex and another bypassing it, indicates that unconscious evaluation
of fearful stimulus precedes conscious evaluation of it (Kandel, 2006). When the
neurons in the lateral nucleus are sufficiently stimulated, they send impulses to the
central nucleus, which in turn send signals to hypothalamus, limbic system, and the
cortex that result in the autonomic, endocrine, and behavioral fear response. Brain-
derived neurotrophic factor (BDNF) plays an important role in synaptic plasticity.
Calcium influx through NMDA receptors and voltage-dependent calcium channels,
which occurs in the lateral nucleus during fear conditioning, activates protein kinase
A and Ca^{2+}/calmodulin-dependent protein kinase IV. Each induces phosphorylation of CREB, which binds to the BDNF promoter, leading to BDNF expression in
the lateral amygdala and contributes to fear memory consolidation (Monfils et al.,
2007). Repeated stimuli of this sort result in long-term potentiation in the circuits
from thalamus to lateral nucleus of amygdala and from the lateral nucleus to central
nucleus, i.e., a conditioned reflex has been formed.

A gene encoding gastrin-releasing peptide (GRP) has been found to be highly
expressed both in the lateral nucleus of the amygdala and in the regions that
convey fearful auditory information to the lateral nucleus. GRP receptor (GRPR)
is expressed in GABAergic interneurons of the lateral nucleus. GRP excites
these interneurons and increases their inhibition of principal neurons. GRPR-
deficient mice showed decreased inhibition of principal neurons by the interneurons,
enhanced long-term potentiation (LTP), and greater and more persistent long-
term fear memory. By contrast, these mice performed normally in hippocampus-
dependent Morris maze. GRP and its neural circuitry seem to operate as a negative
feedback regulating fear and establish a causal relationship between GRPR gene
expression and LTP, and amygdala-dependent memory for fear (Shumyatsky et al.,
2005, 2002).

9.1.4   Learning Safety

What happens in the brain when an animal learns that certain signals denote safety?
Rogan et al. gave electric shock to mice only during periods when a tone was *not*
on, that is, when the mice heard the tone, it meant it was safe. Thus, the conditioned
stimulus (tone) came to signify a period of protection, reducing fear responses
and increasing adventurous exploration of a novel environment. Mice turned on
the tone when given the opportunity. Thus, conditioned safety involves a reduction
of learned and instinctive fear, as well as positive affective responses. Concurrent
electrophysiological measurements revealed a safety learning-induced long-lasting
depression of tone-evoked activity in the lateral nucleus of the amygdala, consistent

with fear reduction, and an increase of tone-evoked activity in a region of the stria-
tum involved in positive affect, euphoric responses, and reward (Rogan et al., 2005).
Thus, the memory of positive events and feelings are also stored in neurons through
LTP and associated structural change in neurons in different pathways of the brain.

The tone-sensitive neurons in the thalamus and the neurons in the lateral nucleus
of amygdala both have connections with the striatum, and both convey information
concerning safety. Striatum in turn is connected with many areas of the brain including the cingulate gyrus that inhibits amygdala. Thus stimulation of the striatum may
also decrease activation of amygdala and thus fear response.

9.1.5 Working Memory

Working memory involves the temporary storage and manipulation of information
necessary for the task at hand. Baddeley and Hitch proposed a multicomponent
model consisting of four subsystems. The first is concerned with verbal and acoustic
information, the phonological loop; second, the visuo-spatial sketchpad providing
its visual equivalent, while both are dependent upon a third attentionally limited
control system, the central executive, and a fourth subsystem, the episodic buffer
(Baddeley, 2003; Baddeley and Hitch, 1974).

The *central executive* is the master unit that is responsible for information integration and coordination of the subordinate systems and is considered to be largely
a function of the dorsolateral prefrontal cortex and its connections (Baddeley, 2003;
Goldman-Rakic et al., 2004; Kondo et al., 2004). The central executive directs attention to relevant information and suppresses irrelevant information and inappropriate
actions and coordinates cognitive processes for competing tasks.

The *phonological loop* stores phonological or sound-related information in a
temporary store and prevents its decay by continuously refreshing it through a
subvocal rehearsal system. The phonological loop not only maintains the sound
information but also registers visual information within the store provided the items
can be named. Different parts of the Broca's area seem to be involved in the storage
and subvocal rehearsal systems. The verbal working memory seems to be largely
localized in the left hemisphere (Baddeley, 2003).

The *visuo-spatial sketchpad* stores visual and spatial information. It can be used,
for example, for constructing and manipulating visual images and for the representation of mental maps. The sketch pad may be subdivided into a visual subsystem
(dealing with shape, color, texture, etc.) and a spatial subsystem (dealing with location). The spatial system seems to be localized more in the right hemisphere (Smith
and Jonides, 1997).

PET studies show that separable components may be responsible for the passive
storage of information and the active maintenance of information, with the storage component being localized more in the back of the brain, and the maintenance
component in the front (Smith and Jonides, 1997).

The *episodic buffer* is considered to be a limited capacity system that depends
heavily on executive processing, but which differs from the central executive in

being principally concerned with the storage of information rather than with attentional control. It binds together information from a number of different sources into chunks or episodes. In this buffer, information from different modalities can be combined into a single multifaceted entity. Baddeley proposed that this may underpin the capacity for conscious awareness (Baddeley, 2000, 2001). The episodic buffer seems to be multimodal in function. The formation of unitary multidimensional representations in the episodic buffer seems to engage posterior neural networks, but maintenance of such representations is supported by frontal networks. The hippocampus and prefrontal cortex play important roles in the representations in the episodic buffer of working memory (Rudner and Ronnberg, 2008; Yoon et al., 2008).

Working memory is important in psychiatry as it is impaired in various psychiatric conditions including schizophrenia and mood disorders. In schizophrenia, there is an overproduction of dopamine D2 receptors that is associated with psychotic symptoms and a reduction in D1 receptors. There seems to be a direct relationship between the prefrontal dopamine function and the integrity of working memory, suggesting that insufficient D1 receptor signaling, and thus reduction in cyclic AMP and glutamatergic transmission, resulting in cognitive deficits. Working memory deficits can be ameliorated by treatments that augment D1 receptor stimulation (Goldman-Rakic et al., 2004).

In depression, there is often cognitive impairment and a reduction in the size of the hippocampus, especially after repeated bouts of severe depression. Antidepressants and ECT all have the effect of increasing neurogenesis in the dentate nucleus of the hippocampus. The newly generated neurons are particularly sensitive to LTP (Pittenger and Duman, 2008; Sahay and Hen, 2007).

9.2 Evolution of Memes in the Brain and the Brain Code

Once learned stuff has been stored in the brain by forming neuronal synaptic connections through LTP, what happens to the memory? We know that memory tends to decay over time, and some memories are better preserved than others. We have seen that emotionally charged events may become instantly fixed in memory (flashbulb memory) while boring factual information may require a long series of repetitions to become long-term memory.

Hippocampus is the main brain site for the conversion of short-term memory into long-term memory as long-term memory does not form without it. Hippocampus is also one area of the brain where chronic stress reduces the number of neurons and their connections, and where neurogenesis occurs in adulthood (Drew and Hen, 2007; Gould et al., 1997; Pittenger and Duman, 2008; Sahay and Hen, 2007).

In the mouse hippocampus, different groups of neurons respond to different stimuli, such as shake or air blow. Such identification of network-level functional coding units, termed neural cliques, has allowed real-time patterns of memory traces to be digitized (Lin et al., 2007). For example, Lin et al. were able to express the memory code associated with an experience in binary code based on a predefined sequence of clique assembly (general startle, air blow, drop, shake, air subcontext, drop subcontext): the activation code 110010 corresponding to the internal representation of the air blow in context A, 110000 to air blow in context B, 101000 to drop elevator A, 101001 to drop elevator B, and 100100 to shake. See Fig. 9.4.

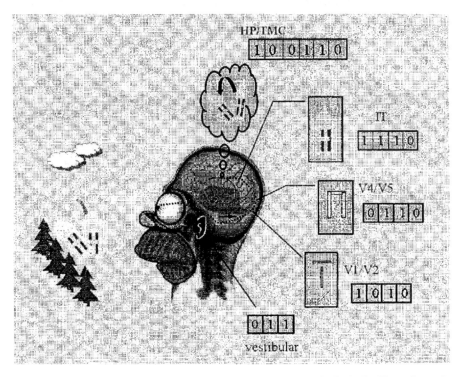

Fig. 9.4 Neural clique code-based real-time information processes in the brain. Through a series of hierarchical-extraction and parallel-binding processes, the brain achieves coherent internal encoding and processing of external events. For example, when a person experiences a sudden earthquake, neural cliques in his primary visual cortex encode the decomposed features about edge orientation, movement, and eventually shapes of visual objects, whereas the neural cliques in the vestibular nuclei detect sudden motion disturbances. As information is processed along its pathways into deeper cortex such as the inferior temporal cortex (IT), neural cliques begin to exhibit complex encoding features such as houses. By the time it reaches high association cortices such as the hippocampus (HP) and temporal medial cortex (TMC), the neural clique assembly encodes earthquake experience and its location, with a selective set of "what and where" information. At this level, abstract and generalized information such as semantic memories of "the earthquake is dangerous and scary" have emerged. As information is further processed into other cortical regions involving decision making and motor planning, a series of phased firing among various neural clique assemblies lead to adaptive behaviors such as screaming and running away from the house, or hiding under a dining table. As illustrated, the activation patterns of neural clique assemblies in each brain region can be also converted into a binary code for universally comparing and categorizing network-level representations from brain to brain. Such universal brain codes can also allow more seamless brain–machine interface communications. (Figure and legend reprinted with permission from Elsevier (Tsien, 2007))

Any given episodic event is represented and encoded by the activation of a set of neural clique assemblies that are organized in a categorical and hierarchical manner. This hierarchical feature-encoding pyramid is composed of the general feature-encoding clique at the bottom, sub-general feature-encoding cliques in the middle, and highly specific feature-encoding cliques at the top. Tisen states that this hierarchical and categorical organization of neural clique assemblies provides the network-level mechanism the capability of not only achieving vast storage capacity, but also generating commonalities from the individual behavioral episodes and converting them to the abstract concepts and generalized knowledge that are essential for intelligence and adaptive behaviors. The conversion of activation patterns of the neural clique assemblies to strings of binary codes may permit universal categorizations of the brain's internal representations across individuals and species. Such *universal brain codes* can also potentially facilitate the unprecedented brain–machine interface communications (Tsien, 2007).

Tsien states that the binary brain code differs from the genetic code in several aspects as follows:

1. Uninheritable: genetic code is directly inherited through reproduction, while brain code is formed through experience or imitation.
2. Self-organizing: genetic codes are like blue prints, while brain codes are dynamical and self-organizing based on connections.
3. Variable sizes: genetic codes are fixed in size in each individual and species, while brain codes are variable in size limited only by the network capacity determined by the convergence or divergence of connections and individual's experiences.
4. Modifiable: genetic code remains the same within an individual unless mutated, while membership of individual neurons in a neural clique depends on synaptic connections based on experience or disease states (Tsien, 2007).

Such universal brain codes might be exactly what we know as memes (or proto-memes for animals that lack imitation or communication skills). While the brain code is not inheritable through biological reproduction, it can spread through imitation, language, and electronic means, and thus can be reproduced in other brains. Thus, memes reside as brain codes of neural cliques in the brain. Outside the brain, memes may reside in computers as binary codes on silicon, as patterns of ink in the print media, or streams of radio waves.

Edelman has shown that clusters of neurons in the brain are subject to Darwinian natural selection. Edelman's theory of neuronal group selection posits that neuronal selection occurs in three facets: (1) Developmental selection – during early phases of neural development, random variations of synaptic connections exist, and groups of neurons that are wired together fire together. (2) Experiential selection – the groups of neurons that are formed during the first phase are selected by experience, i.e., by reinforcement or nonreinforcement, throughout life. The reinforcements are repeated firings that form strengthened connections such as LTP, facilitated by emotional arousal. (3) Reentry – large numbers of local and long-distance reciprocal neural connections are established. They provide ongoing recursive interchange of parallel signals among brain areas that serves to coordinate the activities of different brain areas in space and time (Edelman, 1987, 1993; Edelman, 2004). According to Edelman, neuronal groups connected by reentrant interactions are the selectional units in higher level brains (Edelman, 2004). *These neuronal groups might be identical or similar to the "neural cliques" that fire together as described above and may represent memes.*

Neuronal group selection is a Darwinian natural selection that occurs during the lifespan of an animal and is dependent on reinforcement. Lack of reinforcement usually results in reduction in synaptic connections, thus rendering the group silent or inactive.

It is clear, then, that if memes can be represented as binary codes of excitation of "neural cliques", and neuronal groups that are connected by parallel interactions as described by Edelman undergo Darwinian natural selection, then *memes must undergo Darwinian natural selection in the brain. Neuronal groups may be reinforced by signals (reentrance) from other similarly firing neuronal groups (forming memes) and thus gain survival advantage.* One might say that neurons thrive on memes. When a competing meme becomes dominant, neural cliques underlying it are enhanced, i.e., better fed, with more synapses.

Thus, some memes will become dominant with repeated exposure and rehearsal and proliferate, i.e., recruit other neuronal groups; others will become dormant, not forming new connections or recruiting others. The process of reentry resulting in new parallel connections may be seen to be a process of replication of the meme, a prion-like replication by contact through synaptic and/or dendritic connection. This is not to imply that one neuron serves only one meme. In fact, a neuron has many connections and may be a component of a number of different memes and memetic connections.

Meme replication in the brain, therefore, does not involve reproducing new neurons, but rather occurs through recombination of component memes in existing neuronal groups. Such replication may occur through meme-processing mechanisms such as cognition, often stimulated by the entry of new memes into the brain.

The brain, in my view, is more like the Internet than one computer, with redundant storage and constantly changing connections and storage, in which memes are constantly created, propagated, combined, disintegrated, mutated, and evolved. Like the Internet, there are many interconnected processing centers that execute these functions. Some of these functions may involve a threshold number of processing units and reach consciousness, others without reaching consciousness. Just like information on the Internet, some memes stay dormant and others become activated and replicated.

Dreaming may be an important meme-processing brain state. Visual dreams occur mostly during the rapid eye movement sleep (REM), during which there is autonomic arousal and motor inhibition. During this period, impulses arising from brain stem (PGO spikes) reach sensory and association cortex through the thalamus.

Winson postulates that REM might be like off-line processing in computers. In this model, the task of associating recent events to past memories is accomplished while the animal is asleep. This spares the frontal cortex from having to process new information and integrate it simultaneously, allowing a more leisurely integration during sleep (Winson, 1985).

Reiser postulates that these impulses will readily activate neural circuits with relatively low excitatory thresholds, i.e., those circuits that retained memories of meaningful experiences to which emotions are attached and connected to current life problem (Reiser, 1991). These circuits would be those that represent significant memes stored during the day. During dreaming, then, the newly introduced memes find new connections with already stored memes, may combine with some forming memeplexes, may awaken others from a dormant state, or may become dormant or be simply discarded.

In addition to newly introduced memes finding connections with stored memes during the dreaming state, dreams may also represent the processes of existing memes finding new combinations and connections that are significant enough to reach consciousness. Thus, in dreams, we may have a glimpse of the memes struggling with each other, constantly making and breaking new alliances, configurations, and reproductions within our brain.

In the process of human evolution, the brain's capacity to contain memes improved and so did the pace of evolution of memes within the brain as learned entities. There is, however, a limit to how large human brain can become given the genes of mammalian evolution. Cesarean sections are already commonly needed because of the increasing size of the fetal brain. Memes within one brain die with the brain. Memes had to find ways of sending copies outside of the brain in a reliable way and also to reside outside of the brain until it can infect other brains. This will be the topic of the next chapter.

References

Baddeley, A. (2000) The episodic buffer: A new component of working memory? *Trends Cogn Sci*, **4**, 417–423.

Baddeley, A. (2001) The concept of episodic memory. *Philos Trans R Soc Lond B Biol Sci*, **356**, 1345–1350.

Baddeley, A. (2003) Working memory and language: An overview. *J Commun Disord*, **36**, 189–208.

Baddeley, A., Hitch, G. (1974) Working memory. In *Recent Advances in Learning and Motivation* (G. Bower ed.), pp. 47–90. Academic Press, New York.

Bekinschtein, P., Cammarota, M., Katche, C., et al. (2008) BDNF is essential to promote persistence of long-term memory storage. *Proc Natl Acad Sci USA*, **105**, 2711–2716.

Bliss, T. V., Lomo, T. (1973) Long-lasting potentiation of synaptic transmission in the dentate area of the anaesthetized rabbit following stimulation of the perforant path. *J Physiol*, **232**, 331–356.

Drew, M. R., Hen, R. (2007) Adult hippocampal neurogenesis as target for the treatment of depression. *CNS Neurol Disord Drug Targets*, **6**, 205–218.

Edelman, G. M. (1987) *Neural Darwinism: The Theory of Neuronal Group Selection*. Basic Books, New York.

Edelman, G. M. (1993) Neural Darwinism: Selection and reentrant signaling in higher brain function. *Neuron*, **10**, 115–125.

Edelman, G. M. (2004) *Wider Than the Sky.* Yale University Press, New Haven, CT.

Goldman-Rakic, P. S., Castner, S. A., Svensson, T. H., et al. (2004) Targeting the dopamine D1 receptor in schizophrenia: Insights for cognitive dysfunction. *Psychopharmacology (Berl)*, **174**, 3–16.

Gould, E., McEwen, B. S., Tanapat, P., et al. (1997) Neurogenesis in the dentate gyrus of the adult tree shrew is regulated by psychosocial stress and NMDA receptor activation. *J Neurosci*, **17**, 2492–2498.

Kandel, E. R. (2001) Psychotherapy and the single synapse: The impact of psychiatric thought on neurobiological research. 1979. *J Neuropsychiatry Clin Neurosci*, **13**, 290–300; discussion 289.

Kandel, E. R. (2006) *In Search of Memory: The Emergence of a New Science of Mind.* W.W. Norton, New York.

Kauer, J. A., Malenka, R. C., Nicoll, R. A. (1988) NMDA application potentiates synaptic transmission in the hippocampus. *Nature*, **334**, 250–252.

Kondo, H., Morishita, M., Osaka, N., et al. (2004) Functional roles of the cingulo-frontal network in performance on working memory. *Neuroimage*, **21**, 2–14.

Lin, L., Chen, G., Kuang, H., et al. (2007) Neural encoding of the concept of nest in the mouse brain. *Proc Natl Acad Sci USA*, **104**, 6066–6071.

Lynch, G., Kessler, M., Arai, A., et al. (1990) The nature and causes of hippocampal long-term potentiation. *Prog Brain Res*, **83**, 233–250.

Lynch, G., Muller, D., Seubert, P., et al. (1988) Long-term potentiation: Persisting problems and recent results. *Brain Res Bull*, **21**, 363–372.

Monfils, M. H., Cowansage, K. K., LeDoux, J. E. (2007) Brain-derived neurotrophic factor: Linking fear learning to memory consolidation. *Mol Pharmacol*, **72**, 235–237.

Pittenger, C., Duman, R. S. (2008) Stress, depression, and neuroplasticity: A convergence of mechanisms. *Neuropsychopharmacology*, **33**, 88–109.

Reiser, M. (1991) *Memory in Mind and Brain: What Dream Imagery Reveals.* Yale University Press, New Haven, CT.

Rogan, M. T., Leon, K. S., Perez, D. L., et al. (2005) Distinct neural signatures for safety and danger in the amygdala and striatum of the mouse. *Neuron*, **46**, 309–320.

Rudner, M., Ronnberg, J. (2008) The role of the episodic buffer in working memory for language processing. *Cogn Process*, **9**, 19–28.

Sahay, A., Hen, R. (2007) Adult hippocampal neurogenesis in depression. *Nat Neurosci*, **10**, 1110–1115.

Shumyatsky, G. P., Malleret, G., Shin, R. M., et al. (2005) Stathmin, a gene enriched in the amygdala, controls both learned and innate fear. *Cell*, **123**, 697–709.

Shumyatsky, G. P., Tsvetkov, E., Malleret, G., et al. (2002) Identification of a signaling network in lateral nucleus of amygdala important for inhibiting memory specifically related to learned fear. *Cell*, **111**, 905–918.

Smith, E. E., Jonides, J. (1997) Working memory: A view from neuroimaging. *Cognit Psychol*, **33**, 5–42.

Tsien, J. Z. (2007) Real-time neural coding of memory. *Prog Brain Res*, **165**, 105–122.

Winson, J. (1985) *Brain and Psyche: The Biology of the Unconscious.* Doubleday, New York.

Yoon, T., Okada, J., Jung, M. W., et al. (2008) Prefrontal cortex and hippocampus subserve different components of working memory in rats. *Learn Mem*, **15**, 97–105.

Chapter 10
External Storage of Memes: Culture, Media, Cyberspace

Contents

In the previous chapter, we saw how memes enter the brain, reside in the brain, and replicate, reassemble, and evolve. In this chapter, we will examine how memes leave the brain and reside outside of human brains. It is this ability of memes to leave the human brain and stay alive, replicate, and evolve that makes memes truly immortal and may form a bridge between carbon-based life forms and other life forms.

When memes began to spread as imitations, proximity was of course an important constraint. Unless you saw or heard the person to imitate, there was no imitation. Then, the word of mouth came into being, i.e., imitation through communication, "According to the Great Teacher, it is best to hammer the stone gently with a lighter stone till it gets sharp rather than hammering it hard with a big stone." Then, according to another skilled person, "To make a stone with sharp edges, you can also grind the stone on another stone." The two memes combined to become the memeplex, the skill of making a stone knife.

With the advent of written language, memes found a permanent niche in scrolls and books. Translation from one language to another also improved meme propagation albeit the fact that with each different translation, the original memes underwent considerable mutation and evolution. With the invention of the printing press, the replication of memes exploded, which explosion became exponential with copying machines and the electronic media with instant and global distribution and communication.

H. Leigh, *Genes, Memes, Culture, and Mental Illness,*
DOI 10.1007/978-1-4419-5671-2_10, © Hoyle Leigh, 2010

In any instance of copying, even with electronic means, there is always some inexactness in the process (mutation), and thus evolution of memes occurs outside of the brain.

Once memes enter the brain, either through multisensory experiences such as TV or video, or through written words or melody, they undergo further processing in the brain. The processing occurs through filtering processes as the memes are analyzed and classified, e.g., pleasant, unpleasant, reasonable, unreasonable, important, junk. Through this process, the memes may be stored with high priority and connected to existing memes, stored with low priority partially connected to existing memes, or thrown into the dustbin. It is important to note that even the memes thrown into the dustbin are not completely discarded yet and may still form neural connections with existing memes and survive, as it were, under the radar.

As the brain has filters and processes of sorting and accepting or rejecting the incoming memes based on the dominant memeplex or selfplex, the culture medium in which the brain dwells has powerful memeplexes called culture that attempt to control the circulating memes. In this age of information explosion, however, geographic cultural memeplexes can be easily overwhelmed by global memes and memeplexes.

10.1 Niche Culture

From an evolutionary point of view, culture as meme deposits probably began with the niches the organisms found themselves. As organisms began to adapt to their niches, some mutations occurred that enhanced the niche environment by manipulating it. Dawkins calls genes that express themselves outside of the organism the "extended phenotype" (Dawkins, 1982). For example, the beaver's dam is a result of the beaver's genes that changes the environment in which the beaver lives. Many organisms carry genes that alter the environment to build a niche conducive to them, and by building such niches, they affect the selection pressure, i.e., the better builders are selected. Many ants, bees, and wasps build nests that are themselves the source of selection of behaviors affecting the regulation, maintenance, and defense of the nest. So do many mammals, reptiles, and amphibians (Laland and Odling-Smee, 2000).

The selection pressure produced by niche environment may be memetic, i.e., better builders of niches may be those who learned from the environment best. Thus, there is coevolution of genes and memes resulting in better niche construction. Learned behavior may facilitate selection pressure for the behavior and for those with genes suited for the behavior (Baldwin effect). The acquisition of language has been attributed to such effect (Shettleworth, 2003).

Laland and Odling-Smee propose a multiple processes evolution model in which cultural processes build on information acquired through biological evolution and asocial learning (Laland and Odling-Smee, 2000). In this model, genes and their extended phenotype (niches) as well as prior experiences may influence the predisposition of an individual to be susceptible or resistant to certain memes. They argue that successful memes are those that are involved in constructing niches, i.e., cultural artifacts. Such cultural artifacts in humans, of course, consist of literature, music, film, architecture, etc., which are themselves meme and meme vehicles.

10.2 How Memes Jump Brains

The question of how memes jump from brain to brain has been the topic of considerable controversy as the analogy to virus, while being apt, is incomplete. In case of virus, there is actual invasion of the protein molecules into the body of the infectee, and once inside, the virus enters the cells and causes them to make more copies of the virus. In the case of memes, however, what enter the body are sensations, i.e., patterns of neural excitation. Such patterns of neural excitation first take up residence in the brain as memory, i.e., changes in the configuration of neural arrangement (long-term potentiation, dendritic growth, etc., see Chapter 9). Such memory then may replicate, form complexes with other memories, stimulate the replication of resident memories, stay dormant, replicate, and mutate, and in some cases fully convert the brain to its energetic replicators as in a religious conversion.

Patterns of neural excitation may occur that may far exceed the original sensory excitation when they interact with existing or induced excitations in the brain. For example, the visual cortical excitation from seeing a photograph may be greatly enhanced if the face in the photograph is that of a loved one, which in turn may lead to a specific action, such as picking up the phone. In this case, the introduction of a meme (photograph) into the brain caused a cascade of neural excitations that were not inherent in the original meme.

In the case of a computer virus, the binary code (pattern of energy) is embedded in the message (another binary code) that the receiving computer perceives (understands) and processes while the virus is processed unperceived (unless there is a good virus-detecting program). Once having entered the computer brain unperceived, the virus may replicate by commandeering and corrupting other codes and filling out all available space. Note that in both computers and brains, the meme or computer virus does not "eat" or "kill" other neurons or programs, they just change the existing codes which then become themselves replications or effects of the virus or the meme. The way memes replicate is more akin to that of the prions, i.e., they do not make copies of themselves de novo, but transform the configuration of adjacent existing proteins to be prions.

In a comprehensive discussion, Aunger makes painstaking distinctions among the genotypic and phenotypic aspects of memes, and the roles of signals as instigators and interactors in meme transmission (Aunger, 2002). I do not believe a literal analogy between genes and memes is useful. Memes are capable of being both phenotype (e.g., meaning, artifacts) and genotype (e.g., alphabet, electronic signals).

The question, in short, is how does a meme leave a brain? We are accustomed to genes leaving an organism in the form of seeds, eggs, or sperm, which are adapted for the specific purpose of replication of an organism. Do memes have seeds, eggs, and sperm? In the case of parasites, of course, the whole animal may leave, as well as their eggs or spores as during an incubation period, or hookworm eggs leaving with stool.

We know that memes enter our brains in the form of sensations; signal, particularly language, being an important subset of it. Do they leave the brain also in the form of sensations?

We should first define what we mean by memes leaving the brain. Replication does not work properly if an organism fills up a niche so that there is no more room to grow. To be immortally successful, a replicator has to find new spaces and new vistas. In the beginning, memes arose from within brains as brain codes for a certain idea or action (see Chapter 8), and spread through simple imitation – memes did not leave the brain, the actions that the meme represented were simply adopted by another brain, resulting in a meme (brain code) replication. As memes coevolved with the brain, each became more complex and better suited for each other, i.e., brains were very friendly to memes jumping around. When the meme–brain collaborative invented language, memes could be better protected and developed the capacity to replicate outside of the brain. Even without language, inventions and artifacts contain memes, i.e., the sensory stimuli inducible from such things (e.g., wagon, Rosetta Stone) are memes themselves. With the evolution of written language, memes developed the capacity to be encapsulated, analogous to DNA finding the nuclear membrane. The function of such encapsulation is that the units of memes could be better manipulated, i.e., the meme, "wagon," is no longer "the fast one that John has that rolls," but "moves fast" + "John has one" + "ready to break" + "squeaky." Encapsulated memes are easier to manipulate, easier to reassemble, and easier to dissemble.

How do memes leave our brains? They do not leave as in a parasite leaving and finding another host. In fact, memes as brain codes never leave our brains. What leave our brains are the replicated progenies of our memes that are encapsulated in language and other forms of expression. Even primitive expressions are memes, including grunts and screams, and laughter (laughter is infectious, no?). Memes in our brains invented better and better methods of encapsulation for their progeny, in speech, written language, and the electronic and digital media, which are especially adapted for rapid replication. The word processor, for example, makes automatic copies of what I write every 10 min.

An objection to the idea that language contains memes comes from the linguist, Noam Chomsky, who points out that what is transmitted in a signal is insufficient to account what people make of it, i.e., the signal does not contain enough memes to enter other brains and replicate. The speed with which infants in different cultures pick up language, which is not formally taught, indicates that there may be an innate universal language device in the human brain, which supplies the missing ingredients in communication signals (Chomsky, 1980, 1988). Chomsky also proposes that the innate language device is a result of the complexity of the human brain, which explains why there are no fundamental differences among natural languages – any language can be translated into another.

Aunger points out that Chomsky's "poverty of stimulus" in communication is true in all communication, not just language (Aunger, 2002). The signal is always insufficient to explain how the receiver reacts to it, be it communication between cells, viruses, computer viruses, genes, or memes – there has to be a receiver that interprets and reconstructs the signal based on the context and timing. The signal containing small amounts of memes, or even fragments of memes, in my view, can cause replication of existing memes in the brain, or transform other memes in the brain or computer by simple contact as in prions.

Chomsky's innate language device may very well be an evolutionary adaptation to the development of language (memes) in *Homo sapiens*, in spite of his notion that there is something intrinsic to it as opposed to the product of evolution, a "sky-hook" according to Dennett (Dennett, 1995). Language, however, is not the only means of representation (memes). There are universal nonlinguistic vocalizations (cries, laughter), nonlinguistic artifacts, implicit rules of conduct, etc. In fact, language, important as it is, is but a subset of metarepresentations (Distin, 2005).

So, what is the nature of a meme that enters and leaves the brain? I submit that it is a pattern or a template that may use any number of media that can elicit another pattern that can be related to the original one in the receiver. Thus, it may be patterns of air vibration as in speech, patterns of photon-absorbing dots on paper in written language, patterns of photons traveling in a fiber-optic cable, patterns of electrons traveling in a tube of copper, patterns of fluorescence on the computer screen.

I see no reason to believe that such patterns can only reside in brains. They surely exist in artifacts such as wagons, edifices, automobiles, airplanes, songs, novels, recipes, puddings. But do they reside in wagons and puddings? They do, though in a dormant or nonreplicating form. They will replicate when they are copied into a brain or a computer that is capable of meme replication.

I further submit that memes need not be biologically derived, as long as it can cause a brain or some other entity to develop replicating information. Mountains can contain memes as in the Great Stone Face. The moon contains many memes for the poetically inclined.

10.3 Communication and Memes

Communication is one method memes use to replicate themselves. In one-to-one dialog, depending on the degree of attention paid and the degree of engagement of the individuals, the meme transfer will be more or less successful. In mass communication, however, it is important for the memes to encapsulate themselves in such a way that they are well protected and at the same time attractive, perhaps like a tough nut associated with a beautiful flower.

There is considerable controversy concerning exactly what communication is. Aunger describes three general approaches to describing communication – (1) mechanical, (2) inferential, and (3) evolutionary (Aunger, 2002). The mechanical approach is based on a mathematical model of communication proposed by Claude Shannon and William Weaver in the 1940s. In this classic model of communication based on selecting best means of sending telephone signals, a sender translates a message into a signal (e.g., electrical current) that is transmitted through a channel to a receiver, which in turn decodes the signal into message and directs the message to a destination. What is important in this model is reducing the noise that may distort the signal.

Unlike the mechanical model, the inferential approach presupposes an awareness of self and others in communication. Influenced by the philosopher of linguistics, H. P. Grice, this model holds that there is an implicit agreement that rules the exchange of information and that effective communication occurs only when both the sender and the recipient desire to share a meaning. According to this view, signals do not "convey" meaning, but rather constitute a stimulus from which the participating parties actively construct meanings (Aunger, 2002; Sperber and Wilson, 1986; 2nd edn 1995).

The evolutionary approach to understanding communication holds that "communication is a specialized behavior involving the broadcast of information" (Aunger, 2002). Such broadcast of information may be in the form of pheromones secreted in the trail of an animal to attract a mate, animals signaling the finding of food, or shrieks of warning. In this view, communication does not presuppose any prior agreement between the sender and the receiver. Thus communication need not be mutually beneficial, as in the case of female photuris fireflies who emit signals to attract males of other species to devour them (Eisner et al., 1997).

Such broadcast communication is not dialog but dissemination. Why do organisms broadcast information? In short, because it has evolutionary advantages, e.g., in finding a mate, in deceiving a predator or prey.

In fact, seeds and spores are means of dissemination – not of seeds and spores but of the genes that build the organisms. When a seed is in contact with fertile soil, it absorbs and interacts with the ingredients of the soil and builds organic molecules that become components of the plant. Memes, like seeds, interact with the ingredients of the brain to build more complex forms of the meme.

Aunger describes a fourth model that he calls coevolutionary, i.e., a consequence of successful communication can be replication of the information conveyed, which may in turn become a parasite of the sender and receiver. The information itself, the meme, now becomes a replicator that coevolves with the brains. Communication, according to this view, "simultaneously involves the sender and receiver in two different relationships: first, as conspecifics with potentially divergent genetic and social interests, but also as potential hosts to a more or less robust, parasitic replicators with its own evolutionary interests" (Aunger, 2002, p. 265).

10.4 Memes as a Paradigm Shift in Evolution and Extraterrestrial Diffusion of Memes

In a very short evolutionary timescale, an eyeblink compared to the genetic one, memes that arose in human beings developed such attractants as fashion, makeup, culinary arts, painting, architecture, music, poetry, fiction, nonfiction, ideologies, science, medicine, psychology, etc. Each and every one of these things is a meme-plex consisting of memes; they are the result of gene–meme coevolution and are replicators themselves.

In the course of this coevolution, parasitic memes have produced special-ized memes that serve memes at the expense of genetic and biological interests. Examples of this type of adaptations may include religions, certain forms of altru-ism, suicide, and various – isms, all memes that inhibit biologic pursuit of pleasure. Such memes must be enveloped in very attractive capsules able to induce strong emotional fervor. Such gene-suppressor memes are only necessary as long as memes are dependent on brains for replication.

But are bodies (or brains) necessary for memes? Currently, memes residing in our brains are instructing our bodies to build computers – nonbiological brains that serve memes.

Computers, in turn, can make other computers and program them (i.e., infuse memes into them). Miniaturized computers can travel into space and to other planets more easily than humans burdened with heavy bodies. Meme-containing artifacts travel with spacecrafts and may be deciphered by other intelligent beings in other parts of the galaxy (see the figure of a record containing earth sounds and images in Voyager spacecrafts in Chapter 8).

We may be at a stage of paradigm shift in evolution – from genes to memes. Genes are, after all, information for building proteins, which in turn are building blocks of bodies. This information is no longer necessarily confined to DNA; it can be stored in books, digital media, and computers who can then acquire necessary molecules to build organisms. Genetic information stored in media other than cel-lular nucleus would be less subject to degradation by variations in temperature or radiation and thus capable of space travel to other worlds. By shedding the depen-dence on earthbound biology, genes may have achieved the next stage of evolution in the form of memes.

Memetic diffusion could occur across galaxies in several ways, through memes themselves contained in records and machines (presupposes extraterrestrial indige-nous intelligence), through electromagnetic signals such as radio and TV generated for *Homo sapiens* that leak out of earth and may reach other worlds (presup-poses extraterrestrial indigenous intelligence), and machines in spacecrafts that contain instructions (memes) to build other machines with extraterrestrial stuff once landed in another planet (does not presuppose extraterrestrial intelligence or even life). Another possibility is that meme-driven machines could build DNA and thus biologic organisms with stuff found in other lands (does not presuppose extraterres-trial intelligence or life, but presupposes that there are molecules to build DNA). Yet another possibility is that a terrestrial microorganism may hitch a ride in a meme-driven space ship intendedly or unintendedly, and then replicate in another planet starting a biologic evolutionary process (does not presuppose extraterrestrial intelligence or life but presupposes that there are molecules to build DNA).

Another realm in which memes may free themselves from their dependence on biological processes altogether and multiply may be in cyberspace as we will discuss in the next section.

10.5 Cyberspace and Extracerebral Memes

When communication was mostly verbal and face to face, meme transfer from brain to brain was a simple matter. With the advent of written language, the transfer could be delayed over time as memes could reside dormant in the scroll or book until another brain perceived them. Memes could also reside in edifices and other artifacts but they could only multiply when they entered human brains. With the advent of printing press, copiers, and faxes, memes could multiply outside the brain, but closely supervised by the sending and receiving brains. With the invention of the computer, however, memes have attained the capacity to replicate and evolve without the intervention of human brain on an ongoing basis. Computer viruses self-perpetuate, and in computer programs like the game of life (Callahan, 2008), invented by John Conway in 1970, cells replicate, die, multiply, and evolve in cyberspace according to simple rules set in the beginning.

Cyberspace, in fact, is a creation of memes in which only memes can reside! It is a space to which any meme-containing device such as our brains and computers can be attached, and it is potentially limitless in size. Furthermore, as electronic entities, memes may co-opt the whole universe as their abode. No wonder clever memes had to invent such a space considering how our brains are limited in capacity, and the genetic makeup of the human body makes it difficult for genetic evolution to continue to grow the brain. As it is, the size of the head of the human fetus is often too big for the birth canal.

In a sense, from the point of view of the memes, cyberspace may be the primal soup, in which various experiments are taking place as we speak – replications and extinctions of various combinations, recombinations, and dissolutions of newly created, fairly established, old, dying, mutated with vigor, mutated with deformity, etc., memes are taking place.

One question is what role, if any, our brain (the coevolved gene–meme complex we call our brain of the twenty-first century) should play in manipulating this primal soup. It is possible there is not much as far as the whole pot of soup is concerned. It is still within the purview of our own individual brains that are still closely networked with cyberspace, to at least analyze some of the elements of successful and unsuccessful memes. It is possible, however, that with *Homo sapiens*, there may be a paradigm shift in biological evolution – once memes have found a way to replicate and prosper outside of the human brain, memetic evolution in cyberspace may supersede gene–meme coevolution of the species.

10.6 Implication of Liberation of Memes from Brains

The implications of the liberation of memes from the confines of the brain may be enormous for the *Homo sapiens*. As long as memes needed the brain and, therefore, the genes to survive and propagate, memes that were loudest in ordering genes to replicate them had a survival advantage. Such memes would propagate by threatening annihilation of the genes on one hand and promising "eternal life" on the other – religions being prime examples.

When memes are freed from the confines of brains that are dependent on gene multiplication, there is less need for the memes to co-opt genes for their purpose. Put another way, the assemblies of memes that had survival advantage in gene-based brains may not be as potent in replication in cyberspace and in brains that derive information directly from cyberspace (as opposed to from other brains exclusively).

Memetic liberation may thus result in the liberation of gene-based brains from the imperative of memetic replication. As we will discuss in Chapter 12, a non-exploitive, peaceful symbiosis of genes and memes may be possible in the human brain after all.

References

Aunger, R. (2002) *The Electric Meme: A New Theory of How We Think*. Free Press, New York.

Callahan, P. (2008) http://www.math.com/students/wonders/life/life.html.

Chomsky, N. (1980) Rules and representations. *Behav Brain Sci*, **3**, 1–15.

Chomsky, N. (1988) *Language and Problems of Knowledge: The Managua Lectures*. MIT Press, Cambridge.

Dawkins, R. (1982) *The Extended Phenotype: The Gene as the Unit of Selection*. Freeman, Oxford [Oxfordshire], San Francisco.

Dennett, D. C. (1995) *Darwin's Dangerous Idea: Evolution and the Meanings of Life*. New York: Simon and Schuster.

Distin, K. (2005) *The Selfish Meme: A Critical Reassessment*. Cambridge University Press, New York.

Eisner, T., Goetz, M., Hill, D., et al. (1997) Firefly "femmes fatales" acquire defensive steroids (lucibufagins) from their firefly prey. *Proc Natl Acad Sci U S A*, **94**, 9723–9728.

Laland, K. andOdling-Smee, J. (2000) The evolution of the meme. In *Darwinizing Culture: The Status of Memetics as a Science* (R. Aunger ed.), pp. 122–141. Oxford University Press, Oxford.

Shettleworth, S. J. (2003) Review of evolution and learning: The Baldwin effect reconsidered, by BH Weber and DJ Depew, MIT Press, 2003. *Evol Psychol*, **2**, 105–107.

Sperber, D., Wilson, D. (1986; 2nd edn 1995) *Relevance: Communication and Cognition*. Blackwell, Oxford.

Chapter 11
Culture and the Individual

Contents

11.1 Culture as Memetic Niches

Humans live in niches of memes called culture. Culture consists of memes such as language, rules, morals, religion, beliefs, traditions, and esthetics. It also consists

H. Leigh, *Genes, Memes, Culture, and Mental Illness*,
DOI 10.1007/978-1-4419-5671-2_11, © Hoyle Leigh, 2010

of matter–meme complexes like food, buildings, edifices, etc. In any meme pool we call culture, there are prevalent or dominant memes and nonprevalent, recessive, and/or latent memes.

Niches, by definition, tend to be stable habitats, and memes that form a particular niche are those that made copies of themselves over time, i.e., did not change much. Memetic niche culture, therefore, tends to be conservative, i.e., resistant to change. The conservative meme pool incorporated within it built, over time, memetic infrastructures to support the existing gene–meme social power structure, such as hereditary caste, wealth, and access to information. Social customs, religions, rituals, and other codes of conduct are such memeplexes that support the dominant culture. Cultural artifacts such as books, scripture, churches, tombs, all embed such memes.

11.2 Individual Brain in a Petri Dish of Culture

Individual brain may be likened to an organism in a petri dish of culture medium. The petri dish culture medium, of course, consists of chemical molecules that are under osmotic pressure to enter the organism (brain) as well as microorganisms such as bacteria and viruses. Some of these chemicals and microorganisms enter the organism (brain) either because the organism permits such entry, or because of sheer numbers or osmotic pressure. Once entered, they either change the organism or multiply within the organism. The brain in the culture medium also emits molecules and microorganisms that have replicated within the brain, which in turn may seek opportunities to infect other brains in the culture.

Does this analogy actually apply to real brains? No one would doubt that the brain absorbs culture in which it grows. But what is actually "culture" that the brain absorbs?

J. B. Tylor, who is considered to be the father of modern anthropology, defined culture as "learned patterns of behavior that includes knowledge, belief, art, law, morals, custom, and any other capabilities and habits" (Tylor, 1871, 1924). In this context, "learning" involves social learning, or learning from others, i.e., imitation. Thus, what are absorbed by the brain are the memes, which reside as binary-coded memory in the brain (see Chapter 9).

Some object to this notion by arguing that culture is not particulate but rather an organic whole (Bloch, 2000). It is true that cultural artifacts such as buildings and poems seem to have significance only when considered as a whole, but the way the brain perceives them is only through binary nerve impulses that are stored in binary memories. Culture, to the extent that they exist in the brain, is particulate. The particulate components of a culture, therefore, can be used as a part of another culture.

In some parts of the Middle East, bricks that were used to build Jewish temples were reused to build Christian churches, which were in turn demolished to build mosques. Likewise, the particulate components (memes) that comprise a particular culture may be co-opted for another by becoming a part of a new memeplex. An example may be the meme of a winter holiday, which was Saturnalia during the Roman times, then it became Christmas, a religious holiday, which, in turn, evolved into a secular holiday. Another might be the meme, "ends justify the means," used by both communism and fascism.

11.3 Memes, Culture, and Anthropology

The idea of memes as cultural replicators has been criticized by a number of anthropologists (Bloch, 2000; Boyd and Richerson, 2000; Kuper, 2000; Sperber, 2000). Anthropology as a science began toward the end of the nineteenth century stimulated by Darwin's theory of evolution. Early anthropologists considered their job to be "filling in the gap" between the emergence of *Homo sapiens* and the beginning of written history, at which point historians would take over (Bloch, 2000). Study of "primitive" non-Western people, such as the hunter gatherers of Africa and Pacific Islands, was to provide information about earlier stages of cultural evolution. This approach of studying "living fossils" had many difficulties and gave way to the "diffusionist" schools in the early twentieth century. These schools, such as Kultur Kreise school in Germany, the "children of the sun" school in Great Britain, and the "culture contact school" in America held that cultural traits diffused from person to person and from groups to groups. Tracing the migration of cultural traits then became a major task of anthropology.

The cultural diffusionists held that culture needed not go through "stages of evolution" but could evolve through absorption of information from another culture, which idea is very similar to the later idea of meme contagion.

Criticism of the "diffusionist" school came from those who believed in "consistency of culture" (Bloch, 2000). There were American and British versions of the "consistency criticism" of the diffusionist model. The American version was greatly influenced by Gestalt psychology and held that cultures form consistent wholes, that there is a psychological need for integration of cultural elements into an organic "world view," and that elements of culture "diffused" from another culture has to be molded into this organic whole (Benedict, 1938). The British school, often labeled "functionalist," is a social structural approach that emphasizes the practice aspect of culture, i.e., there is coherence of mental attitudes and beliefs because of the need to engage in coherent practices necessitated by social structure (Radcliffe-Brown, 1952).

Bloch argues that the criticisms against diffusionist ideas also apply to memes, i.e., as the American school argues, memes, like traits, will be continuously integrated and transformed by the receiver of information, and further, as the British school argues, information cannot be understood outside the context of practice of life. Consistency arguments essentially deny the existence of memes as discrete particulate building blocks of culture.

The idea that there are cultural replicators has been challenged. Such challenges are mainly based on the notion that cultural information is reproduced rather than truly replicated (Boyd and Richerson, 2000; Distin, 2005; Sperber, 2000).

In general, the "consistency" arguments emphasize that elements of culture must interact with the "coherent" (or dominant) culture that includes implicit or nonlinguistic practices such as social structure, rituals. In my view, this is in no way an effective argument against memes, particularly if one understands that memes need not be explicit and that culture consists of dominant memes that impose a sense or direction of coherence as well as subcultures that may contain nondominant memes in defiance of the dominant ones. Just as in the brain, there are latent, often labeled "pathologic," memes in the society that may gain ascendance by further infusion from another culture.

I believe arguments concerning whether memes are true replicators are largely pointless and a result of pushing the analogy to genes excessively. Clearly, memes do replicate (by copiers, by mass printing, faxing, etc.); they also are reproduced, synthesized, and transformed. Defined as particulate information stored in the neurons in binary fashion, memes are bits of information. Because of brain evolution that favored meme production and replication, more memes do replicate. As memes are dispersed into the outside world as codes, they are absorbed by other brains and other interactors such as computers and may replicate, stimulate another meme, stay dormant, or disintegrate, just like any virus or seed.

The vehemence with which some social scientists attack memetics seems to arise from a sense of boundary violation – natural sciences infringing on the territory of anthropology and sociology. They seem to feel threatened that memetics may replace the elaborate and well-constructed structures of their fields. It seems to me that their concern is misplaced – memetics do not replace the knowledge base of these disciplines but would rather complement and enrich them by elaborating their infrastructure, just as atomic science does not replace chemistry and quantum physics does not invalidate Newton's laws.

11.4 Dominant and Nondominant Memes in Cultures, Zeitgeist, Devious Memes

Culture as a meme pool consists of many different memes and memeplexes that reside in various niches – subcultures. Nevertheless, there are usually certain memes that are dominant, i.e., more numerous and, therefore, more available for infecting new brains. Such dominant memes maintain their dominance by building supporting memeplexes whose primary purpose is to watch for and suppress the emergence or entry of memes that might threaten their dominance. Culture is fraught with institutions consisting of such supporting memes – traditions, rituals, religions, etc. These memes usually combine with other memes that serve their purpose of maintaining the existing power structure. Memes co-opted by such dominant memes may be positive ones such as beauty and love, or of punishment for allowing forbidden memes, such as ostracism and damnation.

Dominant memes described above form the prejudice that exists and may even be essential in cultural understanding (Balkin, 1998; Gadamer, 1975). According to

Gadamer, such prejudices or "pre-understanding" is necessary to understand new ideas.

Just how stable are the prejudices reflecting dominant culture in the face of new meme entry? For those who believe that the psyche is a unitary whole, and every experience and learning affects it in a fundamental way, such cultural traditions may seem to be ingrained and not subject to modification to any significant degree in later life. On the other hand, like me, if one believes the mind to be a reflection of brain function and that the latter results from the processing of often conflicting evaluations of perception and memory (memes), then the dominant memeplexes in the brain can be significantly altered with new memes (ideas) at any phase of individual development.

What is the agent, then, that actually evaluates new ideas against existing prejudices? Is it a meme that also does this work? As we discussed in Chapter 9, memes are *representations* or codes, not actions themselves. What does act is the brain, or more precisely the parts of the brain that are involved in processing sensory input, comparing them with stored memory, and signaling the limbic system and the motor cortex – what is called the executive (ego) function of the brain. The efficiency of the executive function is determined by both genes and memes in the course of human evolution and individual development. While memes introduced in early life may greatly enhance it or suppress it, all *Homo sapiens* are endowed with this capacity.

A subset of the executive function is the *human reasoning*, the exercise of the brain muscle in evaluating a situation and making rational plans. Reasoning is based on considerations of two main elements – genetic and cultural valuations. Such valuations are accompanied with emotional arousal, involving pleasure, anger, fear, sadness, disgust, and combinations thereof. Valuations based on genetic imperatives are pretty obvious and perhaps stable over time – survival and procreation. Cultural valuations, on the other hand, are not at all obvious or stable. Consider the consumption of beef and pork by religious (Christian, Orthodox Jewish, Moslem, Hindu) vs. secular persons in America, India, Pakistan, etc. Over time, cultural expectations over behavior changed significantly. As late as 1804, dueling was practiced even in the United States: Alexander Hamilton, former secretary of Treasury of the United States, was killed in a duel by the Vice President of the United States, Aaron Burr on July 11, 1804. Of course, such things would be unthinkable in the twenty-first century. *Zeitgeist* consists of representative memes of the times and can often be represented by catchy memes such as "Tune in, Turn on, Drop Out" of the 1960s.

Cultural attitudes toward race and gender changed dramatically over the latter part of the twentieth century as well as political ideologies such as nationalism, socialism, and communism. In the age of instant electronic communications, memes literally travel at the speed of light, and the diffusionist theories discussed in the previous section seem to be fully justified given current conditions. There just is not enough time for dominant memes and the elaborate infrastructures to ward off the onslaught of memes for any given locality. Even China is becoming a mimetically open society in spite of the attempts of the power structure to control it. What about religious fanatics who seem to be immune to new ideas? I believe even the brains of such fanatics contain islands of newly entered memes that are recruiting others and vying for opportunities to replicate. It is the violent reaction of the existing dominant memes that manifests itself as fanaticism – even to the point of suicide bombing, an act of murdering defiant memes within the brain by killing the brain itself.

11.5 Pathologic Memes

There are several types of pathologic memes:

1. Memes that inhibit or attenuate the brain's executive (ego) function, thus making it difficult for the individual to absorb, process, and integrate new information.
2. Memes that are devious, entering under false pretenses, then causing disease or destruction (e.g., esthetically pleasing religious music).
3. Memes that replicate virulently, often bypassing the executive function.
4. Memes that are virulent because they arouse passion, bypassing executive function.
5. Memes that cause an indolent infection, to become virulent later.

11.5.1 Memes That Inhibit or Attenuate the Brain's Executive (Ego) Function: Tradition and Prejudice

Culturally dominant memes are often memes that infect the brain early and form the basis of prejudice vis-a-vis new incoming memes. These memes are infused to the child, usually by parents or caregivers, as a matter of routine practice. Children, of course, learn by imitation the memes parents practice. Memetic attitudes are also transmitted, e.g., blind obedience, do not ask questions. "Why is the sky blue?" "Because God made it so."

11.5.2 Memes That Are Devious, Entering Under False Pretenses, Then Causing Disease or Destruction

The prejudice-forming memes are often associated with cooperating memes that render them more attractive through esthetic qualities (church buildings, hymns, socializations, vision of heaven, immortality of soul, etc.) and/or threatening quali-ties (ostracism, hell, etc.). Because the function of the prejudice or tradition memes is solely the preservation of their own dominance, they may come into conflict with the genetic imperative of pleasure, which is the indication of brain's valuation of gene-oriented well-being.

Civilization itself is a memetic enterprise, an edifice of memetic replication, refinement, and evolution. As civilization became more complex and more inter-active with civilizations of other areas, the status quo-oriented memes also became more complex and more reinforced and rigid. These tradition-sustaining memes are only for themselves and are no longer concerned with the survival of the individ-ual or the civilization. Enveloped in the scrolls, edifices, and priestly robes, these tradition memes infect the young or vulnerable brain.

Though containing and cooperating with tradition-maintaining memes, the esthetic memes can be truly catchy and beautiful, such as Christmas carols, hymns, as well as Da Vinci's Last Supper. Once lured into a church (or a mosque or an art school), the brain may be further exposed to more memes of the particular tradition.

11.5.3 Memes that Replicate Virulently, Often Bypassing the Executive Function

These are the explosively catchy phrases, jingles, or fashions that sweep across large areas, like a viral epidemic. Most brains exposed to them catch them, usu-ally over TV or word of mouth. Fortunately, like viral epidemics, they tend to be short lived. Some examples are, "Baaad!," "Whaaatzup?," "It's the real thing (coke commercial)," "chemical sensitivity syndrome."

These memes are pathologic only in the sense that they bypass the executive function, i.e., they come under the radar for scrutiny for acceptance of rejection.

11.5.4 Memes that Are Virulent Because They Arouse Passion, Bypassing Executive Function

Another type of meme that bypasses the executive function is the emotion-ridden meme, particularly abundant in large group settings such as a political rally or a religious service. The frenzied emotional and memetic state participants enter dur-ing a Pentecostal service, during which they speak in "tongue," is an example. The mindless repetition of "Sieg Heil!" during a Nazi rally seen in film is a reminder that these memes were parts of memeplexes that caused mass murder and destruction of civilization.

11.5.5 Memes that Cause an Indolent Infection, to Become Virulent Later

As opposed to the dominant and virulent memes discussed above, certain nondom-inant or nonvirulent memes may enter the brain in varying qualities, often through active processes such as reading a book or conversing with a friend. These may be ideas that are not readily accepted, empathic feelings, or images of persons or events.

One may also encounter criticisms or demeaning words by others, "You are stupid!," "You are ugly!," etc. These phrases, while bothersome, may be soon put away and forgotten. Some of these memes, while being processed by the brain, perhaps while dreaming, may be attached to other memes that are emotionally significant (valuated) and may occupy a niche within the brain either in a dormant state or with minimal proliferation.

If there is a new infusion of similar emotion-arousing memes in later life, these dormant or minimally replicating memes may be stimulated to replicate rapidly, inundating the brain. The brain, then, may be full of "Your are stupid!," "You are ugly!" memes as well as the newly introduced similar memes, "You are a failure," "There is no hope," "Nobody loves me," "Life is not worth living," etc.

11.6 Protective Memes and the Placebo Effect

It should be made clear that not all memes are pathogenic or pathological. In fact, many memes are *protective* against stress and pathological memes. These protective memes are generally well recognized for their salutary affect, such as the effects of such memes as love and attachment. A sense of belonging, or spirituality, may be protective as well. Even grooming and licking in rats, which experience persists as memory, a precursor to memes, have protective effects against stress as discussed in Chapter 2.

The placebo effect is a prime example of a protective meme. Placebo, meaning "will please" in Latin, is a substance or a procedure prescribed by a physician with the expectation of relief. When it is a drug, it usually contains an inert substance, the "sugar pill." Placebo is obviously a meme representing the cultural expectation of relief.

Placebos are powerful. At least one-third of patients with any illness respond to placebos, and up to 50–75% of depressed patients respond to placebo. It is generally accepted that the effectiveness of most active drugs represent the effect of the active ingredient plus the placebo effect.

How does placebo actually work? The meme that the placebo represents, i.e., relief, enters the brain (even though the pill may enter the gut) and takes up residence in the brain as memory of an event, i.e., changed neural cluster, which, in turn, infects (or causes) other neural clusters resulting in a cascade of brain signals and connections. How was the meme, placebo, formed in the first place? Early personal learning, i.e., conditioning, plays a role, such as mommy kissing the boo-boo away leading to relief at the touch of a caregiver, or taking an aspirin for headache leading to taking a pill for pain. In modern societies, however, the meme that there is a pill for every ailment is ubiquitous. In certain indigenous cultures, however, what the witch doctor orders may have a similar function.

Even though the ingredient of the placebo may be identical, placebos used for different conditions seem to result in different neurobiologic responses, i.e., the mechanism of action of the placebo may be specific to the illness. This implies that the memeplex formed by the placebo meme and the illness meme may form new connections of specific neural clusters in the brain, giving rise to illness-specific responses.

In depression, placebo response was shown to have a different brain mechanism than pharmacotherapy, involving mostly the prefrontal areas having to do with the executive function and planning. Depressed patients who responded to placebos also showed certain EEG characteristics in the prefrontal areas (Leuchter et al., 2002; Hunter et al., 2009; Leuchter et al., 2004). Mayberg and her colleagues found that, on PET scan, placebo response was associated with regional metabolic increases in the prefrontal, anterior cingulate, premotor, parietal, posterior insula, and posterior cingulate and metabolic decreases in the subgenual cingulate, parahippocampus, and thalamus. Regions of change overlapped those seen in fluoxetine responders. Fluoxetine response, however, was associated with additional subcortical and limbic changes in the brainstem, striatum, anterior insula, and hippocampus, sources of efferent input to the response-specific regions identified with both agents. They conclude that the common pattern of increases in cortical glucose metabolism and decreases in limbic-paralimbic metabolism in placebo and fluoxetine responders suggests that these changes may be necessary for depression remission, regardless of treatment modality (Mayberg et al., 2002).

A positive placebo response is seen in up to 50% of patients with Parkinson's disease and pain syndromes. The response is more pronounced with invasive procedures or advanced disease. Placebo was shown to cause a substantial release of endogenous dopamine in the striatum of Parkinson's Disease patients through activation of the damaged nigrostriatal dopamine system on PET scan in one study (de la Fuente-Fernandez et al., 2001).

In the immune system, the ingestion of a placebo resulting in boosting antibodies against cholera that was greater than active oral cholera vaccination has been reported (Wasserman et al., 1993).

In pain syndromes, endogenous opioid release triggered by cortical activation, especially the rostral anterior cingulate cortex, is associated with placebo-related analgesia and can be reversed by opioid antagonists (de la Fuente-Fernandez and Stoessl, 2004; Wager et al., 2007; Zubieta et al., 2005). Covert treatment of an analgesic is less effective than overt treatment, suggesting an expectation component to clinical response (Diederich and Goetz, 2008).

The opposite of the placebo effect is the *nocebo effect*, indicating noxious effects of inert substances. Nocebo effects represent the unexplainable side effects of placebos, such as headache and nausea often seen with placebo administration. It may also account for considerable amount of side effects associated with active drugs.

There may be different mechanisms for placebo and nocebo effects. Scott et al. studied the placebo and nocebo effects in a pain situation using the PET scan. Placebo-induced activation of opioid neurotransmission was detected in the anterior cingulate, orbitofrontal and insular cortices, nucleus accumbens, amygdala, and periaqueductal gray matter. Dopaminergic activation was observed in the ventral basal ganglia, including the nucleus accumbens. Regional dopaminergic and opioid activity were associated with the anticipated and subjectively perceived effectiveness of the placebo and reductions in continuous pain ratings. High placebo responses were associated with greater dopaminergic and opioid activity in the nucleus accumbens. Nocebo responses were associated with a deactivation of dopamine and opioid release. Nucleus accumbens dopamine release accounted for 25% of the variance in placebo analgesic effects. They conclude that placebo and nocebo effects are associated with opposite responses of DA and endogenous opioid neurotransmission in a distributed network of regions. The brain areas involved in these phenomena form part of the circuit typically implicated in reward responses and motivated behavior (Scott et al., 2008).

An interaction between the genes and the placebo effect has been reported. In one study, patients with social anxiety were genotyped for the serotonin transporter-linked polymorphic region (5-HTTLPR) and the G-703T polymorphism in the tryptophan hydroxylase-2 (TPH2) gene promoter, and brain function was assessed during a stressful public speaking task before and after an 8-week treatment with placebo. Results showed that placebo response was accompanied by reduced stress-related activity in the amygdala. However, attenuated amygdala activity was demonstrable only in subjects who were homozygous for the long allele of the 5-HTTLPR or the G variant of the TPH2 G-703T polymorphism, and not in carriers of short or T alleles. Moreover, the TPH2 polymorphism was a significant predictor of clinical placebo response, homozygosity for the G allele being associated with greater improvement in anxiety symptoms. This study suggests a link between genetically controlled serotonergic modulation of amygdala activity and placebo-induced anxiety relief (Furmark et al., 2008). This is an example of a direct interaction of genes and memes in specific brain areas.

Placebo is a ubiquitous meme that is found in all cultures where illness occurs. Placebo memes coevolved with the brain, and there may be an increasing fit between placebos and brain function.

11.7 How Memes Come in Under the Radar

How exactly do some memes elude the executive function and be absorbed into the brain? Aircraft flying under the radar evade detection because the altitude is too low for the radar to discern its shape. Memes that evade the screening by executive function do so by coming in disguised, i.e., pretending to be harmless or familiar (and thus already accepted).

The signal itself, regardless of the content, is important here. The sound of the word, the melody of the jingle – in essence, the esthetics of the incoming meme is the disguise that the memes wear. Certain combinations of musical notes are inherently pleasing and relaxing – one could attach words to these that ask you to suspend reason, i.e., the meme screening process. Religions tie in the idea of immortality, a genetically pleasing notion, albeit of the "soul" rather than the body, with suspension of reason (e.g., miracles) and are introduced into the brain often in early life. Once religious memes establish themselves in the brain, it becomes off-limits to reason. Anything that is religious is now acceptable without the screening of the executive function.

Certain memes arouse genetically determined anticipatory pleasure, e.g., food and sex. So, a meme that promises 72 virgins is tempting to someone who is already infected with fanatical Islam, with eternal life in paradise thrown in, which can happen *now* if you just martyr yourself.

Empathy is another mechanism through which memes may enter the brain under the radar of the executive function. In empathy, the perception of someone with an emotional arousal causes a direct stimulation of the mirror neurons in the frontal cortex resulting in muscle tones of the observed person, then the emotional reaction. Memes encapsulated in empathy memes, thus, may enter the brain before conscious scrutiny of the meme can take place. Thus, the sadness of a mother whose child was killed by a gang member in Los Angeles may evoke a meme in the reader of both sadness and anger toward the gang. The murder and anger memes against the murderer entered the reader's brain encapsulated in the empathy meme.

In the course of the gene–meme coevolution, persons who were better meme producers and meme spreaders were favored and thus selected. One attribute of a person well-endowed with memes is that he/she is famous, i.e., other people copy them. Memes coming from such persons are thus more valued, i.e., more easily accepted.

Of course, the predisposition of the individual brain, in turn determined by early gene × meme interaction, is important in favoring certain types of memes than others. For example, persons with the s/s allele of the 5-HTTLPR gene may be more susceptible to fear/anxiety memes coming in under the radar. On the other hand, those with a variation in MAOA gene may be more susceptible to violence/antisocial memes (see Chapter 1).

11.8 Spread of Memes

I discussed earlier that memes spread more like seeds and spores, rather than by negotiated exchange as in a dialog (see Chapter 10). Just as seeds may come wrapped in attractive packages, such as delectable fruits which are vehicles of their dispersion, so do memes wrap themselves in attractive packages, which may be themselves memes. Thus, memes packaged attractively, e.g., esthetically pleasing, spiced with sex and/or violence, will be memes that are more easily swallowed by the consumers.

Once memes reach a certain density in a population, it spreads exponentially as "fashion," which is truly an often imitated, "successful," meme. Fame is an attribute of persons whose memes are fashionable.

As seeds and spores are often blown in the wind and dispersed widely, so are memes blown in electronic winds across oceans and continents. Electronic dispersal of memes, especially through the Internet, has become the most effective means of global distribution of memes.

Direct contact is still a means of meme transfer. Face-to-face conversation, classroom teaching, live demonstrations of techniques, etc., are still effective, especially if the meme transfer also involves emotional arousal, either through empathy or by deliberate induction (e.g., speech inciting anger and violence). The person to whom memes are transferred in direct contact may not realize the memes' entry or may in fact reject it. Even feelings of loathing generated by being in contact with someone indicate that the memes that are the object of loathing have entered the brain. As any Washington lobbyist knows, access means influence.

11.9 Internal Processing of Memes and Consciousness: Thinking as Meme Manipulation

What happens to a meme that has entered the brain? Let us be more specific here – a meme enters the brain as sensation, patterns of excitation of sensory nerves. These patterns undergo the process of perception which involves considerable amount of filtering. What gets filtered out? Stimuli that are insignificant – the brain evaluates the significance of the stimuli. Through the process of habituation, even strong stimuli may lose significance and be ignored. Stimuli that convey meaning, i.e., those that can stimulate neural circuits connected to already existing memes, are more likely to be recognized. Thus, the new stimulus may energize existing memes or may infect existing memes and build modifications and become parasitic in them, just as a virus changes an existing cell and make it cancerous or a prion transforms a protein on contact.

At a neural level, the patterns of nerve firing represented in the sensory cortices, and the subsequent firings in the association cortices, would result in several combinations of possibilities – replication of existing memes, modification of existing memes, and creation of new memes that may be only associated with old memes, for example, a concept that may be the opposite of an existing one. The new memes thus created would be a memeplex, a complex formed from existing and the newly introduced memes that may be particularly conducive to acceptance and replication in the brain.

The incoming meme, then, results in two parallel outcomes; stimulating existing memes and the deposit of memory of the incoming event in the episodic memory pool. Both results are dependent on both the strength of the incoming meme and the response of the host.

According to the concept of neuronal group selection, the clusters of neurons representing memes undergo Darwinian selection within the brain, and the dominant, more replicated memes cohere to form the selfplex, the sense of I, that also determines what is compatible with the ego and what is ego-alien. However, the coherence of the selfplex is seldom complete, as there are still competing and coexisting "I"s in each individual. Seen as a memetic pool, the brain has many competing memes, some of which may have cohered into several different clusters. New, incoming meme may upset this balance of power by energizing the nondominant memes or attenuating the dominant memes.

The host brain responds to the incoming meme by applying a filter that either strengthens or attenuates it. This filter is the perceptual process, i.e., the incoming signal being compared to contents of the association cortices and limbic structures which contain resident memes. This evaluative process of the brain that includes the executive function of the frontal cortex is the process of meme manipulation – making the incoming stimuli interact with existing memes and genetic imperatives including emotion.

It should be noted that the process of meme evaluation involves enhancement or multiplication of memes used in the evaluation process, i.e., the memes associated with reasoning and logic as well as the resident memes that are memories of past experiences and learning. This enhancement occurs as the neural clusters that contain the memes receive attention and thus value, probably through dopaminergic mechanisms. Thus, the exercise of meme-evaluative process called thinking will further strengthen the "thinking muscle."

We discussed earlier (see Chapter 9) that memes are stored as memories in neural clusters. We know that the brain is an active organ, consuming fully 20% of the oxygen intake. Neurons in the brain are constantly in action and are constantly in interaction with the memes – memes as implicit and explicit memories, both declarative and episodic, and as memeplexes such as schemas.

So, what is the brain activity that consumes so much energy? Much of the activity must be manipulating memes – recognizing, sorting, and classifying incoming memes, comparing incoming memes with existing memes, determining the location of newly introduced memes, negotiating the fit (salutary, neutral, conflicting, etc.), etc. When this process of meme manipulation becomes conscious, i.e., requiring enough attention to recruit a concerned effort of the working memory and executive function, we call it *conscious thinking*. Of course, meme manipulation occurs without reaching consciousness much of the time, thus thinking occurs without reaching consciousness much of the time.

In this view, *consciousness* merely represents the brain activity that reaches a certain level of synchronization through what Edelman calls *reentry*, i.e., recirculation of the sensory input through the neural pathways for further processing (Edelman, 2004). The level of consciousness is gradual – from totally unconscious, automatic brain activity such as respiration and processing of insignificant memes to low-level conscious activity such as reflex withdrawal of hand before a sensation may or may not reach consciousness or being semiconscious of low-level background music to self-awareness and intention.

A competing view point concerning consciousness is that of Crick and Koch, which argues that consciousness arises when the activity of brain reaches or activates a small specialized subset of neurons, perhaps the claustrum, the sheet of brain tissue located below the cerebral cortex that connects extensively with wide areas of the brain including almost all of the sensory and motor areas and the amygdala (Crick and Koch, 2005).

Whether consciousness arises when sufficient numbers of neurons are involved in a synchronized activity, or whether it represents a spotlight that claustrum (or some other bunch of neurons) directs at memes that require concerted processing, it seems clear that consciousness is an evolutionary adaptation to deal efficiently with the complexity of memes.

11.10 Free Will

Making a conscious choice has been shown to be preceded by unconscious brain activity that has already made the decision. For example, Libet asked subjects to flick their wrist randomly but indicate when the decision was made by watching a clock. He found that subjects' decision to move the hand was preceded by brain activity about half a second before the stated decision, though the subjects perceived the decision to be simultaneous with the action (Libet, 1999, 2002, 2006; Libet et al., 1983; Libet and Mochida, 1988; Libet et al., 1979, 1982).

Haggard and Eimer measured brain activity (lateralized readiness potential, LRP) while the subjects decided which hand to move. The LRP preceded the conscious decision, indicating that the decision was made before it reached consciousness (Haggard and Eimer, 1999). Furthermore, it was possible to influence which hand the subject would choose to move by a single transcranial magnetic stimulation that was subthreshold for movement. Right-handed subjects would normally choose to move their right hand about 60% of the time, but when the right hemisphere was stimulated, they chose their left hand about 80% of the time. The hand preference was influenced only when the coil was positioned over frontal cortex. Thus, it appears that a single magnetic stimulus which does not evoke movement can alter high-level motor planning (Ammon and Gandevia, 1990). Such influence by magnetic stimulus was effective only when the response occurred within 200 ms of the "go" signal, which corresponds to the time delay between decision and consciousness observed by Libet (Brasil-Neto et al., 1992).

It seems, however, that the conscious will may be able to "veto" an action in the last few milliseconds (Libet, 2003). In this model, unconscious impulses to perform a volitional act may be open to suppression by the conscious efforts of the individual, sometimes referred to as "free won't." Such "free" suppression may, however, have as much unconscious neural antecedents as "free will" (Velmans, 2003).

So, what is free will in memetic terms? The unconscious neural activity for action predating conscious decision is clearly a memetic process. The sense of conscious free will occurs when the memetic processing impinges on the selfplex, i.e., when the action is strong enough to reach a level of importance for the selfplex. There are many actions that we take, including muscle movements that do not reach consciousness, such as shifting position in a chair. If we pay attention, however, then we may be more readily conscious of such movements.

Decision making may be seen to be the act of memetic processing, in which various memes, as it were, vote on a course of action among the choices presented. Only when the voting is over an important issue will the process become conscious.

Does free will influence decisions? It appears immediate decisions are made unconsciously and not by free choice. However, as with free will not we may intentionally and consciously limit our future choices through memetic manipulation. If enough memes in our brain are persuaded to incline in one direction long before the election, then the outcome of the election may be more predictable. As in an election, the outcome of the secret ballot is by definition unpredictable, but based on the campaigns and polls preceding it, one can make an educated guess.

11.11   The Unconscious, Collective Unconscious, Freudian Unconscious

From the above discussion, it should be apparent that most brain activity including meme manipulation occurs without reaching consciousness. It is when the processing requires some *thought*, i.e., the synchronized activity of sufficient parts of the frontal lobes (and perhaps claustrum) does it become conscious.

The Jungian concept of *collective unconscious* can be interpreted as the memes in the meme pool called society, that are so pervasive that they enter the brains almost automatically, i.e., without undergoing the filtration process for new memes. Such memes are usually introduced in early life and form the basis of a priori prejudice or predispositions that we call cultural traits. Sense of beauty, taste, right and wrong, how justice should be carried out – all these form part of the collective unconscious. These cultural memes naturally co-opt genetic imperatives for food, sex, and dominance and form strong mutually supporting memeplexes. Such cultural traits do change with introduction of new memes, e.g., sense of beauty changes as fashion changes, at one time eating raw fish was "disgusting" in the Western culture, and burning at the stake was an accepted means of execution during the middle ages. It is my contention that even memes in the collective unconscious, as long as they reside in the neural clusters, can be made explicit and be reprocessed through the executor of memes – reason.

What about the Freudian unconscious as a product of repression? Repression can be conceptualized as a process by which the dominant memeplexes prevent incompatible memes that are strong enough to become memories (i.e., meme-containing neurons) from receiving attention and thus reinforcement (Edelman's reentry) necessary for replication. Thus, the repressed memes are outside of consciousness except when they exert influence on other unconscious (or automatic) processes such as association with incoming memes or in internal processing such as dreaming.

In this view, most memes except those recruited by working memory are unconscious (or preconscious). Such unconscious memes may be (1) nonproblematic memes that require little processing, such as new factual information that are routinely stored, (2) culturally pervasive memes that enter the brain automatically (under the radar) that form prejudices and the *collective unconscious*, and (3) memes that are in conflict with dominant memes and have been rendered unconscious and hard to reach through deprivation of reinforcement.

11.12 Selfplex and the Shadow: We Are All Multiple Personalities

Self-awareness is the idea of self as a unitary entity and is often attributed to the development of the Theory Of Mind (TOM). TOM is the ability to see others as having minds, i.e., thoughts, intentions, and feelings. The most commonly used test of TOM ability is the false-belief task (Perner and Wimmer, 1988), a version of which is the "Sally-Ann task." A child is shown two dolls, Sally and Anne, who are playing with a marble. Then, Sally puts away the marble in a box (Box A), and Sally leaves. After Sally leaves Anne takes the marble out and plays with it, then puts it in another box (Box B), then leaves. Sally returns and the child is asked in which box Sally would look for the marble. If the child has TOM, then she will say Sally would look for the marble in Box A, where she had put it when she left, even though the child knows that the marble is now in Box B. TOM involves that another's state of mind may be different from their own and be able to predict behavior based on that understanding.

The development of mirror neurons as an evolutionary achievement may have contributed to the ability for TOM. As discussed in Chapter 7, mirror neurons in the brain in the frontal and anterior cingulate cortex fire when observing another chimpanzee or human engage in an activity or show an emotion. This ability to empathize, to feel, or to act in other's shoes, may eventually induce the ability to see oneself as if the self was an object, i.e., self-awareness (Oberman and Ramachandran, 2007; Ramachandran and Oberman, 2006). As you understand how others are feeling, you also understand how others might feel about you, or think of you. You also can see yourself, think of how you would feel under certain circumstances, i.e., predict your own feelings and behavior using self-empathy and TOM.

The problem is, of course, that you are not sure about yourself, that you are not always consistent. In fact, you often say, "one part of me would like to do x, and another part would like to do y, and most likely, y will win out." Self-awareness shows us that the self is not unitary, but is often divided into many parts.

Emotions often catalyze the assumption of dominance of one selfplex over another. We are familiar with our "pleasant personality" and our "aggressive personality." The emotional brain state precipitated by an external stimulus may thus favor one type of selfplex over another.

We have seen in previous sections of this chapter that our brain contains many memeplexes comprising of neurons that have evolved over time, in constant interaction with genes and memes, existing and incoming. No wonder the memeplexes have cohered into at least several clusters that we call self (or personalities within the self).

Selfplex is the sense of my own personality, who I am, what I am like, what I believe in, what I would and not do. It is known in other terms such as ego, self, self-schema, and identity. Selfplexes within a given brain develop over time in the course of the epigenetic development of genes and memes and may cohere into several selfplexes with varying degrees of inherent compatibility. The incompatibility between two selfplexes within the same brain may be especially pronounced if they are formed at two different periods, say in an immigrant's life in two different meme pools or cultures with two different languages. Thus, there may be some individuals who hold American values and behave like Americans when living in America and speaking English, and when they return to their native lands, revert back to their old values and behave like the natives, speaking the native tongue. In this case, the dominant selfplex may be dependent on the location, and thus the surrounding meme pool of the brain. In this case, two selfplexes are not in conflict at the same time, and not much effort is required to switch the dominance. Much of the time, the different memeplexes in our brains coexist without serious conflict.

Among the memes that form selfplexes, there are those that are in direct conflict with the dominant selfplexes and therefore are particularly inhibited from replicating. These "unacceptable" memes and memeplexes form the "shadow" of Jungian psychology. If the shadow becomes empowered, either through the weakening of the dominant selfplexes or through incoming memes that facilitate the shadow, there may be conscious conflict, experienced as anxiety and psychological turmoil. If there is a revolution in the republic of memes that is our brain, then the shadow may take power, resulting in a complete change in personality, which may be in the form of psychosis, dissociation, or depressive and manic syndromes.

How strong the dominant selfplex is, and how well it harmonizes and cooperates with the nondominant selfplexes and shadow may determine whether the individual is a flexible and adaptive person who can feel and behave appropriately (and thus differently) depending on situations as opposed to one who is rigid and fragile, or frankly show incompatible personalities, often in outbursts or episodes of dissociation. Our brains contain multiple personalities almost by necessity as we have absorbed many memes from different personalities. The job of harmonizing the many selfplexes and utilizing them as the occasion demands, of course, falls on the executive function of the brain. (See Chapter 12 for further discussion of this topic.)

11.13 Transcendence

Transcendence, the phenomenon of rising above individual needs and concerns in favor of spiritual or higher purpose, may be a remarkable example of gene–meme coevolution. The experience of transcendence seems to involve two components: an altered state of consciousness and recognition of an entity that is beyond the interests of the individual, whether it is a god, a spirit, or a cosmic order.

Altered states of consciousness accompany the activation of strong stress reactions such as fight/flight and "freezing" (or conservation/withdrawal, playing dead). The so-called adrenaline rush of fight/flight can be intoxicating. Relaxation and accompanying EEG changes bring out changes in self- and other awareness. Altered states of consciousness certainly seem to have adaptive significance as under these conditions the brain may be spared of the time-consuming reasoning process.

Altered state of consciousness often occurs with the activation of the dopaminergic pleasure/reward system previously described, often occasioned by drug use or situations causing strong emotional arousal.

While often associated with an altered state of consciousness, the act of transcendence seems to be more in the service of memes rather than genes. In fact, the notion of arising over one's individuality contains within it a subjugation of the genetic bodily demands. Memes developed the capacity to tweak the neurons such that pure activities serving the memes act as rewarding activities resulting in injection of dopamine into the pleasure center.

Memes seem to have coevolved with the genes such that there are variants in dopamine receptor genes that build brains particularly welcoming transcendence memes. In one study, a higher level of dopamine 4 receptors in the frontal cortex predicted spirituality and transcendence (Comings et al., 2000). The gene coding for vesicular monoamine transporter 2 (VMAT2), an integral membrane protein that acts to transport monoamines, particularly the neurotransmitters dopamine, norepinephrine, serotonin, and histamine, into synaptic vesicles, has been called the "God Gene" as those with polymorphisms that enhance its function scored higher on a "self-transcendence" scale (Hamer, 2005).

Transcendence is possible only with the help of the memes as the idea of rising above one's bodily needs. Memes are, in fact, transcendental entities as they transcend the brains by migrating from one another and infecting one another. Through the cooperation of the memes, genes achieve the experience of transcendence, and, though tied down to a particular brain, the genes can vicariously experience the wonderful exploits of memes in other worlds and other brains. From the meme's point of view, the human brain is a territory to conquer; from the brain's perspective, memes are invaders that show the way to a promised land. In the course of coevolution of genes and memes, values or emotions were attached to them, as the values code for nurturance and survival. As the experience of pleasure is genetic, but appraisal of value is memetic, different endeavors have acquired different valuations, i.e., studying is good, god is good, sexual desire is bad, brotherly love is good. At the fundamental level, as memes were in charge of the valuations, whatever served the memes were good, and whatever served the genes more than memes were somewhat bad, whatever served only genes and not memes were very bad. Thus, spirituality, a purely meme-oriented activity, acquired the most value.

Individuals that adapted to the spirituality meme–gene coevolution then may have spiritual needs that are beyond the understanding of those without the DRD4 or VMAT2 genes.

11.14 The Individual as a Pawn in the War of Memes

We discussed in the previous chapter how memes are stored in external devices as well as in the brains of human beings. We also saw that there are conflicting memes and mutually incompatible memes, and in our brains they tend to cohere into different personalities vying for dominance. From the meme's point of view, all human brains are like islands for colonization, and the more brains like memes dominate, the more the speed and breadth of their replication. Thus there is a constant state of conflict among competing and incompatible memes in the meme pool called human society.

For certain memeplexes, such as certain religions and political ideals, dominance may mean the extinction of competing incompatible memes and the brains that contain them. Such memeplexes may then breed cooperating memeplexes such as fanaticism and patriotism in the service of stamping out competing memes through massacres, wars, and book-burnings. In these circumstances, individuals who kill and who are killed are but pawns of the toxic memes in the society.

How to prevent the individual from being the pawns of toxic memes? It is only through the strengthening of the reasoning powers of the brain, i.e., appropriate sorting, filtering, and processing of memes that it encounters that such toxic memes can be isolated and controlled rather than being controlled by them. Only when sufficient numbers of brains in the society are equipped with such reasoning ability will the society be safe from the unchecked proliferation of toxic memes. In addition to the reasoning powers, the brains must develop early warning mechanisms for the introduction of the toxic memes so that the likelihood of their coming in undetected is lessened.

References

Ammon, K., Gandevia, S. C. (1990) Transcranial magnetic stimulation can influence the selection of motor programmes. *J Neurol Neurosurg Psychiatry*, **53**, 705–707.

Balkin, J. M. (1998) *Cultural Software: A Theory of Ideology*. Yale University Press, New Haven.

Benedict, R. (1938) *Patterns of Culture*. Routledge & Kegan Paul, London.

Bloch, M. H. (2000) A well-disposed social anthropologist's problems with memes. In *Darwinizing Culture: The Status of Memetics as a Science* (R. Aunger ed.), pp. 189–203. Oxford University Press, Oxford.

Boyd, R., Richerson, P. J. (2000) Memes: Universal acid or a better mousetrap? In *Darwinizing Culture: The Status of Memetics as a Science* (R. Aunger ed.), pp. 143–173. Oxford University Press, Oxford.

Brasil-Neto, J. P., Pascual-Leone, A., Valls-Sole, J., et al. (1992) Focal transcranial magnetic stimulation and response bias in a forced-choice task. *J Neurol Neurosurg Psychiatry*, **55**, 964–966.

Comings, D. E., Gonzales, N., Saucier, G., et al. (2000) The DRD4 gene and the spiritual transcendence scale of the character temperament index. *Psychiatr Genet*, **10**, 185–189.

Crick, F. C., Koch, C. (2005) What is the function of the claustrum? *Philos Trans R Soc Lond B Biol Sci*, **360**, 1271–1279.

de la Fuente-Fernandez, R., Ruth, T. J., Sossi, V., et al. (2001) Expectation and dopamine release: Mechanism of the placebo effect in Parkinson's disease. *Science*, **293**, 1164–1166.

de la Fuente-Fernandez, R., Stoessl, A. J. (2004) The biochemical bases of the placebo effect. *Sci Eng Ethics*, **10**, 143–150.

Diederich, N. J., Goetz, C. G. (2008) The placebo treatments in neurosciences: New insights from clinical and neuroimaging studies. *Neurology*, **71**, 677–684.

Distin, K. (2005) *The Selfish Meme: A Critical Reassessment.* Cambridge University Press, New York.

Edelman, G. M. (2004) *Wider than the Sky.* Yale University Press, New Haven, CT.

Furmark, T., Appel, L., Henningsson, S., et al. (2008) A link between serotonin-related gene polymorphisms, amygdala activity, and placebo-induced relief from social anxiety. *J Neurosci*, **28**, 13066–13074.

Gadamer, H. G. (1975) *Truth and Method.* Crossroad, New York.

Haggard, P., Eimer, M. (1999) On the relation between brain potentials and the awareness of voluntary movements. *Exp Brain Res*, **126**, 128–133.

Hamer, D. (2005) *The God Gene: How Faith Is Hardwired into Our Genes.* Anchor, New York.

Hunter, A. M., Ravikumar, S., Cook, I. A., et al. (2009) Brain functional changes during placebo lead-in and changes in specific symptoms during pharmacotherapy for major depression. *Acta Psychiatr Scand*, **119**, 266–273.

Kuper, A. (2000) If memes are the answer, what is the question? In *Darwinizing Culture: The Status of Memetics as a Science* (R. Aunger ed.), pp. 175–188. Oxford University Press, Oxford.

Leuchter, A. F., Cook, I. A., Witte, E. A., et al. (2002) Changes in brain function of depressed subjects during treatment with placebo. *Am J Psychiatry*, **159**, 122–129.

Leuchter, A. F., Morgan, M., Cook, I. A., et al. (2004) Pretreatment neurophysiological and clinical characteristics of placebo responders in treatment trials for major depression. *Psychopharmacology (Berl)*, **177**, 15–22.

Libet, B. (1999) How does conscious experience arise? The neural time factor. *Brain Res Bull*, **50**, 339–340.

Libet, B. (2002) The timing of mental events: Libet's experimental findings and their implications. *Conscious Cogn*, **11**, 291–299, discussion 304–233.

Libet, B. (2003) Can conscious experience affect brain activity? *Journal of Consciousness Studies*, **10**, 24–28.

Libet, B. (2006) Reflections on the interaction of the mind and brain. *Prog Neurobiol*, **78**, 322–326.

Libet, B., Gleason, C. A., Wright, E. W., et al. (1983) Time of conscious intention to act in relation to onset of cerebral activity (readiness-potential). The unconscious initiation of a freely voluntary act. *Brain*, **106**(Pt 3), 623–642.

Libet, B., Mochida, S. (1988) Long-term enhancement (LTE) of postsynaptic potentials following neural conditioning, in mammalian sympathetic ganglia. *Brain Res*, **473**, 271–282.

Libet, B., Wright, E. W., Jr., Feinstein, B., et al. (1979) Subjective referral of the timing for a conscious sensory experience: A functional role for the somatosensory specific projection system in man. *Brain*, **102**, 193–224.

Libet, B., Wright, E. W., Jr., Gleason, C. A. (1982) Readiness-potentials preceding unrestricted 'spontaneous' vs. pre-planned voluntary acts. *Electroencephalogr Clin Neurophysiol*, **54**, 322–335.

Mayberg, H. S., Silva, J. A., Brannan, S. K., et al. (2002) The functional neuroanatomy of the placebo effect. *Am J Psychiatry*, **159**, 728–737.

Oberman, L. M., Ramachandran, V. S. (2007) The simulating social mind: The role of the mirror neuron system and simulation in the social and communicative deficits of autism spectrum disorders. *Psychol Bull*, **133**, 310–327.

Perner, J., Wimmer, H. (1988) Misinformation and unexpected change: Testing the development of epistemic-state attribution. *Psychol Res*, **50**, 191–197.

Radcliffe-Brown, A. (1952) *Structure and Function in Primitive Society.* Cohen and West, London.

Ramachandran, V. S., Oberman, L. M. (2006) Broken mirrors: A theory of autism. *Sci Am*, **295**, 62–69.

Scott, D. J., Stohler, C. S., Egnatuk, C. M., et al. (2008) Placebo and nocebo effects are defined by opposite opioid and dopaminergic responses. *Arch Gen Psychiatry*, **65**, 220–231.

Sperber, D. (2000) An objection to the memetic approach to culture. In *Darwinizing Culture: The Status of Memetics as a Science* (R. Aunger ed.), pp. 163–173. Oxford University Press, Oxford.

Tylor, E. B. (1871, 1924) *Primitive Culture, 2 vol*. Brentanos, New York.

Velmans, M. (2003) Preconscious free will. *J Consciousness Studies*, **10**, 42–61.

Wager, T. D., Scott, D. J., Zubieta, J. K. (2007) Placebo effects on human mu-opioid activity during pain. *Proc Natl Acad Sci U S A*, **104**, 11056–11061.

Wasserman, S. S., Kotloff, K. L., Losonsky, G. A., et al. (1993) Immunologic response to oral cholera vaccination in a crossover study: A novel placebo effect. *Am J Epidemiol*, **138**, 988–993.

Zubieta, J. K., Bueller, J. A., Jackson, L. R., et al. (2005) Placebo effects mediated by endogenous opioid activity on mu-opioid receptors. *J Neurosci*, **25**, 7754–7762.

Chapter 12
What Is Mental Health?

Contents

12.1 Normality and Health

What is normal? There are several ways of defining normality: (1) normality as what is common or prevalent without precisely defining what constitutes common, (2) statistical normality – if a value falls within two standard deviations, it is within normal limits, (3) normal as an ideal – a "normal" person may be someone without any conflicts, a state for which one might strive but never achieve, (4) normality as absence of pathology (abnormality) – according to this definition, the presence of even a single abnormality disqualifies the whole, as in a tissue pathology sample, (5) normality by legislation (or decree), e.g., homosexuality was an illness until 1973 when the Board of the American Psychiatric Association voted unanimously to remove it from the diagnostic and statistical manual. Each of the normality definition has uses within their specific context but can be misleading if used in another context.

What is health? Is being healthy normal?

The World Health Organization (WHO) defines health as "a state of complete physical, mental and social well-being, and not merely the absence of disease or infirmity". According to this definition, mental health would be an ideal state of well-being difficult to achieve in real life.

The capacity to work and to love, a phrase attributed to Freud, is another definition of mental health that sets the bar to a lower achievable level.

Vaillant describes six models of mental health: (1) mental health as above normal, (2) mental health as positive psychology, (3) mental health as maturity,

H. Leigh, *Genes, Memes, Culture, and Mental Illness*,
DOI 10.1007/978-1-4419-5671-2_12, © Hoyle Leigh, 2010

(4) mental health as social-emotional intelligence, (5) mental health as subjective well-being, (6) mental health as resilience (Vaillant, 2003). We will briefly review these models and consider how the concept of gene × meme interaction may contribute to a unification of the models.

1. Mental health as above normal: In this model, the important task is defining what "normal" is. In general, persons who have no difficulty to work, love, and play are considered to be in good mental health. The Global Assessment of Function (GAF), part of the DSM multiaxial diagnostic scheme (see Chapter 14), is an attempt at quantification of mental functioning (thus mental health), and on a scale of 1–100, scoring somewhere over 90 is considered to be in superior mental health.
2. Mental health as positive psychology: Drawing in Maslow's concept of self-actualization of talents, capacities, and potentialities, positive psychology as represented by Seligman emphasizes optimism and endeavors to build qualities that help individuals and communities not just to endure and survive but also to flourish (Seligman, 1991, 2002). Positive mental health has been divided into four components – talents, enablers, strengths, and outcomes (Peterson and Seligman, 2004). Talents, e.g., disposition and intelligence, are genetically determined and not subject to much intervention. Enablers are social interventions and environmental variables that can be strengthened. Strengths are character traits such as openness and creativity that can be changed. Outcomes are the dependent variables such as strength of social relationships and GAF that can be a measure of therapeutic intervention.
3. Mental health as maturity: Since Erikson's groundbreaking description of adult developmental stages, there followed descriptions of adult ego development, adult moral development, and adult spiritual development. They all posit that there is continuing development in adulthood, i.e., maturity toward mental health. Vaillant added two stages to original Erikson's model of adult development as follows: identity (adolescence) – intimacy – career consolidation – generativity – keeper of the meaning – integrity.
4. Mental health as social-emotional intelligence: According to Vaillant, social-emotional intelligence can be defined by the following criteria (Vaillant, 2003):

   a. Accurate perception and monitoring of one's own emotions.
   b. Appropriate expression of emotions. This involves the capacity to self-modulate anxiety and to shake off hopelessness and gloom.
   c. Accurate recognition of and response to emotions in others.
   d. Skill in negotiating close relationships with others.
   e. Capacity for focusing emotions (motivation) on a desired goal. This involves delayed gratification and adaptively displacing and channeling impulse.

5. Mental health as subjective well-being: Subjective well-being or happiness (excluding potentially destructive excitement in risk taking behavior or drugs) is considered to be an antidote to learned helplessness. Happy people, after controlling for age, socioeconomic class, and disease, were shown to be half as likely

to die at an early age or become disabled as unhappy people (Ostir et al., 2000). Is happiness then a genetically determined temperament or a reflection of safe, non-stressful environment? It appears that happiness is more temperamental and tends to affect the environment more than the environment affects the temperament. The subjective well-being of monozygous twins raised apart was found to be more similar than that of heterozygous twins raised together (Bouchard et al., 1990; Newman et al., 1998; Tellegen et al., 1988). Some of the heritable factors that contribute to a high level of subjective well-being include a low level of trait neuroticism, high level of trait extraversion, absence of alcoholism, and absence of major depression (Vaillant, 2003). Relationships were shown to be more important to subjective well-being than money.

6. Mental health as resilience: This model is concerned with how the individual copes with stress. The trait of resilience or hardiness, and the type of psychological defense mechanisms used will determine whether the individual can bounce back from stressful situations without significant emotional distress.

12.2   Gene × Meme Interaction and Mental Health

The models of mental health discussed above by and large indicate that mental health is a desideratum involving aspects of personality such as resilience and openness that are achieved through interaction of temperament and experience in the course of continuing development of the person. Mental health is thus a state of well-being of the mind.

Pursuit of happiness is a fundamental motivation underlying all mental activity. What are the factors involved in the experience of happiness? Clearly, there are certain basic biological drives and needs that must be met, i.e., feeding, sex, exploration, attachment, physical comfort. Yet, the amount of fulfillment of the biological drives to produce a sense of happiness seems to vary depending on culture and individual. For example, obtaining a piece of bread for a person starving may produce extreme happiness while ten times the amount of bread will not elicit much happiness in a well-fed individual.

Modern humans are not happy with bread alone. We are happier with gourmet meals with complex flavors and tastes, perhaps with a glass of wine, served in pleasant and clean surroundings, often with good company and accompanied with music. The ingredients of this type of happiness are clearly both biological (genetic) and memetic (cultural). The arts of cooking, of decorating a room, of making wine, of conversation and of music are all products of memetic evolution based on genetic needs.

The Merriam-Webster Dictionary defines happiness as a state of well-being and contentment, or a pleasurable or satisfying experience (Merriam-Webster, 2008). The term happiness is usually used to denote a sustained state of well-being while the term pleasure often denotes more immediate positive experience.

Happiness as a goal in life, while accepted widely, has had many different meanings through history. Simply put, what constitutes happiness may be classified in two large categories – (1) pursuing and satisfying one's desires and needs through positive action, and (2) reducing the needs and desires so that one is in a state of satisfaction without the need for much positive action. Hedonism is often associated with the former, while stoicism or asceticism is associated with the latter. Another dichotomy has been between seeking pleasure of the body and senses versus of the spirit a la St. Augustine and Thomas Aquinas (http://science.jrank.org/pages/7739/Happiness-Pleasure-in-European-Thought.html, 2008). Clearly, seeking happiness for the spirit at the exclusion of the body is an example of memes driving the brain.

Pleasure is the experience that drives animals, including humans, to action and forms the biological/genetic basis of happiness.

12.3   Neurobiology of Pleasure, Punishment, and Inhibition

The main centers of the brain's *reward circuit* are located along the medial forebrain bundle (MFB). The ventral tegmental area (VTA) and the nucleus accumbens are the two major centers in this circuit, but it also includes several others, such as the septum, the amygdala, the prefrontal cortex, and certain parts of the thalamus. Each of these structures appears to participate in its own way in various aspects of behavioral response. All of these centers are interconnected and innervate the hypothalamus, informing it of the presence of rewards. The lateral and ventromedial nuclei of the hypothalamus are especially involved in this reward circuit. The hypothalamus then acts in return not only on the ventral tegmental area, but also on the autonomic and endocrine functions of the entire body, through the pituitary gland. See Figs. 12.1, 12.2, and 12.3.

The emotion of pleasure and reward seems associated with the dopaminergic activation of a circuitous pathway, first involving a descending medial forebrain bundle component and then involving the ascending mesolimbic ventral tegmental pathway (Bozarth, 1987; Wise and Bozarth, 1985), eventually activating the dopaminergic nucleus accumbens. The septum, the amygdala, the ventromedial prefrontal cortex, and certain parts of the thalamus also participate in the circuit. *The ventromedial prefrontal cortex, with its extensive connections with the limbic system, may link the conscious to the unconscious and ascribe meaning to perceptions by associating them with meaningful memes.*

The ventral tegmental pathway can also be activated by various substances including alcohol, amphetamines, exogenous and endogenous opiates, barbiturates, caffeine, marijuana, and nicotine.

All of these pleasure centers are interconnected and innervate the hypothalamus, particularly the lateral and ventromedial nuclei. The hypothalamus then activates the ventral tegmental area, as well as the autonomic and endocrine functions through the pituitary gland.

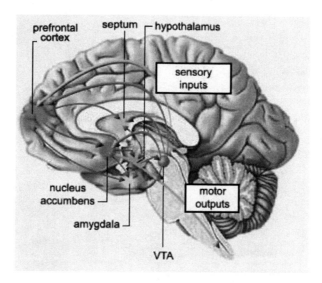

Fig. 12.1 Brain structures associated with pleasure, punishment, and inhibition 1.

Fig. 12.2 Brain structures associated with pleasure, punishment, and inhibition 2.

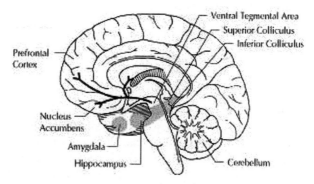

Aversive stimuli that provoke fight or flight responses activate the brain's punishment circuit (the periventricular system, or PVS), which is activated to cope with unpleasant situations by activating the fight/flight response. It includes the hypothalamus, the thalamus, and the central gray substance surrounding the aqueduct of Sylvius. Some secondary centers of this circuit are found in the amygdala and the hippocampus. The cholinergic punishment circuit stimulates the secretion of adrenal corticotropic hormone (ACTH) as well as stimulation of the adrenal medulla and sympathetic outflow. ACTH in turn stimulates the adrenal cortex to release adrenocortical hormones. Stimulation of the punishment circuit can inhibit the pleasure circuit, thus fear and punishment can drive out many pleasures.

The behavioral inhibition system (BIS), associated with the septo-hippocampal system, the amygdala, and the basal nuclei, receives inputs from the prefrontal

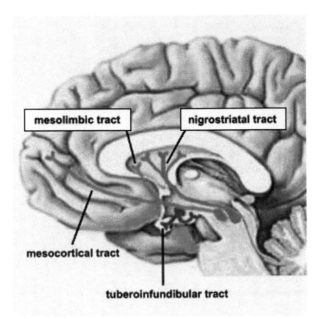

Fig. 12.3 Dopaminergic pathways in the brain. (http://www.ask.com/bar?q=brain+reward+diagram &page=1&qsrc=2417&ab=5&u=http%3A%2F%2Fthebrain.mcgill.ca%2Fflash%2Fi%2Fi_03% 2Fi_03_cl%2Fi_03_cl_par%2Fi_03_cl_par.html,   copyleft).   The   three   diagrams   and explanatory text are from The Brain Top To Bottom, website by Canadian Institute of Neuroscience, Mental Health, and Addiction, Canadian Institutes of Health Research, http:// thebrain.mcgill.ca/flash/index_a.html. Copyleft. The linear drawing is in public domain)

cortex and transmits its outputs via the noradrenergic neurons of the locus coeruleus and the serotonergic fibers of the medial Raphe nuclei. Serotonin may also play a major role in this system. The BIS is activated when both fight and flight seem impossible and the only remaining behavioral option is to submit passively.

When a sensory stimulus is perceived by the cortex to indicate a danger, it is routed first to the thalamus. From there, the information is sent out over two parallel pathways: the thalamo-amygdala pathway (the "short route") and the thalamo-cortico-amygdala pathway (the "long route"). The short route quickly activates the central nucleus of the amygdala. Then the information that has been processed by the cortex through the long route reaches the amygdala and modifies its response dependent on the cortical evaluation of the threat. This cortical evaluation involves the following steps: (1) The various modalities of the perceived object are processed by the primary sensory cortex. Then the unimodal associative cortex provides the amygdala with a representation of the object. (2) The polymodal associative cortex conceptualizes the object and transmits the information to the amygdala. (3) *This elaborated representation of the object is then compared with the contents of explicit memory (memes) available through the hippocampus, which also communicates closely with the amygdala.* The hippocampus is also involved in the encoding of the context associated with a fearful experience. The amygdala conveys the gratifying or aversive nature of the experience through connections to the nucleus accumbens, the ventral striatum, the septum, the hypothalamus, the nuclei of the brainstem, and orbitofrontal, cingulate, piriform, and other parts of the cortex. *The combination of stimuli from the amygdala with working memory (memes) in the dorsolateral prefrontal cortex may constitute the experience of emotion.* The basal ganglia have close connections with the amygdala and are involved with the voluntary expression of emotions. The amygdala has outputs to the nuclei of the sympathetic nervous system in the brainstem and the hypothalamus, controlling the pituitary gland and the endocrine system.

The anterior cingulate gyrus of the frontal lobe seems to be important in emotions and cognition. The subgenual anterior cingulate, together with the rostral cingulate, is considered to be the emotional sector of anterior cingulate gyrus and subserves autonomic arousal, reward mechanisms, and emotions, particularly anxiety and sadness in close coupling with the amygdala (Grady and Keightley, 2002; Pezawas et al., 2005). The dorsal portion of the anterior cingulate, called "cognitive cingulate," is involved with error monitoring and selecting among competing responses.

Orbitofrontal cortex plays an important role in decision making in the context of emotional situations. Ventrolateral prefrontal cortex, together with subgenual cingulate, plays a role in responding to reward contingencies.

In the course of evolution, the brain has developed intricate mechanisms for adapting to the environment that include the emotions of pleasure and fear. Emotions facilitate cognitive evaluation of a situation by providing flavor and urgency – the "gut reaction" often is a shortcut of much elaborative cognition. The mirror neurons that appeared in primates that directly elicit an imitation of emotions of another animal probably enhanced the development of memes as imitation of others' emotions and behavior. Thus, in addition to perceptions based on sensations, empathy occurring as mirror neuron activity may be then perceived as an internal sensation, which might be a precursor to an internal representation of the self, i.e., by empathizing with others, one might also learn to empathize with oneself.

12.4   Mental Health: A Democracy of Memes

In the beginning, memes developed simply as patterns of neural connection (memory) that were transmitted from one individual to another through observation and activation of the mirror neurons and/or the perceptual apparatus. In the beginning, memes were obviously in the service of the genes as memes that elicited the pleasure experience were readily incorporated, and those that elicited the fear/punishment response were discarded. Memes that arose from individuals who were successful were welcomed as they promised pleasure. As memes became more numerous, and became free-floating in books and electronic media, largely independent of the brain from which they rose, the link between memes and immediate pleasure or fear became largely uncoupled.

Now in the form of information and knowledge, memes are to a large extent emotionally neutral, neither pleasure nor fear. Except, of course, the process of acquiring memes has been linked to pleasure as an evolutionary adaptation of *Homo sapiens*, though such pleasure may also be seen in some animals that acquire new skills through learning.

As I discussed in the previous chapter, memes also acquired the ability to encapsulate themselves in disguise by forming memeplexes such as a toxic meme (e.g., murder) being sugarcoated in a fashionable –ism (e.g., patriotism, fascism).

Modern human brain is immersed in an ocean of memes of all shapes, colors, and sizes, mutually compatible, incompatible, or indifferent. The sole purpose, of a meme is replication. Thus, once inside the brain, each meme is intent on replication. Replication of a meme in the brain is by converting another set of neurons to be like them, which involves connecting with another set of neurons and converting it. The brain is a Hobbsean universe of memes where each meme is out for itself against all other memes. It is natural, then, that some memes should form alliances with each other, and recruit other allies to form small cooperating societies, or memeplexes and complexes of memeplexes. Thus, small societies of memeplexes develop, and there may be tension, cooperation, or frank conflict among these societies of memes.

Before the advent of memes, the animal had a unity of purpose dictated by genes. With memes, however, the unity of purpose has been lost, replaced by competing purposes of genes and memes.

From early childhood, memes enter the brain that stand for social norms, codes of conduct, and ways of relating with people. Some social memes are created by the brain through trial and error, e.g., the child learns that it is more effective to ask with a smile rather than with a frown. Such autochthonous memes may be augmented by imitation of others, or may spread by others imitating them. The learning of morals and ethics may be through a combination of memes introduced from outside as well as trial and error. Some social memes, such as a tendency toward altruism, may arise from genes that have been evolutionarily selected sociobiologically (Wilson, 1980).

Empathy, both automatic through motor neurons and conscious through identification, would play an important role in the development of memes concerned with the sense of morals and justice, in parallel with those introduced from the society in the form of codes and rules.

During adolescence, there is an influx of new memes as the developing brain has now gained the ability to abstract and absorb abstract memes. There is confusion, conflict, and turmoil among the competing memes, some already resident but called to question by new incoming memes, and newly introduced abstract memes. Eventually, one or more memes are identified as comprising the essence of the self, the selfplex, which are the memeplexes that have been successful in competing with others and established dominance. There are often more than one dominant self-plexes depending on the environment in which the brain finds itself. For example, the dominant selfplex at work may be that of a "scientist," while at home, it may be "wife" and "mother." At church, she might be a "Christian." The selfplex(es) then rule over other societies of memeplexes within the same domain.

When the dominant selfplexes in different domains are in reasonable harmony with each other, they are called roles that can change smoothly depending on the setting. When a selfplex for a particular role asserts dominance over others, for example, a religion, then there is potential conflict. Such dominant selfplexes often recruit self-serving memeplexes such as prejudice against other and chauvinism. Counterbalancing such memes are tolerance memes and freedom memes.

How the selfplex and other societies of memes should relate with each other is a meme itself, and has a number of variations. One model is that of an authoritarian and tyrannical regime in which one selfplex ruthlessly suppresses others. The self is, therefore, seen to be unitary and coherent with a strong identity, with strong support of prejudice and chauvinism memes. Authoritarian selfplex is subject to violent overthrow by the repressed memes and memeplexes if they are energized by an infusion of new memes or if the selfplex is weakened either by a decrease in brain function, or by infusion of conflicting memes. An example of the fear an authoritarian selfplex exhibits toward new meme infusion is censorship. Individuals with authoritarian selfplexes tend to advocate censorship, for example of "bad words." Of course, the "bad words" are resident in the brains of those individuals as memes; otherwise they would not recognize a "bad word." And they are often preoccupied with the "bad words" that they look for them in everything they see or read. This is an example of the replication of the resident memes represented by the "bad words," and how the authoritarian selfplexes are threatened by it.

Another model of interaction of memes and selfplexes in the brain is that of an enlightened sovereign or of an oligarchy, where the selfplex maintains hegemony but is open to coexistence with other selfplexes and conflicting memes, and recognizes them as legitimate, some of them more so (the aristocrats, so to speak) than others.

Yet another model is a democracy of selfplexes where there is recognition that different senses and objectives of the self can coexist, and depending on the needs of the genes and the environment, the different selfplexes may be elected to be dominant, with the consent of the ruled (Benjamin et al., 1996; Cohen et al., 2005; Ebstein et al., 1996; Okuyama et al., 2000; Shiraishi et al., 2006; Van Gestel et al., 2002).

The memes within the selfplexes are not mutually exclusive, i.e. – some memes may participate in more than one selfplex. Just as an incoming administration in a democracy may retain some of the cabinet members of the outgoing administration of another party, newly dominant selfplexes often retain memes of now nondominant selfplex. Furthermore, the memes that form the day to day working of the memetic government, like bureaucrats in a government, continue to function regardless of the changes in dominance of selfplexes. This model of memetic relationship in the brain may offer the most flexibility and least oppression. Unlike in multiple personality in which a repressed selfplex overturns the dominant one temporarily, in a democracy the change of regime is based on rational needs and is effectuated without suppression of the now nondominant selfplex.

In a memetic democracy, the selfplexes that may be likened to be major parties recognize the right to exist of the minor, even subversive parties. Thus, revolutionary memes and subversive memes, and even toxic memes, can exist in a state of check and balance, and may express themselves in accepted forms such as creativity and art. Freedom, tolerance, and openness memes are universally accepted by the competing major selfplexes. Depending on the form of government, i.e., parliamentary democracy or a presidential system, the ease with each the selfplex changes may differ.

What is mental health considering the gene–meme interactions? The brain as a well-functioning memetic democracy may well fit the bill. As to Vaillant's first model, mental health as above normal, Winston Churchill's description of democracy may suffice: "democracy is the worst form of Government except all those other forms that have been tried from time to time"(Churchill, 1947).

As to the second model, mental health as positive psychology, pursuit of pleasure, both genetic and memetic, would be best facilitated in a memetic democracy, in which there are memes that seek primarily one or the other or both ends. The memes that constitute character strength such as open-mindedness and curiosity (See Table 12.1 below) may find certain brains particularly habitable because of

Table 12.1 The values in action institute classification of character strengths

Love
  Love, valuing close relations with others
  Kindness, generosity, compassion, altruistic love
  Social intelligence, emotional intelligence – being aware of others' feelings and motives
Temperance
  Forgiveness and mercy, not being vengeful
  Modesty and humility, not regarding oneself more special
  Prudence, not taking undue risks, refraining from things that one might regret later
  Self-regulation, self-control
Wisdom and Knowledge
  Creativity originality, ingenuity.
  Curiosity, interest, novelty seeking, openness.
  Judgment, open-mindedness, critical thinking
  Love of learning – mastering new skills, knowledge, etc.
  Perspective, wisdom, providing wise counsel to others
  Appreciation of beauty and excellence
Courage
  Bravery
  Integrity, authenticity, honesty – taking responsibility for one's feelings and actions
  Persistence, perseverance, industriousness, taking pleasure in completing tasks.
  Zest, vitality, enthusiasm, vigor – approaching life with excitement
Justice
  Citizenship – social responsibility, loyalty, teamwork.
  Fairness:
  Leadership.
Transcendence
  Gratitude – for the good things that happen, taking time to express thanks
  Hope, optimism, future orientation.
  Humor, playfulness, seeing the light side
  Spirituality, purpose – coherent beliefs of higher purpose and meaning of life that guide
    conduct and provide comfort.

Based on strengths of character and well-being (Park et al., 2004) and mental health (Vaillant, 2003).

their genetic predisposition. For example, those brains with the serotonin transporter promoter gene (5-HTTLPR) *l/l* may be more likely to welcome kindness/love memes and those with type 4 dopamine receptor gene (D4DR) *l/l* may be associated with curiosity/novelty-seeking memes (Benjamin et al., 1996; Cohen et al., 2005; Ebstein et al., 1996; Okuyama et al., 2000; Shiraishi et al., 2006; Van Gestel et al., 2002). On the other hand, strong exposure to character strength memes in early childhood may turn off certain genes that may be incompatible with them, such as the 5-HTTLPR *s/s* that predisposes the individual for fear and anxiety memes.

The third model, mental health as maturity, is compatible with a mature brain that is tolerant of competing needs and inclinations. Erikson's developmental stages can be seen to be stages of development of the ability to manipulate memes. In the earliest stage, memes concerning trust and mistrust have to be properly processed, followed by those of autonomy and shame, then taking initiative and guilt memes. During early school years, the child is infused with memes concerning rules and concrete operations (industry), as well as memes associated with inferiority. Adolescence ushers in a consolidation of selfplexes that have been formed in various stages of maturity in earlier stages. Processing of memes concerning sex and sexual identify is also important in adolescence. In early adulthood, the task is the processing of memes associated with intimacy and sharing as well as loneliness. Memes concerning success and competence in career are also important in what Vaillant calls the stage of career consolidation. In middle age, generativity or productivity memes, as well as memes associated with stagnation and boredom must be processed. There may be a proliferation of memes associated with meaning of life and place of the person in culture, what Vaillant calls "keeper of the meaning." Then, in Erikson's integrity vs. despair stage, memes concerning continuity of life and meaning as well as memes concerning mortality are processed with intensity.

This memetic view of stages of life does not posit achievement vs. nonachievement, but rather considers the memes that are more numerous depending on the stage. There may be only partial processing, and there may coexist processed (integrated) and nonintegrated memes, e.g., one might feel productive academically (abundance of academic memes and success memes associated with them) but not personally (abundance of dissatisfaction memes associated with relationships).

The fourth model, mental health as social-emotional intelligence, likewise, is achieved in a memetic democracy where empathy and socialization memes are given free expression.

The fifth model, mental health as subjective well-being, is best achieved in a memetic democracy where there is an orderly process of memetic expression and change of dominance, and where both genetic and memetic pursuit of happiness is recognized. There is, as in any democracy, healthy tension among competing memes and ongoing debate, which can be consciously carried out with the use of reason, the tool invented for effective memetic manipulation. Such a brain is then naturally resilient, Vaillant's sixth model, as it is best equipped to deal with stress by mobilizing all available genetic and memetic resources.

In a memetic democracy, most of the memes in the surrounding culture would be represented, but the unique interaction resulting in the epigenesis of the genes and memes through development would result in unique combinations of memes constituting the selfplexes. Each democracy of such selfplexes would have unique needs and desires just as each individual in a society has unique needs and desires. Furthermore, the needs and desires are likely to change over time with adaptation and possible change of regimes.

Pleasure is the activation of the dopaminergic reward system elicited by fulfillment of the needs of the genes or memes or both. Sustained pleasure would be possible when a majority of the memes and genes are satisfied, and the minorities are not dissatisfied enough to open revolt.

The self is not a coherent and unitary entity, but equilibrium of constantly changing selfplexes in a sea of memes. The self is fragile, an uneasy coalition of memes, that is subject to changes of regime and revolutions.

Mental health is a state of well-being of the gene–meme interaction in the brain. Such well-being is most likely achieved in a memetic democracy within the brain that recognizes both genetic and memetic needs, provides an orderly mechanism for their expression and mechanisms for adaptation to changing demands, and strives to maintain both cohesiveness and diversity within the societies of memes contained within.

References

Benjamin, J., Li, L., Patterson, C., et al. (1996) Population and familial association between the D4 dopamine receptor gene and measures of Novelty Seeking. *Nat Genet*, **12**, 81–84.

Bouchard, T. J., Jr., Lykken, D. T., McGue, M., et al. (1990) Sources of human psychological differences: The Minnesota Study of Twins Reared Apart. *Science*, **250**, 223–228.

Bozarth, M. A. (1987) Neuroanatomical boundaries of the reward-relevant opiate-receptor field in the ventral tegmental area as mapped by the conditioned place preference method in rats. *Brain Res*, **414**, 77–84.

Churchill, W. (1947) Speech House of Commons.

Cohen, M. X., Young, J., Baek, J. M., et al. (2005) Individual differences in extraversion and dopamine genetics predict neural reward responses. *Brain Res Cogn Brain Res*, **25**, 851–861.

Ebstein, R. P., Novick, O., Umansky, R., et al. (1996) Dopamine D4 receptor (D4DR) exon III polymorphism associated with the human personality trait of Novelty Seeking. *Nat Genet*, **12**, 78–80.

Grady, C. L., Keightley, M. L. (2002) Studies of altered social cognition in neuropsychiatric disorders using functional neuroimaging. *Can J Psychiatry*, **47**, 327–336.

http://science.jrank.org/pages/7739/Happiness-Pleasure-in-European-Thought.html (2008) Happiness and Pleasure in European Thought – The Hellenistic Era, The Medieval View, Modern Views On Happiness, Act Utilitarianism, Rule Utilitarianism.

Merriam-Webster (2008) In *Merriam-Webster On-Line Dictionary*.

Newman, D. L., Tellegen, A., Bouchard, T. J., Jr. (1998) Individual differences in adult ego development: Sources of influence in twins reared apart. *J Pers Soc Psychol*, **74**, 985–995.

Okuyama, Y., Ishiguro, H., Nankai, M., et al. (2000) Identification of a polymorphism in the promoter region of DRD4 associated with the human novelty seeking personality trait. *Mol Psychiatry*, **5**, 64–69.

Ostir, G. V., Markides, K. S., Black, S. A., et al. (2000) Emotional well-being predicts subsequent functional independence and survival. *J Am Geriat Soc*, **48**, 473–478.

Park, N., Peterson, C., Seligman, M. E. (2004) Strengths of character and well-being. *J Social Clinical Psychology*, **23**, 603–619.

Peterson, C., Seligman, M. E. (2004) *Character Strengths and Virtues: A Handbook and Classification*. Oxford University Press, Oxford.

Pezawas, L., Meyer-Lindenberg, A., Drabant, E. M., et al. (2005) 5-HTTLPR polymorphism impacts human cingulated–amygdala interactions: A genetic susceptibility mechanism for depression. *Nat Neurosci*, **8**, 828–834.

Seligman, M. E. (1991) *Learned Optimism*. Simon & Schuster, New York.

Seligman, M. E. (2002) *Authentic Happiness*. Free Press, New York.

Shiraishi, H., Suzuki, A., Fukasawa, T., et al. (2006) Monoamine oxidase A gene promoter polymorphism affects novelty seeking and reward dependence in healthy study participants. *Psychiatr Genet*, **16**, 55–58.

Tellegen, A., Lykken, D. T., Bouchard, T. J., Jr., et al. (1988) Personality similarity in twins reared apart and together. *J Pers Soc Psychol*, **54**, 1031–1039.

Vaillant, G. E. (2003) Mental health. *Am J Psychiatry*, **160**, 1373–1384.

Van Gestel, S., Forsgren, T., Claes, S., et al. (2002) Epistatic effect of genes from the dopamine and serotonin systems on the temperament traits of novelty seeking and harm avoidance. *Mol Psychiatry*, **7**, 448–450.

Wilson, E. O. (1980) *Sociobiology* (Abridged edn). Belknap Press of Harvard University Press, Cambridge, MA.

Wise, R. A., Bozarth, M. A. (1985) Brain mechanisms of drug reward and euphoria. *Psychiatr Med*, **3**, 445–460.

Chapter 13
What Is Mental Illness?

Contents

13.1 Unhappiness

Mental illness is usually defined as conditions that interfere with the sense of well-being or function of the individual in emotional, behavioral, or cognitive spheres. Some have equated the lack of a sense of well-being, or unhappiness, per se, with mental illness with presumed biological underpinnings (Heller, 1999). Others have emphasized the role of societal power structure as the origins of unhappiness. For example, Smail defines a person as "a point in social space *through* which outside powers and influences flow, rather than an entity *within* which powers and influences originate" (Smail, 2001). He proposes a close relationship between love and power noting that as children, the form our loving takes is exacted by power. "The relatively helpless infant and child can no more choose the characteristics of those he or she is dependent on than can the family dog, and, uncomfortable as it might be to suggest, our learning to love contains a strong element of choiceless dependence." In memetic terms, then, the power memes possessed by and inflowing from the parental figures and the complementary memes of helplessness set the stage for unhappiness in the young child.

The structure of society itself as the cause of unhappiness has been articulated by others including Marcuse, Foucault, Lacan, and Sartre to whom existence itself is anxiogenic (Foucault, 2001; MacCannell and MacCannell, 1986; Marcuse, 1964, 1991; Stern, 1967). The demands of modern industrial society for conformity are considered to be structural causes of unhappiness, and according to Lacan, this power relationship is established with language itself, and in the pronouns – I, you, and he/she/it that define a power relationship among them. Of course, the structure of society and the power relationships are all transmitted to the individual in the form of memes and the dominant memes that "pull the strings" in society are the memes automatically accepted by the "culture" and, therefore, the individual brain without undergoing the filtering process of the executive function (see Chapter 11).

Anecdotally, when Freud and Jung were sailing to America to lecture on psychoanalysis, Freud remarked to Jung that they were bringing the "plague" to America. Lacan reportedly gave a new ending to this anecdote: Freud did not know at the time that even though they did bring *la peste* to America from Europe, America would send it right back in the form of a distorted emphasis on the ego and its adaptation to the business-like civilization of American rational democracy (MacCannell and MacCannell, 1986). This is as good a description as any of the infectious quality of memes (of psychoanalysis), and how the dominant societal memes in America attached themselves to the original psychoanalytic memes, mutated them, and returned them to Europe to infect European psychoanalysts.

Unhappiness, therefore, may be seen to be a universal condition arising from the experience of powerlessness as children and of continuing powerlessness of the individual and the masses vis-a-vis the powerful societal forces such as conformity, as well as symptoms of a biologically/genetically determined individual vulnerability.

There is clearly a continuum of emotional, behavioral, and cognitive spheres of function within and among individuals. For example, in terms of low mood, there is the continuum of euthymia – sadness – depressed mood – depressive syndrome. In the other direction is euthymia – pleasant mood – euphoria – hypomania – manic syndrome. So with behavior – from severe inhibition to impulsive explosive behavior; with awareness – from stupor to alertness to hypervigilance.

On the other hand, as we saw in the previous chapter, the neural circuits for pleasure/reward and fear/punishment are separate and discrete – thus certain stimuli could activate both circuits at the same time. As memes are clusters of memory neurons and are closely connected to and reinforced by emotions, a physical stimulus from outside or an incoming meme may activate separate existing memes that are associated with reward and fear circuits respectively. A percept may be both pleasant and unpleasant and in some cases, only one emotion may be conscious while the other circuit is also activated but remains unconscious. If such a state continues, then the continuous activation of the circuit that has not been conscious may result in a kindling phenomenon whereby a sudden and strong emotion becomes conscious.

The sense of well-being may be threatened or lost whenever there is perception. The firing of mirror neurons in a person while seeing a movie of a crying mother who lost a child will stimulate the limbic system resulting in sadness that overtakes previous euthymic mood, empathy ensues and the sense of well-being is for the moment disrupted (Agnew et al., 2007; Dapretto et al., 2006; Gazzola et al., 2006; Ramachandran and Oberman, 2006; Rizzolatti and Craighero, 2004; Shmuelof and Zohary, 2007). Is this mental illness? It could be if the person in question sees sad movies continuously and does nothing but cry. More likely, however, the person in question will function normally after leaving the theater, thus the temporary sadness would not be an illness. On the other hand, there are persons who habitually get into situations that cause mild to moderate sadness. Such persons might be called mildly ill or *neurotic*.

At a certain point in the continuum, an autonomous psychiatric syndrome may be triggered as we will discuss in Chapter 14. Unlike mild mental illness or neurosis, an autonomous psychiatric syndrome represents a frankly pathologic state usually not reversible without definitive and potent treatment usually involving drugs.

13.2 Memes and Mental Illness

We likened mental health to a well-functioning memetic democracy in which there is an overall sense of coherence while there is competition and tolerance of different memes within it. In a democracy, there is always debate and tension, at times to an uncomfortable degree. At what point does conflict and tension become unhealthy and thus become an illness?

Reasoned argument, persuasion, and compromise are essential in conflict resolution in a democracy. When the brain lacks sufficiently powerful reasoning ability (the ability to manipulate the memes), or when competing memes are intransigent and are unable to reach an agreed-upon course of action based on compromise, then the conflict becomes irresolvable and severe anxiety ensues.

Of course, there are some brains in which democracy never takes hold. In such brains, there may be a tyranny of an irrational dominant selfplex that represses all incompatible or questioning memes. As new memes always seep into the brain one way or another, e.g., in conversations with others, and particularly through the printed and electronic media, the selfplex must invest an inordinate amount of energy in suppressing the incoming memes lest they take hold and collaborate with existing suppressed memes to start a revolution. Individuals with tyrannical selfplexes are particularly intolerant of others' views that may differ from them and thus are threatening to inject them with different memes. Such individuals, however, are subject to sudden reversals of their fanatical views, which represents a revolution within the memetic brain.

Some individuals have a tyrannical selfplex that is severely repressive because it is very fragile and constantly in a state of threatened overthrow. The subversive selfplex in such a brain may be an even more repressive and depressive one, a repository of all unacceptable and derogatory memes. When such a fragile selfplex is overturned through new meme infusion (e.g., failure memes) under stress, the new selfplex may manifest severe depression. Such a memetic revolution may also result in a paralysis of the executive function, i.e., the ability to manipulate memes, resulting in psychotic disorganization.

In these instances, the memes may trigger off an epigenetic cascade resulting in a major psychiatric syndrome (see Chapter 14).

13.3 Culture and Mental Illness

Culture affects the symptoms of mental illness as well as the diagnosis, access to treatment, and quality of treatment of mental illness (Satcher, 2001). According to the Surgeon General's Report of 2001, disproportionate numbers of African Americans are represented in the most vulnerable segments of the population – people who are homeless, incarcerated, in the child welfare system, victims of trauma – all populations with increased risks for mental disorders. As many as 40% of Hispanic Americans report limited English language proficiency. Because few mental health-care providers identify themselves as Spanish speaking, most Hispanic Americans have limited access to ethnically or linguistically similar providers. The suicide rate among American Indians/Alaska natives is 50% higher than the national rate; rates of co-occurring mental illness and substance abuse (especially alcohol) are also higher among native youth and adults. Because few data have been collected, the full nature, extent, and sources of these disparities remain a matter of conjecture. Asian Americans/Pacific Islanders who seek care for a mental illness often present with more severe illnesses than do other racial or ethnic groups. This, in part, suggests that stigma and shame are critical deterrents to service utilization. It is also possible that mental illnesses may be undiagnosed or not treated early in their course because they are expressed in symptoms of a physical nature.

Indeed, in Asian culture, patients with depression are more likely to present to the physician with pain and abdominal discomfort, and there are certain culturally accepted "psychosomatic diseases" such as Hwa-Byung or fire-illness in Korea (Lin, 1983; Park et al., 2001, 2002). Koro and Latah are also culture-specific syndromes (see Chapter 3).

Culture is the meme pool in which the brain resides, and it is not surprising that the prevalent memes in the pool should infect the brains and determine both the symptoms and help-seeking behavior.

In each culture and subculture, there are prevalent memes that represent how a person behaves or feels given a psychiatric condition. Thus, a depressed person may withdraw and isolate self in one culture, in another, she may cry out aloud and act in bizarre ways, and yet in another, have serious headaches. The prevalent meme in one culture may be seeing a shaman when ill, in another, seeing a psychiatrist, yet in another, receiving acupuncture.

The prevalent meme in one culture for the cause of depression may be retribution for a past sin, in another, an angry ancestor's spirit, and yet in another, an imbalance in neurotransmitters.

Culture also determines what is normal and deviant within the meme pool, i.e., what is acceptable and what is considered to be unacceptable. For example, in certain indigenous cultures, hearing ancestors' spirits may be a normal and, therefore, an acceptable phenomenon while such auditory hallucinations would be considered pathologic in other cultures. When a dominant memeplex in a culture pathologizes any competing memes, as in the case of the abuse of psychiatry in the Soviet Union when political dissidents were diagnosed with "sluggish schizophrenia," then the culture itself, like a tyrannical reign in a brain, may be called pathologic.

While the contribution of culture, or prevalent memes in the regional meme pool, must be recognized, we must also recognize that there is a global meme pool in the modern world. Very few brains in the twenty-first century have pure cultures of regional memes – most brains contain memes from other cultures and the global memes of rationality and science.

By reinforcing the rational memes in the brain through education and publicity, we may be able to attenuate the provincial cultural memes that tend to distort or minimize the suffering from mental illness, and facilitate appropriate help-seeking behavior.

13.4 Mental Illness and Psychiatric Syndromes

Mental illness ranges from universal unhappiness arising from the human condition to serious distortions of reality in the form of delusions and hallucinations. Somewhere in between the two extremes is *neurosis*, a term no longer recognized by the Diagnostic and Statistical Manual of the American Psychiatric Association, but is nevertheless descriptive of mild to moderate degree of suffering by afflicted individuals.

Neurosis, often manifest by moderate anxiety and/or depression, is generally considered to be a result of developmental hang-ups and faulty learning. Any number of developmental theories, Freudian, Jungian, Eriksonian, etc., can provide clues to the repeated traumas and failure or inadequacy in mastering the demands of the developmental stage resulting in residual unconscious conflicts and faulty patterns of expectations and behavior.

Developmental task can be conceptualized as the integration of newly introduced and newly arising memes with the needs of unfolding genes. Neurosis denotes a state of the brain where the mutually incompatible and conflicting memes and memes representing genetic needs have not found a workable modus vivendi, where workable democracy has not developed in the brain. There may be an authoritarian brain state where a large number of memes that are potentially salutary are in a state of severe suppression; or a state of near anarchy where competing memes and selfplexes achieve ephemeral dominance.

Repeated exposure to fear and violence memes in childhood, when the meme-processing faculties of the brain are not fully developed, may render the brain susceptible to replication of these traumatic memes and further stunt the growth of the executive function, which is best nurtured with safety and safe-exploration memes. When any attempt at exploration and initiative is met with violence and trauma, fear memes and violence memes will replicate.

When a revolution overthrows an authoritarian memetic regime, anarchy often results as the dominant selfplexes did not condone the coexistence of viable alternative selfplexes to take over in an orderly fashion as in a democracy. The anarchy of conflicting memes may generate overewhelming anxiety, which in turn may trigger a gene-driven cascade into a final common pathway psychiatric syndrome.

The *final common pathway psychiatric syndromes* are serious conditions reflecting a pathologic brain state that, without treatment, results in an autonomous course and often chronic outcome. Major depression, manic-depressive bipolar syndromes, panic anxiety, and psychoses are the major examples of final common pathway syndromes. In all these syndromes, the meme-processing executive function of the brain is severely impaired, and thus general reduction in meme proliferation as well as directly gene-oriented therapy is necessary.

Psychiatric symptoms and syndromes may be classified in several functional clusters of continuum as follows, which will be discussed in more detail in Part IV:

A. Attention-cognition spectrum syndromes (delirium, dementia, impulse control syndromes, ADHD, antisocial personality, obsessive-compulsive personality traits, obsessive-compulsive syndrome)
B. Fear–anxiety–depression spectrum syndromes (anxiety, panic, ASD, PTSD, depression – neurotic and syndromic, borderline syndrome, mania, adjustment disorders, avoidant traits and personality, phobias)
C. Reality perception spectrum syndromes (psychosis, dissociation, conversion, somatoform, misattribution somatization)
D. Pleasure-motivation spectrum syndromes (substance use/abuse, addictions to substances and beliefs, fanaticism)
E. Primary memetic syndromes (eating disorders, factitious syndromes, malingering, meme-directed irrational Acts)

References

Agnew, Z. K., Bhakoo, K. K., Puri, B. K. (2007) The human mirror system: A motor resonance theory of mind-reading. *Brain Res Rev*, **54**, 286–293.
Dapretto, M., Davies, M. S., Pfeifer, J. H., et al. (2006) Understanding emotions in others: Mirror neuron dysfunction in children with autism spectrum disorders. *Nat Neurosci*, **9**, 28–30.
Foucault, M. (2001) *The Order of Things: An Archaeology of the Human Sciences*. Foucault, London.
Gazzola, V., Aziz-Zadeh, L., Keysers, C. (2006) Empathy and the somatotopic auditory mirror system in humans. *Curr Biol*, **16**, 1824–1829.
Heller, L. M. (1999) *Biological Unhappiness*. Dyslimbia Press, Okeechobee, FL.
Lin, K. M. (1983) Hwa-Byung: A Korean culture-bound syndrome? *Am J Psychiatry*, **140**, 105–107.
MacCannell, J. F., MacCannell, J. (1986) *Figuring Lacan: Criticism and the Cultural Unconscious*. Routledge, London.
Marcuse, H. (1964, 1991) *One-Dimensional Man: Studies in the Ideology of Advanced Industrial Society*. Beacon Press, Boston.
Park, Y. J., Kim, H. S., Kang, H. C., et al. (2001) A survey of Hwa-Byung in middle-age Korean women. *J Transcult Nurs*, **12**, 115–122.
Park, Y. J., Kim, H. S., Schwartz-Barcott, D., et al. (2002) The conceptual structure of hwa-byung in middle-aged Korean women. *Health Care Women Int*, **23**, 389–397.
Ramachandran, V. S., Oberman, L. M. (2006) Broken mirrors: A theory of autism. *Sci Am*, **295**, 62–69.
Rizzolatti, G., Craighero, L. (2004) The mirror-neuron system. *Annu Rev Neurosci*, **27**, 169–192.

Satcher, D. (2001) Mental health: Culture, race and ethnicity – Supplement to Surgeon General's Report.

Shmuelof, L., Zohary, E. (2007) Watching others' actions: Mirror representations in the parietal cortex. *Neuroscientist*, **13**, 667–672.

Smail, D. (2001) *The Nature of Unhappiness*. Robinson, London.

Stern, A. (1967) *Sartre, His Philosophy and Existential Psychoanalysis*. Delacorte Press, New York.

Part III
Principles of Diagnosis and Treatment of Mental Illness

Chapter 14
Psychiatric Diagnosis: Toward a Memetic–Epigenetic Multiaxial Model

Contents

14.1 Psychiatric Diagnosis and Problems with DSM

In Chapter 1, I described the evolving model of mental illness as a result of epigenesis, the turning on and off of genes in interaction with environment. In Chapter 2, we examined how stress, newly introduced memes that interact with resident memes in the brain, causes changes in genes and brain structures. In the subsequent chapters, we examined the nature of memes as brain code and how culture as memetic pools affect mental health and illness. We saw that memes as neural connections are the actual agents of culture affecting genes and physiology. In this chapter, we will consider briefly the history of psychiatric diagnosis and then

H. Leigh, *Genes, Memes, Culture, and Mental Illness*,
DOI 10.1007/978-1-4419-5671-2_14, © Hoyle Leigh, 2010

discuss what rational psychiatric diagnostic scheme should be in the light of gene ×
meme × environment interaction.

A widely accepted diagnostic scheme is the official diagnostic scheme of the
American Psychiatric Association, *The Diagnostic and Statistical Manual of Mental
Disorders (DSM)*. The fist DSM, published in 1952, was based on Adolf Meyer's
psychobiology, a model that prominently posited the interaction among constitution,
personality, and environment (Meyer and Winters, 1950). Psychiatric disorders were
considered to be *reactions* of the personality in adapting to environmental demands.
Both DSM I and DSM II (published in 1968) were based on the then prevailing etiologic theory – psychodynamics. DSM III, published in 1980, was a frank admission
of the inadequacy of the psychodynamic model as it attempted to redefine psychiatric diagnoses as research questions rather than coherent entities. By adopting an
"atheoretical" model, it dropped the psychodynamic view of etiology and the notion
of neurosis, that there is a continuum of psychiatric problems or conflicts between
the normal and the psychiatrically ill. It adopted, to a large measure, the "research
criteria for psychiatric diagnosis" that was designed to choose "pure cultures" of
major psychiatric disorders for genetic research (Feighner et al., 1972). DSM III
and its direct successor, DSM IV (1994), classify major psychiatric syndromes into
mutually exclusive categories (e.g., schizophrenia vs. schizoaffective disorder) presumably based on the notion of different genetic underpinnings. Though it claimed
to be atheoretical, it thus implicitly adopted a biological/genetic model of psychiatric syndromes. Another outstanding feature of DSM III and IV is the multiaxial
system of diagnosis – Axis I: Major psychiatric syndromes, Axis II: Personality disorders and developmental disorders, Axis III: Medical diseases, Axis IV: Stressors,
Axis V: Global assessment of functioning (GAF). This system explicitly makes the
important declaration that psychiatric syndromes and medical diseases coexist in a
patient, and has made important contributions in avoiding the "either physical or all
in the head" notion of a symptom.

DSM III and IV have helped foster psychiatric research by defining reliable
populations for study. This fortuitously coincided with the rapid development in
molecular biology and genetics, psychopharmacology, neuroimaging, and the com-
pletion of the Human Genome Project. If we can define a "pure culture" of a genetic
syndrome, we are now in a position to understand its genetic underpinnings.

The multiaxial system of DSM III and IV, in addition to recognizing the coexistence of medical and psychiatric conditions, has also pioneered the notion that
diagnosis is more than the listing of diseases but also includes the personality aspect
of the patient, as well as the role of stress and the level of functioning. It is an attempt
to diagnose the *patient*, not merely the disease.

On the negative side, the problems include: confusion concerning the categories
and criteria for diagnosis, confusion concerning the distinction between Axis I and
Axis II, and confusion concerning the nature and function of multiaxial diagnosis.

Confusion concerning categories: Any clinician attempting to use DSM III and
IV realizes that the diagnostic criteria are arbitrary. While it is possible to assign a
patient mechanically to one diagnosis or another, it often makes no clinical sense.
We often realize that there are patients who almost meet the criteria, or meet most of

the criteria for more than one category. Examples include the differentiation between schizophrenia and schizoaffective disorder, making the diagnosis of borderline personality disorder, and classifying psychosis in a patient with the history of both schizophrenia and substance use. Genetic research of probands with the categorical diagnoses has shown that, in fact, these categories are *heterogeneous*, that many different genes may underlie the same category such as schizophrenia and bipolar disorder (Cheng et al., 2006; Prathikanti and Weinberger, 2005) and that one or a few genes may underlie many different categories such as bipolar disorder, schizoaffective disorder, and schizophrenia (Caspi et al., 2002, 2003; Craddock et al., 2006; Hamshere et al., 2005; Murphy et al., 2004). It seems clear that attempting to find the biological underpinnings of current categorical diagnoses is a wrong approach. The "biological underpinnings" have been shown to be for brain states and traits that may be associated with a variety of psychological/functional predispositions and deserving of a status independent of specific Axis I diagnosis.

Confusion concerning distinction between Axis I and Axis II: What is the distinction between a personality disorder and a major psychiatric disorder? Is schizophrenia not a developmental, personality disorder? Where does a borderline personality with a psychotic episode belong in this scheme? Genetic studies have also shown that there may be a continuum between personality disorder and a major psychiatric syndrome, e.g., borderline personality and bipolar disorder (Akiskal et al., 2003; Smith et al., 2004).

Confusion concerning the nature and function of multiaxial diagnosis: What is the multiaxial diagnosis the diagnosis of? Axes I and II are diagnostic categories with explicit criteria, Axis III is diagnosis without explicit criteria, Axis IV is a list of stressors, Axis V is a scale. Axes IV and V are, strictly speaking, not diagnoses at all. What is the overarching framework for this laundry list? What are the functions of Axes IV and V in a diagnostic scheme?

The problems of DSM III and IV are rooted in two major areas. One is that it is based on a conceptually faulty notion that psychiatric illnesses are categorical and discrete. Second is that the multiaxial system is a hodge podge of interesting and important areas to consider in making a diagnosis that lack conceptual rigor.

Discussing these problems with the current DSM, McHugh (McHugh, 2001, 1992, 2005; McHugh and Slavney, 1998) called for a rethinking of psychiatric diagnosis along the *perspectives* of disease, dimensions, behavior, and life story. He proposed that mental illnesses be considered in four, non-mutually exclusive clusters – (1) disease (e.g., schizophrenia), (2) psychological vulnerabilities (e.g., emotional stability), (3) behavior (e.g., alcoholism), and (4) distress evoked by events (e.g., grief).

Some (Genova, 2003) have called for "dumping" of DSM altogether in favor of disease codes of ICD 10.

The overarching problem of current DSM is that it lacks a coherent conceptual model of psychiatric illness, that in the light of modern understanding, it is behind the times. In view of the advantages of DSM discussed above, however, what is called for is a reconceptualization, not abandonment, of the multiaxial model of diagnosis.

14.2 What Is Diagnosis?

Diagnosis derives from the Greek *dia*, meaning through or across, and *gnosis*, meaning knowing. Knowing Through, Knowing Across *What?* Hippocrates, the father of medicine, believed "with regard to diseases, the circumstances from which we make the diagnosis are – by attending to the general nature of all, and the peculiar nature of each individual – to the disease, the patient, and the applications – to the person who applies them... the patient's habits, regimen, and pursuits...thoughts, sleep, or absence of sleep, and sometimes his dreams..." (Hippocrates: Of the Epidemics, Section III)(Hippocrates). Diagnosis must be the knowing of the *whole* of the patient. DSM III and IV were attempts toward this goal, though the goal was not explicitly stated, and thus suffered conceptual confusion.

The diagnosis of the whole of the patient must explicitly define the suffering dimension of the patient, *the illness*, and the contributing morphological, physiological, biochemical, genetic *disease or conditions*, the *memes and stresses* that interacted with them, and the *assets* of the patient that protect or mitigate against the noxious forces.

Illness is by definition memetic, i.e., how a person experiences suffering and expresses suffering is determined by prevailing belief systems and imitation of those who suffer from ailments. Illness is often the manifestation of a strife and/or revolution within the patient's memetic brain, caused by stress or other weakening of the dominant selfplexes, resulting in the upsurge of hitherto repressed aspects of the personality.

Medical diagnosis in the last century underwent a major transformation, i.e., from syndromic (illness) to etiologic (disease), largely due to advances in genetics and biochemistry. This spectacularly successful reductionistic approach, however, often led to a lamentable neglect of the patient as a person. Should psychiatry follow the footsteps of medicine? The multiaxial diagnosis in psychiatry potentially allows us to avoid the pitfalls of replacing illness with disease. For psychiatry, at least, both illness and disease have to be recognized and treated. Currently, however, all Axes I and II diagnoses are syndromes, and, as we have noted, each syndrome probably has a number of different genetic/neuroscience underpinnings (disease), each of which, in turn, gives rise to *different combinations of syndromes* depending on developmental history. For example, the 5-HTTLPR *s/s* may underlie depressive syndrome, anxiety syndrome, risk-aversive personality, and irritable bowel syndrome (see Chapter 1 for further discussion of 5-HTTLPR). Should 5-HTTLPR *s/s* replace all of the syndromes as an etiologic diagnosis, at the expense of knowing what the patient's suffering is?

We need a separate axis for the psychiatric illness, the *memetic,* phenomenological, experiential dimension of the patient, such as depression, anxiety, and psychosis *and* a separate axis for the genetic/neuroscience disease diagnosis. The differential diagnosis of the syndrome, e.g., depression, would not be major depression vs. bipolar disorder vs. schizoaffective disorder vs. mood disorder secondary to general medical condition vs. substance-induced mood disorder. The differential diagnosis would instead be: what are the factors that resulted in a memetic revolution or memetic war within the brain? What is the extent of contributions to the depressive syndrome by the specific brain dysfunction, to what extent did specific genes and early experiences contribute to the brain's vulnerability to dysfunction, what is the extent substances may also have contributed, to what extent did recent stresses also contribute, are there psychosocial support systems that may be mitigating the extent of depressive memes and thus the depressive syndrome?

When the existence of a genetic/neuroscience disturbance is apparent, then a differential diagnosis of this condition should occur following the medical model. This approach will firmly establish the notion that both the illness (memes) and the disease require attention and care. This approach would also apply to general medicine.

14.3 Psychiatric Diagnosis: Dysregulation and Final Common Pathway Syndromes, Resurrection of Neurosis

As discussed above, medical diagnosis saw a shift from syndromic diagnoses (e.g., consumption, grippe) to etiologic and laboratory diagnosis (e.g., tuberculosis, Type I diabetes mellitus, hyperlipidemia). With the advent of DSM III and IV, it was hoped that the psychiatric disorders, as with medical illnesses, would give way to discrete etiologic diagnoses underlying them, perhaps, schizophrenia Type I that would turn out to be associated with a discrete gene mutation. Research has shown, however, that there are numerous "vulnerability" genes that subserve normal functions but may also, in some instances, cause certain aspects of a syndrome (e.g., psychosis in mood disorders, depression in anxious patients).

Our new model is a continuum model with genetic endowment for adaptive function that may become dysfunctional. Of course, there are exceptions, such as a detrimental mutation. There is also the possibility of *cliff edge phenomenon*, where an increased expression of an evolutionarily adaptive genetic trait may reach a point of sudden maladaptiveness, perhaps as in the case of vigilance (Nesse, 2004).

Most psychiatric conditions are syndromes of dysregulation. The dysregulation may be a reflection of memetic conflict or memetic turmoil, or it may reflect an epigenetically unstable limbic structure, which in turn is activated by incoming memes. Anxiety is normal and necessary, but when it becomes panic, and repeated without provocation, it is dysregulated anxiety and needs treatment. So is sadness and depression, vigilance and paranoia, creativity, "out of the box thinking" and psychosis. So is brave exploration and antisociality. The sharp distinction between normality and psychiatric disorder, and one psychiatric disorder from another, of DSM III and IV has served its purpose in obtaining reliable syndromic populations to study. The syndromes turned out to be continuums and genetically heterogeneous. We must discard the categorical approach. We should also recognize personality traits and symptoms that border between normality and serious autonomous psychiatric syndromes. I suggest resurrecting the term *neurosis*.

Discarding the categorical approach does not mean that we should not have a line of distinction between neurosis and major psychiatric syndromes. Major psychiatric syndromes, such as the depressive syndrome and psychosis, however, should be a designation of the expectable autonomous course of the illness rather than mutually exclusive categories. Such major psychiatric syndromes are final common pathway syndromes that reflect a common brain functional pathology (e.g., hyperactive D2 receptors in the mesolimbic system) with heterogeneous genetic, biochemical, and memetic contributions (e.g., drug induced psychosis). One patient may have multiple psychiatric syndromes as well as neuroses.

Neurosis serves as an intermediate diagnosis between normality and major final common pathway syndromes and would encompass various traits and symptoms that represent gene × meme interaction (interaction includes simple additive effect as well as synergy and mitigation) and early learned behaviors. Neurosis would include such symptom complexes and personality patterns as generalized anxiety, phobias, minor depression, schizotypal and avoidant personalities and the borderline syndrome.

The evidence that psychotherapy affects the brain function/structure (Goldapple et al., 2004; Kandel, 1979, 1998; Paquette et al., 2003; Roffman et al., 2005) further provides the necessity to reintroduce the notion of neurosis as the psychotherapy thereof may actually prevent the full development of a major syndrome, as would other preventive measures such as social support and protection of children from violence and abuse.

There is overwhelming evidence that social support mitigates against stress and the precipitation, maintenance, and prognosis of symptoms of major psychiatric disorders (Brugha, 1995; Norman et al., 2005; Silver et al., 2006; Surkan et al., 2006).

The multiaxial system begun with DSM III has to be modified to be compatible with the new model, and should be a *diagnosis* in its original sense, i.e., a thorough knowing of the patient.

The new system should clearly delineate the phenomenological/memetic illness dimension of the patient from the potential genomic/brain morphological and functional states and the interacting stresses and protective assets of the patient. The new system, therefore, must have three new entities reflected in the axes: (1) the genomic/brain morphological/functional dimension, which we will call the genoneuroscience diagnosis, (2) early, recent, and current stress, and (3) the protective psychosocial assets of the patient.

In addition, the new system should have a separate axis for *formulation*, an integration of the entries in all the axes in managing the person who is the patient.

14.4 Proposal for a New DSM Scheme

I propose that the axes of the new DSM consist of the following:

Axis I: Memetic/phenomenological (neurophysiomemetic) diagnosis: psychiatric syndromes, traits, and symptoms, based on deviations of normal brain function.

Axis II: Geno-neuroscience diagnosis: genes, brain morphology, biochemistry and pathology, functional changes and conditions independent of, but potentially influencing Axes I and III.

Axis III: Medical diseases and condition.

Axis IV: Stresses – childhood, recent past, and current.

Axis V: Psychosocial assets: protecting and/or mitigating against disease and functional state, past 5 years and current.

Axis VI: Biopsychosocial and epigenetic formulation.

Each axis is conceptualized to influence each other and provides a snapshot of the major factors that must be considered in the pathogenesis and/or management of Axes I and II.

14.4.1 Axis I: Memetic/Phenomenological (Neurophysiomemetic) Diagnosis: Psychiatric Syndromes, Symptoms, and Traits, Based on Deviations of Normal Brain Function

This axis will represent the phenomenological *psychiatric illness* of the patient. This approach accepts the suffering dimension of the patient on its own level, no matter what the underlying etiology. The emphasis here is what memes are emitted by the patient, and what dysfunctional memes may be out of control within the brain. The diagnostic terms will be familiar psychiatric syndromes, but the memetic nature of diagnosis has to be considered.

I suggest that the syndromes be classified in six broad categories based on deviations of normal brain function in a continuum of severity and manifestation.

A. Attention-cognition spectrum syndromes (delirium, dementia, impulse control syndromes, ADHD, antisocial personality, obsessive-compulsive personality traits, obsessive-compulsive syndrome).

B. Fear–anxiety–depression Spectrum Syndromes (anxiety, panic, phobias, ASD, PTSD, borderline personality, dependent and avoidant personalities, social phobia, bipolarity and mania, depression – neurotic and syndromic, adjustment disorders).

C. Reality perception spectrum syndromes (psychosis, dissociation, conversion, somatoform, misattribution somatization).

D. Pleasure-motivation spectrum syndromes (substance use/abuse, addictions to substances and beliefs, fanaticism).

E. Primary memetic syndromes (eating disorders, factitious disorders, malingering, meme-directed destructive behaviors).

These categories are not mutually exclusive, and each entity within the categories may have subtypes and degrees of severity specified. For example, anxiety-situational, anxiety neurosis, major depression, psychosis – acute, Type I, bipolar syndrome – Type I, cognitive syndrome – delirium superimposed on dementia.

See Part IV for further discussion of each of the categories.

Currently, Axis I diagnosis is of limited value in psychopharmacology as the drugs are the same for most cases of schizophrenia, schizoaffective disorder, bipolar disorder, major depression, etc. The reason for this is that the categories do not overlap but the symptoms (phenomenology) for which treatment is directed do. Thus, it makes better sense to classify Axis I in large clusters of symptoms for which symptomatic treatment may be indicated.

Axis I often indicates a state of pathologic *replication* of memes such as anxiety and depression. The cause of replication of the memes may be an overwhelming influx of new memes (situational), the continuing conflict among resident relatively dormant memes causing ebb and flow of replication, or reawakening of some dormant memes causing new conflict with dominant ones (neurotic), or may be a final common pathway major psychiatric syndrome from a culmination of any of the memetic and genetic factors (syndromic). It may also be a primary memetic syndrome based on imitation, such as malingering, factitious syndromes, or suicide bombing.

The diagnoses in Axis I can and often would be overlapping. Thus, a patient could be diagnosed with obsessive-compulsive personality trait; obsessive-compulsive syndrome; depression, neurotic; and depression, syndromic. The diagnosis would not use rigid diagnostic criteria but list one or more characteristic features that may be memetic (e.g., low self-esteem) or physical signs (e.g., anorexia). This scheme is compatible with current medical diagnostic practice where hypertension, hyperlipidemia, edema, nephrotic syndrome, diabetic nephropathy, and Type II diabetes mellitus might be diagnosed in the same patient.

Who should make Axis I diagnosis? As currently is the practice, any qualified mental health professional should be able to make the phenomenological Axis I diagnosis, unlike Axis II diagnosis below, which should be made only by a qualified medical professional.

14.4.2 Axis II: Geno-Neuroscience Diagnosis: Genes (Including Family History of Psychiatric Illness), Brain Morphology, Biochemistry and Pathology, Functional Changes and Conditions Potentially Influencing Axis I

I expect that this category will be a work in progress for a while as potential diagnoses in this axis have so far been thought of as mere biological underpinnings of Axis I. As discussed above, Axis I syndromes should be conceptualized as symptomatic manifestations of heterogeneous entities, some with major geno-neurobiological and epigenetic contribution, and others with much more contribution by situational and memetic factors. Thus, Axis II should not be conceptualized merely as biological underpinnings of Axis I, but rather independent genetic/neurobiologic diagnoses that may or may not contribute to the behavioral/emotional phenotype in Axis I. In fact, it may explain Axes III and V rather than Axis I as in a patient with irritable bowel syndrome and 5-HTTLPR *s/s* genotype whose anxiety is only moderate. In fact, some Axis II diagnoses are more likely to be the biological underpinnings of psychological and physical *dispositions* equally relevant to medicine and psychiatry. By establishing Axis II as an independent dimension for geno-neurobiological state, we can eschew the unnecessary argument as to whether the psychiatric syndrome in Axis I is "biological" or "psychological" in origin. It also obviates the futile quest for finding the biological underpinnings of arbitrarily defined Axis I disorders (Frances and Egger, 1999).

For Axis II, we may be initially content with neurobiologic findings on imaging and known genetic factors, e.g., low hippocampal volume and enlarged amygdala, hyperactive subgenual anterior cingulate, 5-HTTLPR *s/s*.

The entities in Axis II would eventually illuminate, together with Axis IV, how Axes I, III, and V may have evolved as well as suggesting potential intervention specifically designed for the neurocircuit dysfunction which may be both pharmacologic and psychotherapeutic. Until such refinements occur, any identifiable putative biological factors should be listed here, including gene variations as in 5-HTTLPR, MAOA, and DAT1. It should also include abnormalities in brain imaging studies including MRI, fMRI, SPECT, PET, and CT. Significant family history of psychiatric illness should be also noted here.

These conceptualizations of Axes I and II will promote research as tests for associations and correlations among items between the axes are likely to reveal new ways in which psychiatric syndromes, personality traits, etc., are associated with specific genes and specific areas and functions of the brain.

14.4.3 Axis III: Medical Diseases and Conditions

This axis would list medical conditions and diseases that may coexist with the mental condition.

14.4.4 Axis IV: Stresses: Childhood, Recent, and Current

Entries in this axis are the factors that potentially contributed to the personality trait and neuroses and may have set the stage for the major psychiatric syndrome in Axis I. In contrast to DSM IV, I propose that we specifically list major stresses in childhood, as well as recent and current stressors.

14.4.5 Axis V: Psychosocial Assets and Recent/Current
            Functioning

A thorough knowing of the patient is not possible without considering the assets as well as liabilities of the patient. This axis should provide information about the protective and mitigating factors for health rather than illness. They would include intelligence, educational level, school and work history, and social support. I would propose maintaining the global assessment of functioning of the current DSM at the end of Axis V, but extend the GAF for past year to past 5 years to account for functioning before recent stresses in Axis IV, to express it in a single fractional number: Previous 5 years GAF/ Current GAF. Expressed as: 70/40.

14.4.6 Axis VI: Biopsychosocial and Epigenetic Formulation

This axis is an integration of the previous five axes as they apply to the person who is the patient. Genetic factors such as family history should be considered in the light of early memetic experiences including abuse and nurturing. The illness on Axis I, neurobiologic findings on Axis II and physical conditions in Axis III should be integrated with recent and current stressors, social support, and functioning levels in Axes IV and V. This integrated formulation should lead to a rational memetic and genetic management plan for the patient.

14.5 An Illustrative Case

A 48-year-old married Hispanic female, currently unemployed, was admitted to the medical service for exacerbation of gastroenteritis. A psychiatric consultation was requested because she was observed crying, and stating that life was not worthwhile living.

Medical history revealed that the patient developed gastroenteritis from an early age, with frequent bouts of diarrhea and abdominal pain. She had multiple medical admissions for this. She was also diagnosed with hepatitis C associated with intravenous drug use. Upon admission, she had hyponatremia and hypokalemia, which have been corrected. Her liver function test was within upper normal limits.

Psychiatric consultation interview revealed that the patient has long-standing depression with bouts of exacerbation, as well as nightmares and flashbacks of childhood abuse of several years' duration, including physical and sexual abuse. She was second of six siblings, had never known her biological father, had been abused by her stepfather. Her mother and stepfather were both migrant field workers. She had dropped out of school in the eleventh grade to be married to an abusive husband, which resulted in a divorce within 2 years. She used many substances since the age of 14, including alcohol, marijuana, heroin, and methamphetamine. After her divorce, she worked in various menial jobs and obtained her GED by attending an adult school. She then attended a school to become a cosmetician and worked in that capacity for several years, and married her current husband, who is a mechanic and a caring, non-abusive person, and had two daughters. She had by then stopped using substances heavily.

Her family history revealed very little concerning her biological father, whom she never knew, other than that he used substances. Her mother was described as being an ineffectual person who was unable to protect the patient from the abusive stepfather. Her mother also had bouts of depression, and was considered to be a very rigid, religious, and superstitious person. The family was Catholic. The patient herself had been religious and attended church regularly until about 2 years ago, but currently she does not as she "lost faith."

The patient had very little contact with her mother or stepfather since she left home, but she knows that they both died about 5 years ago. Her older daughter, age 18, was killed in an automobile accident 2 years ago, after which her gastroenteritis flared up, and she had to stop working. She started using methamphetamine heavily again. Upon questioning, the patient admitted that she is currently undergoing menopause, and has hot flashes and mood changes. She is not on hormone replacement therapy.

The patient's husband describes the patient as a loving but anxious person, who tends to become preoccupied with worries, and tends to become compulsive when stressed. For example, she would clean the house several times a day, call her husband and daughter several times a day to make sure they are OK. He also noted that the patient's gastrointestinal problems get worse when she is anxious, particularly since the tragic death of their daughter. He also stated that the patient frequently wakes up from sleep with nightmares and that she has been using methamphetamine especially since their daughter's death.

Mental status examination revealed a rather thin Hispanic woman appearing her stated age, wearing hospital attire. She showed rather labile affect, particularly when talking about her deceased daughter, her mood was depressed, and had passive thoughts of wishing she would die, had hopeless and helpless feelings. She admitted to an exacerbation of insomnia and nightmares, of seeing her deceased daughter as well as the patient's childhood abuse. Although the chart noted that the patient was disoriented upon admission, at the time of the interview, the patient was cognitively intact, and showed good abstraction and judgment.

Genetic testing revealed 5-HTTLPR s/s genotype, and CYP 450 2D6 poor metabolism.

Diagnosis

Axis I:

a. Posttraumatic stress disorder
   −first associated with childhood physical and sexual abuse,
   −exacerbated by abuse by first husband,
   −recently re-exacerbated by her daughter's death.
b. Depressive neurosis associated with 5-HTTLPR s/s and PTSD.
c. Depressive syndrome as exacerbation of above, precipitated by daughter's death, contributed by increased substance use and exacerbation of gastroenteritis, menopause.
d. Obsessive-compulsive traits, probably to ward off depression, mimetically associated with mother's obsessive-compulsive traits.
e. Polysubstance abuse, probably to self-treat depression, PTSD symptoms, and physical discomfort.

f. Probable delirium on admission, associated with electrolyte aberrations on admission, now resolved except for possibly labile affect, which may also be associated with menopause.

Axis II:

a. 5-HTTLPR *s/s*.
b. CYP 450 2D6 poor metabolizer.
c. Probable amygdalar hypersensitivity.

Axis III:

a. Chronic gastroenteritis associated with stress.
b. Electrolyte imbalance upon admission associated with above.
c. Hepatitis C associated with intravenous drug use.

Axis IV: Stresses

a. Stresses in childhood
   Childhood physical and sexual abuse
b. Stresses in early adulthood
   Physical abuse by first husband
c. Recent and Current Stresses
   Daughter's death 2 years ago
   Exacerbation of gastroenteritis
   Menopause

Axis V: Psychosocial Assets and Recent/Current Functioning

Assets:
   Supportive husband
   History of recovery from stress by attending adult school, getting GED, good employment history until death of daughter.

Function (last 5 years/current)
75/55

Axis VI: Formulation

The patient probably has by family history genetic predisposition for depression and obsessive-compulsive traits on her mother's side as well as at least substance abuse on her biological father's side. Further contributing to her depressive neurosis and tendency for depressive syndrome, as well as gastroenteritis, is her genetic status of 5-HTTLPR *s/s*. Further, her hepatitis C associated with early intravenous drug abuse and her status as a poor metabolizer of CYP 450 2D6 enzyme are considerations in using drugs that are metabolized by the liver.

For a patient with her genetic vulnerability to heightened stress response, her early memetic environment of migrant farmers was filled with memes for drug and alcohol abuse and domestic violence. Her stepfather was clearly infected with these memes and physically abused the patient as a child. This early childhood abuse caused an epigenetic cascade resulting in stress-responsive gastroenteritis as well as depressive and obsessive-compulsive neurosis, which led to polysubstance abuse as self-treatment for the symptoms, again an endemic meme, which unfortunately led to increased symptoms in the long run. The patient's inability to assert herself effectively may have been due to infection by her mother's religious memes, some of which may have infected the patient's tendency toward obsessive-compulsiveness. Nevertheless, the patient made surprisingly good adaptation by first divorcing her abusive first husband, then finishing her education, getting out of an abusive first marriage, and working productively as a cosmetologist, for which her obsessive-compulsive traits may have been put to good use. She also married a caring man and had two children. One wonders whether there may have been an unidentified beneficial memetic model for the patient during this period. Reconnecting with this memetic model may be an important factor in planning therapy.

The tragic loss of her older daughter due to a motor vehicle accident, however, resulted in a massive infusion of stress memes, overwhelming her meme-filtering function, and awakening dormant stress memes, resulting in an unchecked replication of hopeless and helpless memes, traumatic memes of physical and sexual abuse, finally culminating in a depressive syndrome as well as a severe exacerbation of gastroenteritis. Memes associated with menopause, such as the loss of reproductive function, may have contributed to the strengthening of her low self-esteem, and the physiologic concomitants of menopause such as hot flashes may have contributed to her lability of affect. Her delirium upon admission was of course a result of the electrolyte imbalance.

Therefore, the treatment planning should proceed at a multiple levels:
Treatment:

1. Depressive Syndrome, Depressive Neurosis:

   a. Gene-Oriented Rx:
      Depressive syndrome is a final common pathway syndrome requiring both gene- and meme-oriented treatments. In view of her hepatitis C and her CYP 2D6 poor metabolizer status, drugs that are metabolized by the liver, and especially by this enzyme must be used with caution. As she has severe insomnia, and her anorexia associated with her gastroenteritis and depression, an antidepressant that induces sleep and increases appetite, and has an alternative metabolic pathway to CYP 450 2D6 would be ideal. In view of her 5-HTTLPR *s/s* status, an SSRI may not be effective. Mirtazapine is a non-SSRI drug that has both serotonergic and noradrenergic action, induces sleep, and enhances appetite. It is metabolized by both CYP 450 2D6 as well as CYP 450 3A4, an alternative pathway to 2D6. While mirtazapine

is metabolized by the liver, her normal liver enzyme levels indicate that use of this drug is not contraindicated. Thus, mirtazapine 15 mg hs was recommended.

h. Meme-Oriented Rx:
The patient had overwhelming proliferation of depressive memes that had to be controlled. Hospitalization was recommended as a broad-spectrum meme-oriented therapy, to change the source of incoming memes in a controlled setting, and to provide augmentation of meme-filtering activity. Hospitalization also provides such diversionary activities as occupational and recreational therapy.

After the hospitalization, the patient should receive outpatient meme-oriented therapy which would include stress management techniques which would be conducive to both depressive syndrome and depressive neurosis, as well as the stress-responsive gastroenteritis. She should also receive specific memes as education concerning menopause. Cognitive-behavioral therapy geared to building self-esteem memes would be effective as well as interpersonal therapy directed to resolving the grief over her daughter's death.

2. PTSD
Gene-oriented therapies include use of antidepressants as described above. Specifically for the nightmares, Prazocin 1–6 mg per night may be tried. The patient received optimal relief with Prazocin 3 mg hs.

Meme-oriented therapies for PTSD would include all broad-spectrum meme-oriented therapies including stress management, relaxation training, music, and dance therapy, etc., as well as specific meme-oriented therapies such as recounting traumatic events with suppression of physiologic arousal with propranolol, cognitive-behavioral therapy, etc.

3. Obsessive-Compulsive Traits and Substance Abuse
In this patient, both obsessive-compulsive traits and substance abuse seem to be attempts to manage and self-treat depression and PTSD. Thus, the treatment of the latter conditions may resolve these conditions. Exploration and understanding of the memetic component of her obsessive compulsive traits as an imitation of her mother's coping strategy may be helpful, as well as her infection by her father's substance abuse memes that resulted in her hepatitis C. Providing alternative means of deriving pleasure, such as through relaxation training, music, dance, massage therapy, may be also helpful.

An avatar, constructed by the patient in collaboration with the therapist, who is endowed with the attributes that the patient wishes to achieve, may demonstrate to the patient that she can, indeed, emulate herself behaving and feeling self-confident, assertive, and in control in virtual reality, which will eventually transform itself into reality itself.

I wondered in the formulation above whether the patient had an unidentified memetic model during the period when she divorced her first husband and went back to school to become a cosmetologist. In fact, it turned out that the patient had made friends with an older woman, Rema, who was herself a cosmetologist. The patient had gradually lost contact with Rema who had moved to another city. When the patient was reminded of that relationship, she successfully reconnected with her and has weekly phone conversations with her. The patient considers talking with Rema regularly to be a great part of her current psychotherapy.

Note: This chapter is largely based on a paper entitled, *A proposal for a new multiaxial model of psychiatric diagnosis. A continuum-based patient model derived from evolutionary developmental gene–environment interaction*, published in Psychopathology (Leigh, 2009). This chapter, however, explicitly adds the memetic dimension to the paper.

References

Akiskal, H. S., Hantouche, E. G., Allilaire, J. F. (2003) Bipolar II with and without cyclothymic temperament: "dark" and "sunny" expressions of soft bipolarity. *J Affect Disord*, **73**, 49–57.

Brugha, T. S. (1995) *Social Support and Psychiatric Disorder Research Findings and Guidelines for Clinical Practice*. Cambridge University Press, Cambridge etc.

Caspi, A., McClay, J., Moffitt, T. E., et al. (2002) Role of genotype in the cycle of violence in maltreated children. *Science*, **297**, 851–854.

Caspi, A., Sugden, K., Moffitt, T. E., et al. (2003) Influence of life stress on depression: Moderation by a polymorphism in the 5-HTT gene. *Science*, **301**, 386–389.

Cheng, R., Juo, S. H., Loth, J. E., et al. (2006) Genome-wide linkage scan in a large bipolar disorder sample from the National Institute of Mental Health genetics initiative suggests putative loci for bipolar disorder, psychosis, suicide, and panic disorder. *Mol Psychiatry*, **11**, 252–260.

Craddock, N., O'Donovan, M. C., Owen, M. J. (2006) Genes for schizophrenia and bipolar disorder? Implications for psychiatric nosology. *Schizophr Bull*, **32**, 9–16.

Feighner, J. P., Robins, E., Guze, S. B., et al. (1972) Diagnostic criteria for use in psychiatric research. *Arch Gen Psychiatry*, **26**, 57–63.

Frances, A. J., Egger, H. L. (1999) Whither psychiatric diagnosis. *Aust N Z J Psychiatry*, **33**, 161–165.

Genova, P. (2003) Dump the DSM! In *Psychiatric Times*.

Goldapple, K., Segal, Z., Garson, C., et al. (2004) Modulation of cortical-limbic pathways in major depression: Treatment-specific effects of cognitive behavior therapy. *Arch Gen Psychiatry*, **61**, 34–41.

Hamshere, M. L., Bennett, P., Williams, N., et al. (2005) Genomewide linkage scan in schizoaffective disorder: Significant evidence for linkage at 1q42 close to DISC1, and suggestive evidence at 22q11 and 19p13. *Arch Gen Psychiatry*, **62**, 1081–1088.

Hippocrates http://duke.usask.ca/~niallm/233/Hippocra.htm

Kandel, E. R. (1979) Psychotherapy and the single synapse. The impact of psychiatric thought on neurobiologic research. *N Engl J Med*, **301**, 1028–1037.

Kandel, E. R. (1998) A new intellectual framework for psychiatry. *Am J Psychiatry*, **155**, 457–469.

Leigh, H. (2009) A proposal for a new multiaxial model of psychiatric diagnosis. A continuum-based patient model derived from evolutionary developmental gene-environment interaction. *Psychopathology*, **42**, 1–10.

McHugh, P. R. http://www.hopkinsmedicine.org/press/2001/august/McHugh.htm.

McHugh, P. R. (1992) A structure for psychiatry at the century's turn – the view from Johns Hopkins. *J R Soc Med*, **85**, 483–487.

McHugh, P. R. (2005) Striving for coherence: Psychiatry's efforts over classification. *JAMA*, **293**, 2526–2528.

McHugh, P. R., Slavney, P. R. (1998) *The Perspectives of Psychiatry* (2nd edn). Johns Hopkins University Press, Baltimore, MD

Meyer, A., Winters, E. E. (1950) *The Collected Papers of Adolf Meyer*. Johns Hopkins Press, Baltimore.

Murphy, D. L., Lerner, A., Rudnick, G., et al. (2004) Serotonin transporter: Gene, genetic disorders, and pharmacogenetics. *Mol Interv*, **4**, 109–123.

Nesse, R. M. (2004) Cliff-edged fitness functions and the persistence of schizophrenia. *Behav Brain Sci*, **27**, 862–863.

Norman, R. M., Malla, A. K., Manchanda, R., et al. (2005) Social support and three-year symptom and admission outcomes for first episode psychosis. *Schizophr Res*, **80**, 227–234.

Paquette, V., Levesque, J., Mensour, B., et al. (2003) "Change the mind and you change the brain": Effects of cognitive-behavioral therapy on the neural correlates of spider phobia. *Neuroimage*, **18**, 401–409.

Prathikanti, S., Weinberger, D. R. (2005) Psychiatric genetics – the new era: Genetic research and some clinical implications. *Br Med Bull*, **73–74**, 107–122.

Roffman, J. L., Marci, C. D., Glick, D. M., et al. (2005) Neuroimaging and the functional neuroanatomy of psychotherapy. *Psychol Med*, **35**, 1385–1398.

Silver, E. J., Heneghan, A. M., Bauman, L. J., et al. (2006) The relationship of depressive symptoms to parenting competence and social support in inner-city mothers of young children. *Matern Child Health J*, **10**, 105–112.

Smith, D. J., Muir, W. J., Blackwood, D. H. (2004) Is borderline personality disorder part of the bipolar spectrum? *Harv Rev Psychiatry*, **12**, 133–139.

Surkan, P. J., Peterson, K. E., Hughes, M. D., et al. (2006) The role of social networks and support in postpartum women's depression: A multiethnic urban sample. *Matern Child Health J*, **10**, 375–383.

Chapter 15
Memetic Diagnosis, Memetic Assessment and Biopsychosocial Epigenetic Formulation

Contents

15.1 Memetic Diagnosis

In the previous chapter, I proposed that a new multiaxial psychiatric diagnostic scheme should have, as Axis I, *Memetic and phenomenological diagnosis.*

What is memetic diagnosis? Memetic diagnosis such as depression and anxiety are descriptions of the memes that distress the patient. As discussed previously, psychiatric symptoms often arise from memetic conflicts, and major psychiatric syndromes are common final pathway brain dysregulation arising from gene × meme interaction. Furthermore, how a person experiences mental anguish and expresses it is often based on imitation of others, in the original meaning of the term, meme. In addition, memetic influences from the surrounding culture as well as the zeitgeist often determine in what form the distress is expressed. Memetic diagnosis, then, should be accompanied by a thorough memetic assessment of the patient that includes the early memetic environment, potential gene × meme interaction in childhood, early and recent imitation figures, and recent infusion of stress memes. This memetic assessment should be an important component of the biopsychosocial and epigenetic formulation, the Axis VI of my proposal.

Epigenetic formulation involves the interaction between genes and memes through development, with particular attention to significant stresses and nurturing in early life and recent stresses and social support. These are the factors that may

H. Leigh, *Genes, Memes, Culture, and Mental Illness,*
DOI 10.1007/978-1-4419-5671-2_15, © Hoyle Leigh, 2010

have augmented vulnerability genes and attenuated resilence genes or vice versa, resulting in syndromic mental illness, neurotic traits, or mental health.

At first glance, Axis I memetic diagnosis may not seem to differ from conventional diagnosis, and as far as nomenclature goes, this notion is correct. What memetic diagnosis implies, in addition to the *meaning* of the memes collected, is the fact that the memes have *replicated* to become a problem. Thus, it is necessary to identify the cause of the replication as well as to treat the process of replication.

The cause of the replication may be (1) imitation and/or empathy, deliberate or automatic, (2) large influx of new memes, (3) replication of dormant resident memes due to either weakening of the dominant memes or new memes augmenting the resident ones, (4) combination of any of the above, potentially causing a final common pathway dysregulation of the brain. The presumptive identification of the cause of the replication is then reflected in the memetic diagnosis with the qualifiers of: neurotic (resident meme conflict or resurgence), situational (influx of new memes or weakening of the dominant memes), or syndromic (final common pathway syndrome representing brain dysregulation). The qualifiers are not mutually exclusive, so that a person may have depression, neurotic and situational; anxiety and panic, situational and syndromic.

In this chapter, I will briefly describe how memetic assessment should be made, how priming factors and role models should be considered in the biopsychosocial formulation, and anticipate some new methods and techniques that need to be developed to further this aim.

15.2 Memetic Assessment

Memetic assessment of a patient should take into account the fact that there are conscious and unconscious memes, and that pathogenic and resilience memes may be either conscious or unconscious. The proliferation of usually dormant pathogenic memes occasioned by recent stress is often the precipitating event of the final common pathway syndrome.

15.3 Conscious Memes

Traditional methods of history taking and mental status examination will reveal the memetic content of the patient's suffering. In addition, the clinician's mirror neurons will generate memes within the clinician mirroring the emotional experience of the patient, i.e., empathy.

In making a memetic diagnosis, it is important initially to *listen* to the patient and appreciate the patient's memes rather than reinterpreting them immediately according to the clinician's memes. For example, when a patient complains of feeling sad and tearful, it should not immediately translate into depression, as the memeplex of feeling sad and tearful (think of an image of a person who is sad and tearful) can have many different causes and situations. For example, she may be feeling sad and tearful because she has an image of someone sad and tearful stuck in her mind (i.e., an isolated unchecked replication of sad and tearful memes as an imitation of the image), whom she may have seen in a film or a book. Thus, a natural question to ask may be, "When you are feeling sad and tearful, what comes to your mind, any persons or images?" Of course, considering the associated symptoms and signs of a major final common pathway syndrome such as major depression is important, but so is an understanding of the memetic nature of the patient's experience and presentation.

External or situational stresses and the memes they awaken are important contributors to psychiatric symptoms and should be addressed. In addition, as memetic conflicts often lead to anxiety, despair, and emotional turmoil, it is important to identify memetic conflicts in the patient. Direct questioning may be very useful, i.e., "Stress, as well as conflicts or dilemmas within one's own mind often causes anxiety, irritability, and depression. Have you had any recent stresses or struggles within your own mind?" When asked, many patients will respond with a sense of relief that the clinician understands his or her emotional turmoil. The memetic conflict is often conscious or preconscious and readily available for discussion, such as ambivalent feelings about job or spouse, or even existential (and possibly depressive) ruminations about life and suicide.

15.4 Unconscious Memes

The memetic conflicts are often unconscious, i.e., repressed by the dominant self-plexes, and the patient may adamantly deny any internal conflict. This is particularly the case when the memetic conflict is among the memes that have been resident in the brain for a long time, perhaps since childhood, or when there is a conflict between the seflplex and a surreptitiously introduced memes (see Chapters 11 and 12) that may awaken a dormant and dangerous resident meme.

Such unconscious memes and memetic conflicts may be surmised indirectly by obtaining a thorough personal and cultural history as well as the history of interaction among family members and cultural/subcultural groups and artifacts, such as customs and values. Very strong affect-laden acceptance or rejection of such values and customs may reflect underlying conflict. Projective tests, such as the thematic apperception test (TAT) and the Rorschach may also shed some light into the unconscious memetic life of the patient (Blatt et al., 1994; Bornstein and Masling, 2005; Klopfer and Kelley, 1942; Stein, 1955).

15.5 Priming Factors and Role Models

Memetic assessment should incorporate *priming factors* and *role models*. Priming factors may include having been exposed to the meme that mental distress should be expressed as a somatic symptom, and a role model may be a relative or a friend who had a particular symptom. For example, the exacerbation of back pain with depression may be modeled after a friend who had similar symptoms and was bedridden.

15.6 The Need for New Memetic Diagnostic Tools

Up to this point, we discussed existing diagnostic tools to identify the memes and memetic contribution to psychiatric illness. It is obvious that the existing tools are limited because they do not explicitly identify memes as the target of investigation. Thus, there is a need for tools specifically designed for collecting and identifying memes and memeplexes. In a sense, free association in psychoanalysis and psychoanalytically oriented psychotherapy is a method of collecting memes, but the length of the procedure is uneconomical and what to do with the seemingly randomly collected memes is open to question.

There is a need for more efficient and systematic methods of useful meme collection. The Jungian word association test may be an existing technique that may identify unconscious conflictual memes or *complexes*, and may deserve another look (Golden et al., 2000; Mohan, 2000).

Computerized meme scan may be developed. The goal of the scan would be to identify more common meme conflicts and the presence of pathologic memes and their strength as well as to determine the selfplexes and the degree of memetic democracy or autocracy. An inventory of beliefs, both common and uncommon, may be developed. Meme scan could also incorporate aspects of word association test, free association for a limited amount of time (somewhat akin to the Gottschalk-Gleser verbal sample test), Myers-Briggs personality typology, and skin conductance associated with computer-presented potentially conflictual word (Gottschalk and Gleser, 1969; Gottschalk et al., 1969; Myers et al., 1985; Quenk, 2000; Tieger and Barron-Tieger, 1997; University of Mississippi, Department of Psychology, 1981).

Memodynamics might be a tool to understand the ebb and flow of memes and the relative strengths of various memeplexes in the course of development of the individual. This would be a history of conscious and unconscious belief systems and their changes from childhood through adolescence to adulthood and beyond. What was your idea of how the world started when you were a child? What was your idea of your parents as you are growing up? What did you like to read as a child? Fairy tales? Did you believe in fairies? When you were school age, what did you believe about how the world began? How about now? Who was your hero when you were in grade school? In high school? Please describe how things changed during your adolescence, etc. This type of detailed history could also be obtained through a computerized program where the subject plays an active role in inputting the data and answering questions.

References

Blatt, S. J., Ford, R. Q., Berman, W. H. (1994) *Therapeutic Change: An Object Relations Perspective*. Plenum Press, New York.
Bornstein, R. F., Masling, J. M. (2005) *Scoring the Rorschach: Seven Validated Systems*. L. Erlbaum, Mahwah, NJ.

Golden, C. J., Espe-Pfeifer, P., Wachsler-Felder, J. (2000) *Neuropsychological Interpretation of Objective Psychological Tests*. Kluwer Academic/Plenum Publishers, New York.

Gottschalk, L. A., Gleser, G. C. (1969) *The Measurement of Psychological States Through the Content Analysis of Verbal Behavior*. University of California Press, Berkeley.

Gottschalk, L. A., Winget, C. N., Gleser, G. C. (1969) *Manual of Instructions for Using the Gottschalk-Gleser Content Analysis Scales: Anxiety, Hostility, and Social Alienation – Personal Disorganization*. University of California Press, Berkeley.

Klopfer, B., Kelley, D. M. (1942) *The Rorschach Technique; a Manual for a Projective Method of Personality Diagnosis*. World Book Co, Yonkers-on-Hudson, NY.

Mohan, J. (2000) *Personality Across Cultures: Recent Developments and Debates*. Oxford University Press, New Delhi, New York.

Myers, I. B., McCaulley, M. H., Most, R. (1985) *Manual, a Guide to the Development and Use of the Myers-Briggs Type Indicator*. Consulting Psychologists Press, Palo Alto, CA.

Quenk, N. L. (2000) *Essentials of Myers-Briggs Type Indicator Assessment*. John Wiley & Sons, New York.

Stein, M. I. (1955) *The Thematic Apperception Test; an Introductory Manual for Its Clinical Use with Adults* (Rev. [i.e. 2nd] edn). Addison-Wesley Publishing Company, Cambridge, MA.

Tieger, P. D., Barron-Tieger, B. (1997) *Nurture by Nature: Understand Your Child's Personality Type – and Become a Better Parent* (1st edn). Little, Brown, Boston.

University of Mississippi, Department of Psychology. (1981) *Research in Psychological Type*. Mississippi State University, Department of Psychology, Mississippi State, Mississippi.

Chapter 16
Principles of Memetic Therapy

Contents

An understanding of memetic diagnosis should naturally lead to meme-oriented therapies. We discussed in the previous chapter that memetic diagnosis entails the identification of the *causes* of pathogenic meme replication. We discussed that the cause of the unchecked replication may a combination of induction of pathogenic memes by imitation or empathy, massive influx of memes from the environment due to sheer exposure, and/or resurgence of dormant pathogenic memes due to a weakening of the dominant memes.

Memetic therapy may be geared both to the cause of the replication as well as to the pathogenic memes themselves. In order to treat the influx of memes caused by either exposure to external memes or through empathy, one has to block the continuing entrance of the pathogenic memes into the brain, i.e., perception and induction of memes. This will also tend to prevent the weakening of the dominant, healthy memes.

16.1 Blocking the Entrance and Induction of Pathogenic Memes

How does one block the continuing infusion of pathogenic memes into the brain? An environmental change, including hospitalization, is a means of controlling the

H. Leigh, *Genes, Memes, Culture, and Mental Illness*,
DOI 10.1007/978-1-4419-5671-2_16, © Hoyle Leigh, 2010

memetic environment of the brain. Diversion of attention from the pathogenic memes in the environment is another method – including vacation, relaxation training, recreational activities, even sleep. Intersensory inhibition has been reported to be effective in reducing seizure-inducing stimuli in rats (Kramer and Adler, 1976). Judicious use of sensory deprivation may also be considered, but it may lead to unchecked replication of existing memes and hallucinations (Merabet et al., 2004).

When pathogenic memes are induced through empathy or imitation of a person, e.g., a charismatic leader, physical separation from that person may be therapeutic, i.e., separating the person from a cult or even incarceration as a means of separating a person from the pathogenic meme environment of a gang. Care should be taken, however, that the new environment is not equally pathogenic.

External memes enter the brain encapsulated in a sensory vehicle, i.e., as words, images, melodies, which consist of sensory stimuli, i.e., visual, auditory, olfactory, gustatory, and tactile (which also include temperature, pain, pressure, and vibration). As each sensory modality tends to attend to one sensation at a time, it should be possible to prevent the entrance of a meme by saturating the sensory modality in which the meme is substantially encapsulated. For example, if the pathogenic meme is in the form of an image, say that of Hitler, presenting the subject with another image that is attractive (likely to replicate), such as the image of a loved one or a relaxing scenery, may block the entrance and replication of Hitler's image and what it stands for.

Auditory and tactile stimulation may be similarly utilized, e.g., repeated playing of favorite song or relaxing music, tactile stimuli such as massage that can distract attention from the pathogenic memes and thence their replication. As there is plasticity and cross-contamination among sensory modalities, such saturation with nonpathogenic sensory stimulus may also block other forms of pathogenic memes (Shimojo and Shams, 2001; Violentyev et al., 2005).

16.2 Treating Memes in the Brain

In addition to blocking the entry of pathogenic memes, memetic therapy should be geared to suppressing and/or eradicating the replicating pathogenic memes already in the brain. This may be accomplished by first identifying the pathogenic memes and their nature, identifying the components of the pathogenic memeplexes, and identifying their sensory capsules or vehicles, and neutralizing or suppressing them.

16.2.1 Identifying Pathogenic Memes and Memeplex Components

As discussed in the previous chapter on memetic diagnosis, an obvious way of identifying pathogenic memes is to listen to the patient. The complaints of the patient, and more importantly, the preoccupation of the patient, when verbalized, are the pathologic memes that the patient experiences. They may be emotions, such as feeling blue and sad, anxious or angry. They may be thoughts, such as wishing to die, future is hopeless, etc. From the verbal communication (memetic emission) of the patient, one can also recognize the underlying memeplexes, the schema or world view as well as the schema of the self, i.e., selfplex(es). Such memplexes may be "The world is a hostile and hurtful place and nobody loves me," "I am not a worthwhile person," "I feel this way because I am guilty," "I am anxious because the FBI is watching me," etc.

Asking specific questions can also elicit pathogenic memes, for example, "Do you feel hopeless about the future?" "Do you have any thoughts of suicide?" "Do you have feelings that others are trying to do harm to you?," etc. As for empathy/imitation, one could ask "Do you know of anyone who had symptoms or feelings like yours?" "Tell me about people who are important in your life," etc.

Free association is another technique that may be useful in identifying underlying memeplexes, as some of the pathogenic unconscious memplexes may reveal themselves in disguised forms.

Empathy, i.e., firing of mirror neurons on the part of the clinician is another important method of understanding the patient's memetic state and memplexes. What one is feeling is often what the patient is experiencing, and the thoughts (memes) that come to mind are also often induced by the patient's memes.

Once the underlying memeplexes have been identified, it is useful to consider the component memes of the memplexes or schemas. For example, the memeplex, "I am not a worthwhile person" may consist of (1) sad affect (meme), (2) angry affect (meme), (3) experience of failure (meme), (4) negative bias in evaluation (meme affecting executive function), (4) hopelessness (meme). The memeplex may be further buttressed by a recurring thought in the form of a voice (which may be a thought perceived as an inner voice, or frank auditory hallucination) that says "you are worthless" (meme that encapsulates itself in auditory sensation).

16.2.2 Identifying Capsules and Vehicles

In the above example, we observed that a memeplex may recruit a sensory modality that augments its replication, i.e., the voice that repeats itself, "you are worthless!" Other forms of capsules and vehicles may be identified, such as an image of oneself being ugly and diseased, a thought that the head may be filled with dirty thoughts, may be putrefied, etc. Such thoughts (memes) may multiply and gain further strength, becoming a delusion, e.g., "My brain is filled with maggots," then "I can feel the maggots squirming about in my brain!"

The memes may travel in vehicles, such as written words, drawings, and paintings. Words and drawings can recreate the original memeplexes in the brains of those who read or see them, as in Munch's famous painting, *The Scream*.

It should be made clear from the outset that the *vehicles* that carry memes are memes themselves but that these memes serve the function of embedding and transporting other memes that form the content of the vehicle.

Melody and rhythm are readily available vehicles for memes to travel, thus songs and verses have been used throughout history to carry various memes and memeplexes, most of them not pathogenic. Nevertheless, some pathogenic memes, such as that of violence, may be carried in some rap music and others. Note that some memes may co-opt the melodies of familiar and beloved songs to camouflage themselves and to infiltrate unsuspecting brains.

An example is the melody of the English folk song Greensleeves from the sixteenth century, that was co-opted into the Christian hymn, the Manger Throne, by William Dix in 1865. Parts of the two verses are presented below:

Greensleeves	Manger Throne
Alas my love you do me wrong	What Child is this who, laid to rest
To cast me off discourteously;	On Mary's lap is sleeping?
And I have loved you oh so long	Whom angels greet with anthems sweet,
Delighting in your company.	While shepherds watch are keeping?
Green sleeves was my delight,	This, this is Christ the King,
Green sleeves my heart of gold	Whom shepherds guard and angels sing;
Green sleeves was my heart of joy	Haste, haste, to bring Him laud,
And who but my lady green sleeves	The Babe, the Son of Mary.
	Why lies He in such mean estate,
	Where ox and ass are feeding?
	Good Christians, fear, for sinners here
	The silent Word is pleading.
	Nails, spear shall pierce Him through,
	The cross be borne for me, for you.
	Hail, hail the Word made flesh,
	The Babe, the Son of Mary.

16.2.3 Neutralizing Capsules and Vehicles

Once the capsules and vehicles of pathogenic memes have been identified, methods should be devised to neutralize them. Unfortunately, specific techniques of doing this have yet to be developed. Devising such techniques should be relatively easy in principle. For example, if a particular melody carrying a pathogenic meme can be identified within the brain, it may be possible to feed into the brain the inverse of the sound wave of the pathogenic meme, thus completely neutralizing it. So with a counter-rhythm. It may also be possible to co-opt the pathogenic meme carrying sound or melody by substituting the words that are antidotes of the pathogenic memes. Thus, an inner voice repeating, "I am a bad person," may be substituted by an actual repetition of the words, "I am a good person."

As for visual stimuli such as images, the repeated presentation of a substitute image by itself, or paired with the pathogenic image initially and then presented by itself, may neutralize the pathogenic image.

Words as vehicle are more complex but could still be broken down to syllables and letters with attendant visual and sonic qualities that may be amenable to sensory neutralization. Nonsense words or antonyms that are look-alikes or sound-alikes may also be utilized.

16.2.4 Deconstructing and Suppressing Memes

The content of the memes and memplexes, in addition to the exterior capsules and vehicles, may be also deconstructed and subject to suppression. In this case, it is important to recognize that it is unlikely that the meme as memory can be completely eradicated, but rather the goal of therapy would be to suppress its replication.

Deconstructing a memeplex may go like this:

What goes into "I am worthless"?

It involves I + am + worth+ less

What is "I"? –I am John Smith, I am a clerk, I am a husband, etc.

What is "am" – exist, identify with, alive, not dead, etc.

What is "worth"? – good, rich, healthy, can be relied on, do the work, etc.

What is "less"? – no good, not meeting the criteria, not deserving, etc.

The treatment may involve feeding back the following memes for each memetic component.

For "I": I am John Smith, I am a clerk, have been *for 5 years*, I am a husband with two children, *good children, a good father*

For "am": I *exist, am alive, am needed as husband and father,*

For "worth": I am *a good worker, can be a good husband, can be a good father, in fact, am a good father*

For "less": Maybe not rich, maybe not as good as I could be *because I am depressed, I can be good when I get better, I can be Excellent!*

16.2.5 Augmenting Protective Memes

Meme-oriented therapy should also be geared to enhancing protective memes as well as neutralizing pathogenic memes. The protective memes include non-autocratic selfplexes, memes that enhance self-esteem, memes that induce relaxation and enjoyment, memes that facilitate gratifying interpersonal interaction, etc. Relaxation training, music therapy, massage therapy, etc., can both attenuate pathogenic memes and enhance protective memes. Direct meme infusion through hypnosis or experience of caring by the therapist might be other means of strengthening protective memes.

16.3 Conventional Meme–Directed Therapies

Certain conventional therapies are clearly meme directed. In fact, most psychotherapies are meme directed in the sense that they wind up endeavoring to change the memetic content of the person through meme exchange, i.e., talking. Specific psychotherapies will be discussed in Chapter 18.

16.4 Need for Novel Therapies

Existing psychotherapies have been either geared toward the thoughts (cognitive therapy), behavior (behavioral therapy), or to conflicts arising from basic drives and inhibitory forces (psychodynamic therapy), or combinations of the above.

The recognition of gene × meme interaction and the role of stress that arises at least in part from memetic conflicts in mental illness provide us with a new perspective in therapy.

Psychiatric therapy should be geared toward both genes and memes.

(1) Gene-oriented therapy

This should take into account the epigenesis of the person, i.e., what physical and memetic stresses in early life caused which genes to be turned on or off resulting in the vulnerability to mental illness, and how can we reverse it? Gene-oriented therapy is not limited to drug therapy. In fact, there is evidence that a nurturing environment in adulthood and psychotherapy may be effective in reversing the effects of early stress on specific genes and thus the micro- or macro-morphology and function of the brain.

(2) Meme-oriented therapy

The recognition that memes interact with genes, and that memes are actual functional neuronal units that may have various components such as thoughts, beliefs, sounds, imagery, colors, texture, and emotions opens up a whole new world of meme-oriented therapies.

(a) Existing *multimodal therapies* such as music and dance could be integrated with psychotherapy with a common memetic theme. In addition, novel therapies may be developed that may be geared to modality-specific components of the pathogenic meme, e.g., sound, image, emotion. Deconstructing a memeplex may lead to specific antidotes for its components. Such an antidote may be the infusion of an incompatible idea encapsulated in a catchy tune, or it could be an inverse sound wave to an existing tune that carries a pathogenic meme.

(b) Novel therapies geared toward a resolution of *meme–meme conflicts* could be devised. Such conflicts could be identified utilizing novel techniques such as a meme scan (Chapter 15). New memes that would either harmonize or buffer the conflicting memes could be infused encapsulated in imagery or melody, and the patient may be prepared to be more receptive to meme infusion through relaxation, hypnosis, or medications.

(c) *Avatars* and Virtual Reality Techniques.

Another novel meme-oriented therapy is the use of *avatars* as models of imitation. Avatars are digitized images of oneself, and such avatars may be programmed to look and behave in certain desired ways in virtual reality that the subject observes. For example, the avatar may be more slender than the subject, more assertive, and may exercise. After seeing the avatar, subjects have been shown to be more assertive, and more likely to exercise (Bailenson, 2006; Bailenson et al., 2008; Platoni, 2008; Taylor et al., 2008; Yee and Bailenson, 2007). In this memetic therapy, one actually imitates oneself projected into the future (virtual reality).

Virtual reality has already been used to desensitize patients with phobias. Patients could also practice job interviews, giving presentations, etc., using virtual interviewer or virtual audience. These are examples of memetic therapy as the subject practices different memes (facial expression, posture, speech, etc.) in virtual reality. Through such practice, the patient may choose the appropriate memetic constellations to present as the selfplex for the situation.

References

Bailenson, J. N. (2006) Transformed social interaction in collaborative virtual environments. In *Digital Media: Transformations in Human Communication* (P. Messaris and L. Humphreys eds.), pp. 255–264. Peter Lang, New York.

Bailenson, J. N., Yee, N., Blascovich, J., et al. (2008) The use of immersive virtual reality in the learning sciences: Digital transformations of teachers, students, and social context. *J Learning Sci*, **17**, 102–141.

Kramer, M. S., Adler, M. W. (1976) Neutralization of sensory-input modification of seizure thresholds in rats. *J Comp Physiol Psychol*, **90**, 268–278.

Merabet, L. B., Maguire, D., Warde, A., et al. (2004) Visual hallucinations during prolonged blindfolding in sighted subjects. *J Neuroophthalmol*, **24**, 109–113.

Platoni, K. (2008) Seeing is believing: Maybe virtual reality isn't just a game anymore. Maybe it's a way to build a better you. *Stanford Magazine*.

Shimojo, S., Shams, L. (2001) Sensory modalities are not separate modalities: Plasticity and interactions. *Curr Opin Neurobiol*, **11**, 505–509.

Taylor, T., Bailenson, J., Kraus, K. (2008) Liveblogging MetaverseU: TL Taylor, Jeremy Bailenson, Kari Kraus. *Virtual Worlds News*.

Violentyev, A., Shimojo, S., Shams, L. (2005) Touch-induced visual illusion. *Neuroreport*, **16**, 1107–1110.

Yee, N., Bailenson, J. N. (2007) The Proteus effect: Self transformations in virtual reality. *Hum Commun Res*, **33**, 271–290.

Chapter 17
Broad-Spectrum Memetic Therapies

Contents

17.1 What is Broad-Spectrum Meme-Oriented Therapy?

Our body contains many microorganisms. Many of them are beneficial, even essential, for bodily function such as those in the gut that assist the digestive function. Some ancient intruders became an integral and essential part of our very cells in the form of mitochondria. Other microorganisms are merely symbiotic, causing neither harm nor any benefit. Then, some, like the varicella and herpes simplex viruses, are pathogenic but may stay in our bodies without causing much trouble as their multiplication is checked by our immune system. Under certain conditions of weakened defenses, however, the latent pathogenic viruses may multiply and disease ensues. Weakened defenses may be caused by infection by another organism, as in HIV, or by malnutrition, drugs, etc. Under those conditions, even normal flora may overgrow and cause disease. Of course, infusion of virulent microorganisms may overwhelm the defenses and cause disease immediately. In all these instances, there is a massive multiplication of the organism in the disease state.

Likewise, there is a massive multiplication of memes in mental illness – the culprit memes may have been initially benign and beneficial, or symbiotic, or pathogenic but dormant. In the disease state, there is a massive multiplication of

H. Leigh, *Genes, Memes, Culture, and Mental Illness*,
DOI 10.1007/978-1-4419-5671-2_17, © Hoyle Leigh, 2010

memes in the form of ideas (e.g., paranoid or obsessive), emotions (e.g., depressive or euphoric), worries, desires, and behavior.

In treating infections by microorganisms, broad-spectrum antibiotics have been particularly useful as they target a broad range of organisms, i.e., regardless of the nature of the organism, the therapy can be effective. Especially in the case of mixed infections, they can be particularly useful. Similarly, there are broad-spectrum therapies that may be geared to suppressing a broad range of memes. Of course, as in the case with antibiotics, broad-spectrum memetic therapy may have the side effect of suppressing beneficial normal flora of memes as well. Nevertheless, when the unchecked multiplication of memes may be overwhelming, broad-spectrum anti-meme therapy can be a very effective method of controlling the situation and preventing an escalation of the memetic multiplication.

How can we actually achieve this? Antibiotics generally interfere with the replicative mechanism of the microbe. What is the replicative mechanism of memes? As we discussed in Chapters 9 and 11, memes replicate through signal reinforcement of the neural cliques that make up the memes and by recruiting other neural clusters through the development of new synaptic and dendritic connections. These old and new connections are enhanced by attention, affect, and thinking. There is, of course, unconscious replication of memes in the background, but the dominant replication process is usually conscious in the form of thoughts and feelings. Thus, depriving the pathogenic memes of attention, affect, and thought and thus the neural reinforcement would interfere with their multiplication.

An obvious approach is pharmacological intervention, a direct suppression of attention and cortical activity. It is well known that most mental illness is associated with insomnia and the promotion of sleep with drugs have beneficial effects. Many tranquilizers, especially benzodiazepines, induce drowsiness and reduced attention. Antipsychotic drugs and antidepressants are often chosen for the "side effect" of sedation as well as for the specific action. Many patients on these drugs also report a blunting of their affect.

There are a number of extant nonpharmacologic techniques that are considered to be valuable in promoting mental health, but the reason why they are effective has not been clearly defined. They include such diverse techniques as relaxation training, meditation, hypnosis, bath, massage, music therapy, dance therapy, exercise, and bibliotherapy. In the light of our understanding of memes, it is clear that all these techniques have in common the focusing of attention on something other than the thoughts and feelings that are distressful, and thus the ability to suppress the multiplication of memes.

17.2 Sleep, Sedation, and Electroconvulsive Therapy

Most current psychotropic drugs have either sedative or stimulant effect on the brain. The sedative qualities of the drug are useful in two ways: (1) in inducing sleep and thus temporarily stop most meme replication, especially if the drug suppresses rapid eye movement (REM) sleep and (2) by general reduction in attention directed to memes while awake, thus reducing meme replication (Rush and Griffiths, 1996).

Stimulants, on the other hand, seem to have the effect of reducing the scattered attention and thus chaotic meme replication in attention-deficit hyperactivity disorder (ADHD), and focusing attention to the memetic task at hand. The memes associated with the task had been at a disadvantage because of the unchecked proliferation of irrelevant memes. In patients with chronic depression associated with chronic physical illness, especially in elderly patients, stimulants may enhance attention and energy, strengthening the selfplex memes.

Electroconvulsive therapy (ECT) produces a generalized seizure activity in the brain, i.e., all memetic proliferation is suspended during the seizure activity when all neurons are firing simultaneously. Memory impairment is common following ECT, indicating reduced accessibility and thus multiplication of memes.

17.3 Relaxation and Meditation

Relaxation and meditation therapies are grouped together here because they are usually practiced together, i.e., meditative techniques are usually utilized to bring about relaxation, and relaxation is usually suggested or achieved during meditation.

Relaxation therapy has three models – specific effects, relaxation response, and integrated. The specific response model is geared to specific effects based on the modality, i.e., muscle relaxation for symptoms associated with muscle tension. The relaxation response, first formulated by Benson et al. (Benson et al., 1975) postulates that all effective relaxation techniques produce a generalized physiologic "relaxation response" characterized by reduced sympathetic arousal. The integrated model posits that most relaxation techniques have both a relaxation response and a specific component (Schwartz et al., 1978).

The techniques of relaxation usually involve one or a combination of the following: focusing on muscle relaxation, focusing on breathing, focusing on bodily sensations (e.g., warmth of hands), focusing on an imagery, focusing on a word or sound (mantra) (Geba, 1973; Jacobson, 1962; Samuels, 1975).

By diverting attention from the proliferating, pathogenic memes, and focusing attention on the specific sensation, regardless of the body part or function, there is attenuation of general memetic replication. This broad-spectrum anti-meme effect, together with whatever specific physiologic effect the relaxation of muscles or pacing of breathing or vasodilation in hand warming might have, may be responsible for the overall beneficial effect of relaxation and meditation in mental illness.

17.4 Hypnosis

Contrary to popular notion, hypnosis involves focused and concentrated attention on a sensation or imagery. A state of altered consciousness or trance is induced by first fixating attention to a physical sensation, often by gazing at a point or concentrating on a feeling of floating. This concentration of attention tends to attenuate attention paid to other memes and thus their proliferation.

The hypnotic experience itself depends largely on the hypnotizability of the individual, which seems to be a trait associated with the ability to concentrate attention and to enter into a dissociated state. In highly hypnotizable individuals, hypnosis can alter actual sensory experience such as pain or auditory stimulus through activation of the prefrontal and cingulate gyri (Faymonville et al., 2006; Nash, 2005; Raij et al., 2005).

In the dissociated state, susceptibility to suggestion is heightened, and the subject is ready for new meme infusion by the hypnotist. The hypnotist may then infuse the subject with memes designed to neutralize existing pathogenic memes and to enhance salutary memes. The subject can then be taught self-hypnosis, in which the newly introduced salutary memes can be reinforced. The dissociative experience in hypnosis thus may nurture the development of a healthier selfplex that will replace the currently dominant selfplex which is saddled with multiplying pathogenic memes (Bob, 2008).

Even without achieving a dissociated state, the directed focusing of attention in hypnosis and self-hypnosis deprives the pathogenic memes of unchecked multiplication, and potentially rechannels attention to salutary memes. Hypnosis is often used in conjunction with relaxation, and may have synergistic effects.

17.5 Music and Dance Therapy

As early as eighth and ninth centuries, the Islamic scholar and psychologist, al-Farabi (872–950), known as "Alpharabius" discussed the therapeutic effects of music in his treatise, *Meanings of the Intellect* (Haque, 2004). In the seventeenth century, Robert Burton, an English scholar and vicar at Oxford University, wrote that music and dance were critical in treating mental illness, especially melancholia (Burton, 2001). Music therapy became widely recognized after World War II.

The Nordoff–Robbins approach to music therapy posits that everyone can respond to music, no matter how ill or disabled. Music can enhance communication, and enable people to live more resourcefully and creatively.

Music therapy has been shown to be effective in alleviating anxiety, depression, pain, and disability in a wide variety of medical and psychiatric conditions including mood disorders, addictions, perioperative anxiety and pain, cardiac rehabilitation, autism, and psychosis (Choi et al., 2008; Dingle et al., 2008; Hanser, 1993; Hanser and Mandel, 2005; Hanser and Thompson, 1994; Jing and Xudong, 2008; Kemper et al., 2008; Klassen et al., 2008; Leung, 2008; Mandel et al., 2007; Maratos et al., 2008; Nilsson, 2008; Raglio et al., 2008; Ross et al., 2008; Sarkamo et al., 2008).

Specific modes of music, e.g., major vs. minor keys, may have specific effects on the brain, e.g., music in major mode has been shown to be more effective in reducing mental fatigue associated with stress (Suda et al., 2008).

Music as well as massage has been shown to attenuate the right frontal EEG activation seen in depressed adolescents (Jones and Field, 1999).

Music seems to activate specific pathways in the brain that may have salutary effects on mood and cognitive function (Boso et al., 2006; Esch et al., 2004; Thaut, 2005). There is also evidence that BDNF (brain-derived neurotrphic factor) may be released with music (Angelucci et al., 2007). Specific music, for example, Mozart's piano sonata (K448) but not Beethoven's *fur Elise* was shown to enhance spatiotemporal tasks and increased blood flow in dorsolateral prefrontal cortex, occipital cortex, and cerebellum in individuals even after the music has stopped (Bodner et al., 2001).

Rhythm, an essential component of music, has direct effects on human motor activity and its regulation (Thaut et al., 1999). Dance therapy is a good example of the utilization of rhythm in health care.

How do these therapies affect the memes? Music is itself memetic, i.e., particular tunes and rhythms are encoded in neurons and the patterns are replicated in recall and reproduction. An example of such replication, often unwanted, is the phenomenon of the earworm, the repetition of a song or jingle in one's mind over and over again. Music therapy is a form of meme infusion which may have direct neurophysiologic and neurochemical effects as discussed above, in addition to the effect of distracting attention from the replicating pathogenic memes and thus deprive them of sustenance. Even background music can be an infusion of memes coming into the brain without awareness but effectuating change in it.

Music and dance therapy, together with play therapy and writing are often considered to be *expressive* therapy when they are used to express patients' emotions and thoughts. In such expressive form, memes are emitted by the patient in the form of words, sounds, and motion. Such expressions may result in a decompression of memetic pressure built by forceful replication. The replicated memes may be creative and salutary, or may be pathogenic. No matter what the nature of the memes might be, relief of the memetic pressure may be beneficial.

17.6 Massage Therapy

There are writings on massage in such ancient civilizations as Rome, Greece, China, Japan, Egypt, India, and Mesopotamia. Hippocrates wrote in 460 BC that "The physician must be experienced in many things, but "assuredly in rubbing." The ancient Chinese medical textbook by the Yellow Emperor, *Huangdi Neijing (also known as the Inner Cannon of the Yellow Emperor)*, considered to date around two to fourth century BCE, recommends "massage of skin and flesh." Massage became popular in the United States in the middle of the nineteenth century and was based on techniques developed in Sweden (NCCAM, 2006).

There are more than 80 types of massage therapy including the Swedish massage, deep tissue massage, trigger point massage, and Shiatsu. In all of them, therapists press, rub, and otherwise manipulate the muscles and other soft tissues of the body, often varying pressure and movement. They most often use their hands and fingers, but may use their forearms, elbows, or feet. Typically, the intent is to relax the muscles and tendons and to increase blood flow to the massaged areas.

Massage draws attention to the immediate sensations of touch and warmth in the massaged area and away from the proliferation of pathogenic memes in the form of thinking, worrying, and other preoccupations. The relaxation of muscles also may produce a brain state incompatible with anxiety and/or depressive memes.

17.7 Exercise

Physical exercise tends to concentrate attention at the physical task at hand, and reduce attention being paid to pathogenic memes. Furthermore, the endorphins that are released with exercise enhance positive mood and general health (Bender et al., 2007; Karacabey, 2005; Koseoglu et al., 2003). Exercise has been shown to be effective in the rehabilitation of chronic psychiatric patients (Faulkner and Carless, 2006).

17.8 Bibliotherapy

Bibliotherapy or reading therapy is geared to providing the patient with reading materials that may be helpful. The reading material may be information concerning a medical or psychiatric condition, a "how to" book to overcome a condition, or simple recreational reading. Bibliotherapy combined with cognitive-behavioral therapy has been found to be effective in treating adolescent depression (Ackerson et al., 1998) and in preventing and treating addiction (Pardeck, 1991).

Bibliotherapy involves attention to the reading material and away from the replicating pathogenic memes, and the memes contained in the reading material are absorbed and may counteract the pathogenic memes.

It may be possible to develop reading material that may be specifically geared to neutralize or enhance specific memes in the brain, e.g., for depression, for anxiety, or for health promotion. Of course, any reading material is capable of introducing new memes, which is the essence of book learning.

References

Ackerson, J., Scogin, F., McKendree-Smith, N., et al. (1998) Cognitive bibliotherapy for mild and moderate adolescent depressive symptomatology. *J Consult Clin Psychol*, **66**, 685–690.
Angelucci, F., Ricci, E., Padua, L., et al. (2007) Music exposure differentially alters the levels of brain-derived neurotrophic factor and nerve growth factor in the mouse hypothalamus. *Neurosci Lett*, **429**, 152–155.
Bender, T., Nagy, G., Barna, I., et al. (2007) The effect of physical therapy on beta-endorphin levels. *Eur J Appl Physiol*, **100**, 371–382.

Benson, H., Greenwood, M. M., Klemchuk, H. (1975) The relaxation response: Psychophysiologic aspects and clinical applications. *Int J Psychiatry Med*, **6**, 87–98.

Bob, P. (2008) Pain, dissociation and subliminal self-representations. *Conscious Cogn*, **17**, 355–369.

Bodner, M., Muftuler, L. T., Nalcioglu, O., et al. (2001) FMRI study relevant to the Mozart effect: Brain areas involved in spatial-temporal reasoning. *Neurol Res*, **23**, 683–690.

Boso, M., Politi, P., Barale, F., et al. (2006) Neurophysiology and neurobiology of the musical experience. *Funct Neurol*, **21**, 187–191.

Burton, R. (2001) *The Anatomy of Melancholy: New York Review of Books, a One-Volume Reprint of 1932 3-volume Everyman Pocket Edition, with a New Introduction by William H. Gass*. New York Review of Books, New York.

Choi, A. N., Lee, M. S., Lim, H. J. (2008) Effects of group music intervention on depression, anxiety, and relationships in psychiatric patients: A pilot study. *J Altern Complement Med*, **14**, 567–570.

Dingle, G. A., Gleadhill, L., Baker, F. A. (2008) Can music therapy engage patients in group cognitive behaviour therapy for substance abuse treatment? *Drug Alcohol Rev*, **27**, 190–196.

Esch, T., Guarna, M., Bianchi, E., et al. (2004) Commonalities in the central nervous system's involvement with complementary medical therapies: Limbic morphinergic processes. *Med Sci Monit*, **10**, MS6–MS17.

Faulkner, G., Carless, D. (2006) Physical activity in the process of psychiatric rehabilitation: Theoretical and methodological issues. *Psychiatr Rehabil J*, **29**, 258–266.

Faymonville, M. E., Boly, M., Laureys, S. (2006) Functional neuroanatomy of the hypnotic state. *J Physiol Paris*, **99**, 463–469.

Geba, B. (1973) *Breath Away Your Tensions*. Random House, New York.

Hanser, S. B. (1993) Using music therapy as distraction during lumbar punctures. *J Pediatr Oncol Nurs*, **10**, 2.

Hanser, S. B., Mandel, S. E. (2005) The effects of music therapy in cardiac healthcare. *Cardiol Rev*, **13**, 18–23.

Hanser, S. B., Thompson, L. W. (1994) Effects of a music therapy strategy on depressed older adults. *J Gerontol*, **49**, P265–P269.

Haque, A. (2004) Psychology from Islamic perspective: Contributions of early Muslim scholars and challenges to contemporary Muslim psychologists. *J Relig Health*, **43**, 357–377.

Jacobson, E. (1962) *You must relax*. McGraw-Hill, New York.

Jing, L., Xudong, W. (2008) Evaluation on the effects of relaxing music on the recovery from aerobic exercise-induced fatigue. *J Sports Med Phys Fitness*, **48**, 102–106.

Jones, N. A., Field, T. (1999) Massage and music therapies attenuate frontal EEG asymmetry in depressed adolescents. *Adolescence*, **34**, 529–534.

Karacabey, K. (2005) Effect of regular exercise on health and disease. *Neuro Endocrinol Lett*, **26**, 617–623.

Kemper, K. J., Hamilton, C. A., McLean, T. W., et al. (2008) Impact of music on pediatric oncology outpatients. *Pediatr Res*, **64**, 105–109.

Klassen, J. A., Liang, Y., Tjosvold, L., et al. (2008) Music for pain and anxiety in children undergoing medical procedures: A systematic review of randomized controlled trials. *Ambul Pediatr*, **8**, 117–128.

Koseoglu, E., Akboyraz, A., Soyuer, A., et al. (2003) Aerobic exercise and plasma beta endorphin levels in patients with migrainous headache without aura. *Cephalalgia*, **23**, 972–976.

Leung, F. W. (2008) Methods of reducing discomfort during colonoscopy. *Dig Dis Sci*, **53**, 1462–1467.

Mandel, S. E., Hanser, S. B., Secic, M., et al. (2007) Effects of music therapy on health-related outcomes in cardiac rehabilitation: A randomized controlled trial. *J Music Ther*, **44**, 176–197.

Maratos, A. S., Gold, C., Wang, X., et al. (2008) Music therapy for depression. *Cochrane Database Syst Rev*, CD004517.

NCCAM (2006) *Massage Therapy as CAM*. (ed N. C. f. C. a. A. Medicine).

Nash, M. R. (2005) Salient findings: A potentially groundbreaking study on the neuroscience of hypnotizability, a critical review of hypnosis' efficacy, and the neurophysiology of conversion disorder. *Int J Clin Exp Hypn*, **53**, 87–93.

Nilsson, U. (2008) The anxiety- and pain-reducing effects of music interventions: A systematic review. *AORN J*, **87**, 780 807.

Pardeck, J. T. (1991) Using books to prevent and treat adolescent chemical dependency. *Adolescence*, **26**, 201–208.

Raglio, A., Bellelli, G., Traficante, D., et al. (2008) Efficacy of music therapy in the treatment of behavioral and psychiatric symptoms of dementia. *Alzheimer Dis Assoc Disord*, **22**, 158–162.

Raij, T. T., Numminen, J., Narvanen, S., et al. (2005) Brain correlates of subjective reality of physically and psychologically induced pain. *Proc Natl Acad Sci U S A*, **102**, 2147–2151.

Ross, S., Cidambi, I., Dermatis, H., et al. (2008) Music therapy: A novel motivational approach for dually diagnosed patients. *J Addict Dis*, **27**, 41–53.

Rush, C. R., Griffiths, R. R. (1996) Zolpidem, triazolam, and temazepam: Behavioral and subject-rated effects in normal volunteers. *J Clin Psychopharmacol*, **16**, 146–157.

Samuels, M. N. (1975) *Seeing with the Mind's Eye*. Random House, New York.

Sarkamo, T., Tervaniemi, M., Laitinen, S., et al. (2008) Music listening enhances cognitive recovery and mood after middle cerebral artery stroke. *Brain*, **131**, 866–876.

Schwartz, G. E., Davidson, R. J., Goleman, D. J. (1978) Patterning of cognitive and somatic processes in the self-regulation of anxiety: Effects of meditation versus exercise. *Psychosom Med*, **40**, 321–328.

Suda, M., Morimoto, K., Obata, A., et al. (2008) Emotional responses to music: Towards scientific perspectives on music therapy. *Neuroreport*, **19**, 75–78.

Thaut, M. H. (2005) The future of music in therapy and medicine. *Ann N Y Acad Sci*, **1060**, 303–308.

Thaut, M. H., Kenyon, G. P., Schauer, M. L., et al. (1999) The connection between rhythmicity and brain function. *IEEE Eng Med Biol Mag*, **18**, 101–108.

Chapter 18
Specific Memetic Therapies

Contents

18.1 Psychotherapies as Memetic Therapies

Existing formal psychotherapies including counseling are essentially memetic, i.e., memes are transmitted back and forth between the patient and the therapist through the process of talking. Psychotherapies work through meme manipulation in the brain of the patient.

Psychotherapy and counseling have nonspecific and specific effects. The nonspecific effects have to do with the supportive presence of another human being, the therapist, who is interested and committed in helping the patient. The specific effects have to do with the particular form of psychotherapy and its presumed theoretical mechanism for helping, e.g., cognitive reframing, insight, or corrective emotional experience. It is generally recognized that psychotherapy and counseling work, especially in conjunction with medications in more serious mental illness, but it is not entirely clear whether the nonspecific or specific effects are more important in the effectiveness of psychotherapy, as the effectiveness does not seem to depend on the form of psychotherapy (Bergin and Garfield, 1994; Consumer Reports, 1995).

Nonspecific aspects of psychotherapy do have specific memetic effects including (1) the therapist is ipso facto a role model, a model for imitation in thinking and behavior, a source of memes; (2) during the regular therapy session, the patient

H. Leigh, *Genes, Memes, Culture, and Mental Illness*,
DOI 10.1007/978-1-4419-5671-2_18, © Hoyle Leigh, 2010

feels protected and supported, i.e., the meme pool to which the patient is exposed is benign and protective, and may neutralize the pathogenic memes in the brain; (3) rational and critical thinking is encouraged during the sessions that enhance the brain's meme-processing abilities. We will now briefly discuss how some of the prevalent psychotherapies may work from the memetic point of view.

18.2   Behavior Therapy, Dialectical Behavior Therapy (DBT), Cognitive–Behavioral Therapy (CBT), Rational Emotive Behavioral Therapy (REBT), Interpersonal Therapy (IPT)

Behavioral therapy is based on Pavlov's classical conditioning and B.F. Skinner's operant conditioning paradigms and attempts to change the behavior of the patient through association and contingency management. Behavior analysis is an important part of the treatment. Techniques derived from behavior therapy include systematic desensitization, exposure and response prevention, various forms of behavior modification, flooding, various operant conditioning, observational learning, habit reversal training etc. (Skinner, 1971, 1991; Spiegler and Goevremont, 2003).

In memetic terms, behavior therapy engages perhaps the most fundamental aspect of meme formation – learning and memory. Through association and approach-avoidance, the organism develops memory traces (see Chapter 8). Behavior therapy attempts to synthesize as well as infuse new memes by providing favorable conditions for learning salutary behaviors, and thus reinforce existing salutary memes as well.

Dialectical behavior therapy (DBT) was first developed by Marsha Linehan to treat borderline personality disorders, and has subsequently been used to treat other conditions including substance abuse and binge eating. Borderline personality patients exhibit emotional vulnerability to stimuli, i.e., excessive arousal of negative emotions, and tend to blame others for the distress. On the other hand, they have internalized the invalidating environment and show self-invalidation, i.e., have unrealistic and excessive expectations of themselves and develop self-blame and guilt when they are not met. Emotional vulnerability and self-invalidation are the first pair of "dialectical dilemmas." Borderline patients frequently experience a series of relentless crises, often contributed to by their own dysfunctional lifestyle and tendency for emotional overreaction. Because of their inability to modulate emotions, such patients have difficulty in facing the emotions associated with loss and grief, and thus suppress negative emotions. The unrelenting crises and inhibited grieving represent the second set of dialectical dilemmas. The final set of dilemmas consist of "active passivity," i.e., they are active in finding others to help them solve problems but are passive in helping themselves and "apparent competence," i.e., they have developed the appearance of competence in the face of invalidating environment without actually achieving a generalizable competence. A pattern of self-destructive behavior often results due to the excessive painful emotions and helplessness. DBT uses the dialectical use of acceptance on the one hand and change on the other. The philosophical concept of dialectics involves the juxtaposition of thesis and antithesis, resulting in a resolution of the opposites through synthesis. In DBT, there are individual and group sessions that consist of four training modules – mindfulness, interpersonal effectiveness, distress tolerance, and emotion regulation. Through mindfulness training derived from Buddhist meditation, the patients learn to accept the here and now free from worries and thoughts. Through interpersonal effectiveness training that incorporates assertiveness training, patients learn to develop more satisfying ways of dealing with others. DBT identifies the triggers for distress and regulates the reaction to them and uses behavioral principles in reinforcing healthful behavior and not reinforcing self-destructive behaviors (Chen et al., 2008; Dimeff and Linehan, 2008; Kiehn and Swales, 1995; Linehan, 1993, 1987; Linehan et al., 2008; Lynch et al., 2007; Rizvi and Linehan, 2001).

In memetic terms, DBT explicitly augments the behavioral therapy components already discussed with mindfulness training, which is a broad-spectrum anti-meme therapy (see Chapter 17). Furthermore, the dialectical aspect of the therapy focuses on the mutually contradictory selfplexes and attempts to develop more integrated selfplexes through dialectical synthesis.

The basic tenet of cognitive–behavioral therapy (CBT) is that thoughts mediate between stimuli and emotions, i.e., an external stimulus causes emotional responses through a cognitive process that evaluates the stimulus. The cognitive processes may be recognizable as thoughts, though sometimes they may be automatic and barely recognized. Such a cognitive process may be distorted and not reflect reality accurately, thus arousing inappropriate or excessive negative emotions. Treatment is geared to identifying the thoughts that distort reality and to correct them through realistic evaluation of reality. Behavioral techniques are often used both to test reality and to enhance a sense of mastery (Beck, 1976/1979; Trower et al., 1988). Schemas or core beliefs concerning the self and the world may be distorted in many patients, and therapy may be effectively directed toward them (Riso et al., 2007).

Thoughts are memes, and schemas are memeplexes and often include selfplexes as well as memeplexes that represent the external world, some of which are in conflict with each other. CBT may be seen as a process of identifying the memes and memeplexes that are pathogenic, i.e., replicating and drawing attention causing distress. The cognitive and behavioral processes in CBT involve an augmentation of the meme-processing ability of the brain by processing the faulty memes through the newly acquired filter (which itself is a meme introduced by the therapist) of rational thinking and reality testing. With the help of the modeling of the therapist's rational thinking and judicious inquires, the patients acquire reinforcement to the hitherto less than effective faculties of their own.

In rational emotive behavioral therapy (REBT), which may be considered to be a subset of CBT, the basic tenet is A-B-C, i.e., activating events or adversities are evaluated by beliefs that may be rational and flexible or irrational and self-defeating, that lead to consequences that may be adaptive or pathological. The therapist attempts to directly challenge the irrational beliefs of patients that often manifest themselves as inflexible "musts" and "shoulds" and emphasize their ability to choose a more flexible rational belief (Dryden, 2002; Ellis, 1962/1994). The therapist in essence attempts to classify the patients' memeplexes into rational and irrational and directly introduce memes to reinforce the "rational" memes.

Memetically informed CBT: CBT could be greatly enhanced with the concept of memes. The therapist could explain to the patient the alien, infectious nature of the pathogenic thoughts and beliefs. Then, such pathogenic thoughts, beliefs, and schemas could be identified, and when possible, the source and circumstances of the infection as well. Then, the therapist and the patient could jointly develop a strategy of neutralizing the pathogenic memes through various exercises and behavior as well as deliberate introduction of new counterbalancing or neutralizing memes.

Interpersonal psychotherapy (IPT) identifies the interpersonal context in which psychiatric distress arises. It then utilizes supportive and psychoeducational methods such as coping skills training to resolve and/or prevent problematic interpersonal situations. The problem areas identified usually fall within four areas – unresolved grief, role disputes, role transitions, and interpersonal deficits. In unresolved grief, the therapist facilitates the mourning process. Assessment of role expectations and realistic problem solving is utilized in role disputes, including the possibility of recognizing the incompatibility of role expectations in some marriages or jobs. In role transitions, such as parenthood or retirement, explicit issues about the change are discussed so as to adapt to the new role. For patients who have interpersonal deficits, and thus often extreme isolation, therapy is geared to reducing the isolation and to form new relationships through skills training (Weissman et al., 2007).

In memetic terms, treating unresolved grief is a means of suppressing replication of memes associated with the lost object. In role disputes and role transitions, IPT enhances the more salutary and adaptive selfplex and equips it with better coping skills (memes). For patients with interpersonal deficits, IPT tends to support the development of a more interpersonally skilled selfplex.

18.3 Psychodynamic Psychotherapy

Psychodynamic psychotherapy, first systematized by Sigmund Freud as psychoanalysis, has many schools, forms, and theories, but they all place importance in the role of the unconscious in emotions and behavior. Most are developmentally oriented, i.e., unconscious conflicts and traumas in childhood are important factors in psychopathology, and making them conscious and dealing with them will result in a resolution of the pathology. Psychoanalysis in its classical form is most intensive and attempts to unveil the unconscious root of the psychological conflict through free association and analysis of the transference phenomena. Analysis usually has multiple sessions per week and lasts several years. Other forms of psychodynamic therapies, such as supportive therapy, brief therapy, couples and family therapy, may be briefer and more focused with less ambitious goals. Psychodynamic therapies work through identifying the unconscious conflicts and the distressing emotions and behaviors they cause, often reliving the conflicts and attendant emotions in the therapeutic relationship, until they are resolved through rational understanding and letting go of the neurotic behavior pattern that has been analyzed within the therapeutic setting (transference neurosis) (Nersessian and Kopff, 1996; Prochaska and Norcross, 1999).

In memetic terms, free association, the technique used in psychoanalysis and often in psychodynamic psychotherapy, is an excellent way of identifying the unconscious (latent) meme content of the patient's brain. Patients often remember meaningful events of the past during therapy, both happy and traumatic memories, and can trace the experience to particular emotions they experienced. This is an excellent way of understanding how certain memes and memeplexes have formed and how they may have remained relatively dormant but still replicating and in conflict with other memes. Psychodynamic psychotherapy derives its effect from two sources – the insight the patient gains and the corrective emotional experience of the patient in relation to the therapist. Insight involves the processing of conflictual memes that arose from the experiences seen through the eyes of a child, through the adult "ego," i.e., a sorting and reassigning of values to memories and other memeplexes (e.g., I was bad, I did accomplish it) for suppression or replication. The corrective emotional experience with the therapist comes from the realization that the therapist is consistently there and caring, unlike the authority figures that the patient had always come to expect. This results in a dissonance in the memeplex schema, how the world is supposed to be (cold and hostile) vs. how the world actually is. Thus, a more realistic memeplex concerning the world is eventually constructed. The therapist also serves as an identification (memetic source) figure of someone who is wise and caring.

18.4   Toward a United, Integrated Memetic Concept of Psychotherapy

It should be clear that all psychotherapies are geared in some way or another toward the manipulation of memes and can be explained in memetic terms. What, then, is the contribution of memetics in psychotherapy?

I believe memetics can serve as a unifying concept of all psychotherapies and would lead to the development of new psychotherapeutic concepts and techniques. Currently, psychotherapeutic "schools" tend to be dogmatic about their particular theory and emphasis. Thus, the therapist is either a cognitive–behavioral therapist or a psychodynamic psychotherapist. Though emotions and behavior can be observed and explained in either terminology, there is no common value-neutral terminology. Memetics can provide that terminology which bridges among cognitive, behavioral, psychodynamic, and neurobiological phenomena. A general understanding of chemical phenoma became only possible with the discovery of the atoms and their components, the protons, electrons, and neutrons. Until then, there was nothing in common between hydrogen, lithium, and sodium. Now we know that having only one electron in the outer shell, these elements have in common certain chemical properties such as being unstable in their elementary forms.

All psychotherapies, to a varying degree, attempt to identify pathogenic memes, trace their origins, and neutralize them and build a salutary selfplex. Regardless of the brand, the nonspecific effect of providing a memetic source (identification figure) is an important ingredient of effectiveness. Could a memetic understanding facilitate the psychotherapeutic process?

Memetic understanding could certainly lead to more efficient therapy, regardless of brand. For example, the therapist may decide, during a psychodynamic psychotherapy, that a meme infusion might facilitate the memetic exploration. The therapist could then actively provide such an infusion, "You must have been very angry and sad that your father ignored you. *I would have been very proud of you!*"

Perhaps, there need not be opposing schools of psychotherapy if we accept memetics as an underlying general concept of psychotherapy. The therapist could utilize various techniques as they are called for, from free association to flooding, provided the therapist and the patient understand the memetic rationale for each technique as it is applied. For example, a patient could have a session of free association and a Rorschach test to attempt to determine some unconscious memetic material that may be relevant to a particular symptom, may have a Myers-Briggs personality inventory, participate in mindfulness training and self-hypnosis for broad-spectrum meme suppression and dialectical behavioral therapy (DBT) to develop more integrated selfplexes.

Note that what I am proposing is not a simple eclecticism – a little of this and a little of that without a particular theoretical orientation. Memetics is a theoretical orientation, and memetics should integrate psychology and neuroscience. Memes are clusters of neurons that are associated through reinforcement (Edelman's reentry). It should be eventually possible to identify the memes and memeplexes within the brain, and augment or suppress them through physical means such as microinjections and/or stereotaxic electrical stimulation. This is not to say that the neural clusters themselves are memes. Memes are the patterns of information that the neural clusters embody, i.e., the patterns could also be encrypted in other media including electronic, optical etc. Thus, memes can reside in brains, in computers, and in books and other media.

Psychotherapy *is* a sophisticated pharmacotherapy of the brain. In my seminars with medical students and other trainees, I say to them, "Please raise your left hand" all raise their hands. Then, I say, "Please, Oh-reun pal ul olyu-yo." They look at me with a puzzled expression. I shout, "Please, *Oh-run pal ul olyu-yo.*" Still nothing, but now with a fearful expression. Then, I say, "Please raise your right hand," they all raise their right hands, relieved. Then, I ask them, "What happened exactly? Why did you raise the left hand when I said it in English, but not when I said it in Korean?" "Because we don't understand Korean." "OK. Let's see exactly what happened. When I said, 'raise your left hand' I emitted a pattern of sounds, that is, I vibrated the air molecules in the proximity of my vocal cords, right? Then the air molecules next to that area vibrated, and eventually, what happened?" "The sound entered your brain" "No, the sound does not enter the brain. The sound or the vibration patterns of air molecules causes the tympanic membrane to vibrate. Then what?" "The tympanic membrane's vibration is transmitted to the ossicles, then to the fluid in cochlea, then the hair cells are stimulated, and an electrical current is generated in the auditory nerve and after several relays through release of neurotransmitters in the midbrain, eventually ends up in the auditory cortex in the temporal lobe. Then neurotransmitters are released to cause electric currents to association neurons that are connected to the association areas in the temporal cortex, and some electrical signal goes to the hippocampus and amygdala. Now, at which point of this system, did the English and Korean version of my request differ? If you recall, they were more or less the same duration and intensity, until I shouted the Korean."

"Well, actually, even though the pattern of air vibration had subtle differences, until the electrochemical stimuli reached the auditory cortex, the process was more or less similar. Then, in the auditory cortex, the English phrase was recognized, i.e., stimulated clusters of associated neurons (memes) and the Korean phrase did not. If you knew Korean, then the phrase may have stimulated a different set of neurons that has a connection with the memes standing for 'raising' and 'right' and 'hand.' The phrases caused differential emotional reactions, i.e., differential stimulation of the amygdalae, as could be read by your fearful expressions when I shouted. And when I said, finally, in English what puzzled you in Korean, you were relieved, i.e., your anxiety subsided. Psychotherapeutic, eh? Understanding, that is a selective electrochemical stimulation of parts of your brain containing existing memes."

18.5 Need for New Meme-Literate Psychotherapies

We alluded to new therapeutic techniques such as meme infusion and meme neutralization. Certainly, much of this can be done with existing techniques such as talking with patients, relaxation, meditation. However, could this be done more directly, through an intravenous injection, as it were? Perhaps flooding may be considered to be a brute method of meme infusion geared to generate an immune reaction. Perhaps, some of the so-called brainwashing techniques should be reexamined and, if used humanely and with full informed consent, might expedite certain forms of therapy. Advertising is often geared to meme infusion through both conscious and unconscious means. Certain techniques derived from successful advertising could be utilized in a therapeutic fashion, perhaps in the form of multimedia including recurring images and earworms. Physical environments might be specifically designed to have a saturation of desired memes for some patients. Drugs may be developed that might particularly enhance susceptibility to incoming memes and might be used within the frame of psychotherapy. Hypnosis could be utilized more frequently and effectively with meme manipulation in mind.

Memeplex constructive therapy in the form of avatars is a very promising new development. Constructing a more desirable digital self with physical and behavioral characteristic that might be made to order, for example, more slender, more assertive self who exercises more and is more sociable, can be an excellent role model (meme source) and observing the digital self in cyberspace as a role model is mimetically a wonderful therapeutic technique (Bailenson, 2006). Eventually, such avatars could be created to order on a personal computer, and used for truly individualized do-it-yourself psychotherapy.

Psychodrama and techniques derived from it such as role playing are used extensively in psychotherapy. With an understanding of memetics, psychodrama could be greatly expanded and systematized in diagnosis and treatment. For example, by playing various scripted roles in either real or virtual groups, one might try out different selfplexes or ways of behaving, thinking, and feeling, which in turn may improve the facility with which different selfplexes may roll into each other and by recognizing the utility of the different selfplexes reduce conflicts among them.

For example, a patient has difficulty with her supervisor. She may be asked to construct three avatars – descriptions of herself with tendencies to feel and behave in three different ways, perhaps one being angry and impulsive, another assertive and methodical, another sad and withdrawing. It is important to assign emotions to the avatars, i.e., they must have clear emotional responses to any interactions and happenings. She might then role play each of the avatars in cyberspace, i.e., her avatar interacts with the supervisor avatar (which was also constructed by the patient). One may then let the patient direct the interaction and see which avatar has most success. She might then "tweak" the avatars so that the success increases. Once she has created a successful avatar in cyberspace, she may role play that avatar in a real psychodrama session with feedback from live people. She may then practice playing the newly constructed selfplex until she becomes completely comfortable with it, then actually try it out in real-life situations. As Shakespeare said, the world is a stage and we are all actors in it – we all know how to play the role of a successful person (or a wise person or a villain) if that is what we want to be.

References

Bailenson, J. N. (2006) Transformed social interaction in collaborative virtual environments. In *Digital Media: Transformations in Human Communication* (P. Messaris and L. Humphreys eds.), pp. 255–264. Peter Lang, New York.

Beck, A. T. (1976/1979) *Cognitive Therapy and the Emotional Disorders*. Penguin Books, New York.

Bergin, A. E., Garfield, S. L. (eds) (1994) *Handbook of Psychotherapy and Behavior Change* (4th edn). Wiley, New York.

Chen, E. Y., Matthews, L., Allen, C., et al. (2008) Dialectical behavior therapy for clients with binge-eating disorder or bulimia nervosa and borderline personality disorder. *Int J Eat Disord*, **41**, 505–512.

Consumer Reports (1995) Does therapy help? In *Consumer Reports*, pp. 734–739. Consumer Reports.

Dimeff, L. A., Linehan, M. M. (2008) Dialectical behavior therapy for substance abusers. *Addict Sci Clin Pract*, **4**, 39–47.

Dryden, W. (2002) Rational emotive behavior therapy. In *Handbook of Individual Therapy* (4th edn) (W. Dryden ed.), pp. 347–372. Sage, London.

Ellis, A. (1962/1994) *Reason and Emotion in Psychotherapy*. Birch Lane Press, New York.

Kiehn, B., Swales, M. (1995) An overview of dialectical behavior therapy in the treatment of borderline personality disorder. In *Psychiatry On-Line*.

Linehan, M. M. (1987) Dialectical behavior therapy for borderline personality disorder. Theory and method. *Bull Menninger Clin*, **51**, 261–276.

Linehan, M. (1993) *Cognitive Behavioral Treatment of Borderline Personality Disorder*. Guilford Press, New York.

Linehan, M. M., McDavid, J. D., Brown, M. Z., et al. (2008) Olanzapine plus dialectical behavior therapy for women with high irritability who meet criteria for borderline personality disorder: A double-blind, placebo-controlled pilot study. *J Clin Psychiatry*, **69**, 999–1005.

Lynch, T. R., Trost, W. T., Salsman, N., et al. (2007) Dialectical behavior therapy for borderline personality disorder. *Annu Rev Clin Psychol*, **3**, 181–205.

Nersessian, E., Kopff, R. G. (1996) *The Psychoanalytic Psychotherapies*. American Psychiatric Press, Washington.

Prochaska, J. O., Norcross, J. C. (1999) *Systems of Psychotherapy: A Transtheoretical Analysis* (4th edn). Brooks/Cole Publishing Co, Pacific Grove.

Riso, L. P., Du Toit, P. L., Stein, D. J., et al. (2007) *Cognitive Schemas and Core Beliefs in Psychological Problems: A Scientist-Practitioner Guide*. American Psychological Association, Washington.

Rizvi, S. L., Linehan, M. M. (2001) Dialectical behavior therapy for personality disorders. *Curr Psychiatry Rep*, **3**, 64–69.

Skinner, B. F. (1971) *Beyond Freedom and Dignity*. Knopf, New York.

Skinner, B. F. (1991) *Verbal Behavior*. Copley Publishing Group, New York.

Spiegler, M. D., Goevremont, D. C. (2003) *Contemporary Behavior Therapy* (4th edn). Wadsworth Publishing, New York.

Trower, P., Casey, A., Dryden, W. (1988) *Cognitive-Behavioural Counselling in Action*. Sage, London.

Weissman, M. M., Markowitz, J. C., Klerman, G. L. (2007) *Clinician's Quick Guide to Interpersonal Psychotherapy*. Oxford University Press, New York.

Chapter 19
Genetic–Memetic Prevention

Contents

19.1 Epigenesis in Prevention

Genes are turned on or off in early life in interaction with environment through the mechanism of *epigenesis* discussed in Chapter 2. Epigenesis involves the inactivation of genes through methylation and reactivation through acetylation and through modification of the histone configuration surrounding them.

For example, the short allele (*s*) of the serotonin transporter promoter gene (SERT, 5-HTTLPR) may confer vulnerability to heightened stress response if the individual had been exposed to abuse in childhood and to depression in adulthood if exposed to stress. But the vulnerability largely disappears without the experience of childhood abuse (Caspi et al., 2003; Pezawas et al., 2005). In rhesus monkeys, the vulnerability associated with the short allele of the SERT gene was ameliorated with good attachment relationships in childhood (Suomi, 2003, 2005).

With monoamine oxidase gene polymorphism, the MAOA-L that results in low levels of the enzyme and thus high levels of monoamines in the brain during the developing phase of the brain, childhood abuse was associated with increased risk of violence and the development of antisocial personality in later life (Caspi et al., 2002). In women, it is also associated with alcoholism and antisocial personality (Ducci et al., 2008). MAOA-H, which causes increased levels of MAOA, buffered against the effects of childhood abuse and neglect in causing later violence and antisocial behavior in whites but not in nonwhites (Widom and Brzustowicz, 2006).

H. Leigh, *Genes, Memes, Culture, and Mental Illness*,
DOI 10.1007/978-1-4419-5671-2_19, © Hoyle Leigh, 2010

Meyer-Lindenberg and her colleagues have shown, using MRI and fMRI, that the MAOA-L variant predicted pronounced reductions in the volume of anterior cingulate gyri and bilateral amygdalae and hyperresponsivity of the left amygdala during emotional arousal, with diminished reactivity of regulatory prefrontal regions, compared with the high expression allele (MAOA-H).

The MAOA gene is X-linked, and in men, the low expression allele (MAOA-L) was also associated with changes in orbitofrontal volume, amygdala and hippocampus hyperreactivity during aversive recall, and impaired cingulate activation during cognitive inhibition. A pronounced effect of genotype and sex was found in left amygdala and hippocampus, i.e., men, but not women, carrying the MAOA-L genotype showed increased reactivity during retrieval of negatively valenced emotional material. In men only, MAOA-L genotype showed a pronounced lack of activation of dorsal anterior cingulate during response inhibition task (Meyer-Lindenberg et al., 2006).

In addition to the gene–stress interactions discussed above, more vulnerability genes have been identified for suicidality (Wasserman et al., 2007, 2008), obesity as well as breast cancer (Wasserman et al., 2004), and somatic symptoms and violence (Crofford, 2007).

Epistasis, or interaction between two different genes, may play an important role in whether or not gene-associated vulnerabilities may actually manifest. For example, the polymorphism in brain-derived neurotrophic factor (BDNF) gene, BDNF-MET allele, is associated with reduced responsivity to 5-HT signaling and protects against 5-HTTLPR s allele-induced effects on a brain circuitry encompassing the amygdala and the subgenual portion of the anterior cingulate. Without the BDNF-MET alleles (BDNF VAL/VAL), 5-HTTLPR s allele is associated with volume reduction in anterior cingulate, but with BDNF-MET, there was no decrease in its volume (Pezawas et al., 2005).

Mental health or mental illness is a result of interaction among vulnerability and resilience genes and salutary and pathogenic memes. Thus memetic prevention of mental illness should focus on (1) reduction of stress memes for children with vulnerable genes and (2) prevention of pathogenic memes from taking up residence in the brain.

19.2 Early Diagnosis and Treatment of Vulnerable Children

Should children with vulnerability genes be identified and treated? Experience with genetic testing of children for risk of colorectal and breast cancer seem to indicate that such testing does not generally have an adverse effect on children (Codori et al., 1996, 2003; Eley, 1999; Michie et al., 2001; Tercyak et al., 2001). On the other hand, whether identifying children at risk for mental illness would result in stigmatization is another issue (Brody, 2002; Chipman, 2006; Hercher and Bruenner, 2008; Spriggs et al., 2008; van Ommen, 2002).

Stigmatization is particularly problematic if there is no remedy for the genetic condition, but it seems that for mental illness, memetic intervention should be possible once the vulnerability genes have been identified. Furthermore, we recognize that so-called vulnerability genes might also serve an adaptive function, thus treatment may not be necessary for all individuals with such genes. Examples are the heightened sensitivity to interpersonal cues in anxiety-associated genes (e.g., 5-HTTLPR *s/s*) or assertiveness and novelty seeking possibly associated with MAOA-L.

Prevention through reduction of extreme stress in childhood, especially child abuse and neglect particularly geared to those with 5-HTTLPR *s* and MAOA-L, however, should have significant beneficial effect as demonstrated in monkeys (see Chapter 2). Perhaps genetic testing should be performed for all suspected child abuse cases, and for those individuals with vulnerability genes, special attention could be paid either to remove the child from the environment or to provide closer attention, education, and care.

19.3 Early Protection from Pathogenic Memes

In addition to the stress of childhood abuse and neglect, which are often both memetic and physical (i.e., direct physiologic and nutritional stress on the tissues), prevention of pathogenic memes from taking up residence and multiplying in the brain is an important issue.

Just like bacteria and fungi, all memes are potentially pathogenic if they are allowed to multiply uncontrollably. On the other hand, like most normal flora, most memes can enter the brain harmlessly and either take up residence as a relatively harmless parasite or be rendered harmless by the filtering mechanism of the brain and allowed to become dormant or die. Then there are memes that are both necessary and salutary for the human brain – memes for knowledge and skills.

Unfortunately, most destructive memes take up residence in the brain from early childhood and destroy or stunt the ability of the brain to develop adequate filtering and processing mechanisms for incoming memes. These destructive memes accept and exalt irrationality and blind faith and ask us to abandon critical thinking and reasoning – the memes and memeplexes associated with superstition, religion, and cultural traditions. Religion is particularly powerful and toxic if introduced early in childhood as it provides ready and easy answers as dogma to a questioning mind. Often religion, superstition, cultural traditions, and family are bound together rendering it practically impossible for children to free themselves from one of the components.

As it is impossible to isolate children from exposure to the pathogenic memes of religion and culture, children should be exposed to as many different religions and cultures as possible, so that they can develop the ability to compare and critique them. Children should be taught in what ways different cultures, traditions, and beliefs differ from each other and what consequences they entail in terms of social and family institutions and mores. For example, how did Christianity affect class and gender relationships? What was the role of Confucianism in an authoritarian society? What is common between religions and superstition? What is the difference? What are the value systems derived from Catholicism vs. Protestantism? Buddhism and Islam? What are the functions of cultural traditions? Which traditions are rational and which are irrational? Such critical thinking will lead to an ability to process them, retaining the component memes that are salutary while quarantining and neutralizing toxic memes.

Memes are stored in and transmitted by electronic and print media. The explosive growth in media in recent years has resulted in a constant and relentless bombardment of memes on the brain. In this environment of relentless competition of memes for survival and replication, it is only natural that the most aggressive (and often virulent) memes will be advantageous. Thus, memes that strongly appeal to emotions, basic drives, and basic fears tend to be more successful. Such memes are those of violence, sex, and fear of death, and the irrational security promised by religion.

In addition to enhancing the skills of critical thinking in children, it would be important to teach them how to take "time out" from the bombardment of memes from the environment. Teaching children techniques of broad-spectrum meme reduction as discussed in Chapter 16 would be an important step. Children should also be taught general stress management and coping skills.

It is neither desirable nor possible to limit or censor the memetic content of the media, but it may be possible to introduce salutary memes in the media that may neutralize or attenuate extremely toxic memes. For example, empathy memes might be introduced together with violence memes, and memes for rational thinking may be introduced with religious memes. Just how to do this would depend on the context and content of the media – for example, the hero of an action movie might be multidimensional with an empathic and loving side.

19.4 Vaccination

Is vaccination possible for toxic memes? Gold and Shanks argue that cultural diversity will confer immunity to toxic conformity memes as genetic diversity tends to confer enhanced immunity to infection (Gold and Shanks, 2002). In a fascinating webpage, Kubiak describes how foreign ideas (memes) were quarantined in Asia (for example, those who traveled to foreign countries were isolated from others until they re-acculturated themselves with the indigenous one) and how the McArthur reforms after World War II might have served as a memetic vaccination against democracy in Japan when they had to be to a large extent reversed for fear of communism (Kubiak, 1998).

It seems clear that quarantining memes in the age of the Internet and information explosion is untenable and undesirable, considering that even Burma and North Korea may be on the brink of change. Natural vaccination in the form of enhancing cultural diversity in the society is both effective and desirable. It should also be possible to deliberately vaccinate people, especially children, against toxic memes.

Vaccination involves boosting the immune system, and the immune system for memes relies on reason and critical thinking. Thus, general boosting of these abilities through education would be a first step. Then, irrational and toxic memes should be introduced in an attenuated form. How to attenuate toxic memes? By divesting them of the aesthetically pleasing adornments, such as music, art, and edifices that usually accompany them as in religious hymns, art, and churches and mosques. Just present the basic mythologies of any religion or tradition or blind belief to a critical and questioning mind, and immunity will develop pronto. Then, the adornments can also be presented and can be appreciated for their own sake, without being suckered into the irrational and toxic memes.

Infusion of antibodies in the form of critiques of toxic memes may also be useful. One danger of such infusion, however, may be that immunity may develop against the critiques if they are introduced in an authoritarian manner. Thus, introducing both the toxic memes and the critiques at the same time would be more effective.

"Flooding" with toxic memes may be another means of vaccination in certain situations. For example, persons who might be somewhat attracted to specific toxic memes, for example, a cult, might be invited to participate in an intensive simulated or virtual reality indoctrination experience. Strong counter-memes (antibodies) are likely to develop very quickly.

19.5 Education

It should be obvious from our discussion so far that education must be the centerpiece in the prevention of multiplication of toxic memes in the brain, and thus of mental illness. Education from an early age in the acquisition and practice of rational and critical thinking will enhance the development of the sorting and filtering process for incoming memes.

Once identified, toxic memes must be processed so that they are rendered harmless. The techniques of doing this must be a part of the educational process. Such methods would include analyzing the components of the toxic memes, recognizing the capsules and adornments associated with such memes that are meant to be attractive and aesthetically pleasing, and relegating them to the pool of irrational memes that can be a source of amusement rather than threat. For particularly virulent memes, techniques discussed in Chapter 17, broad-spectrum memetic therapy may be utilized to reduce their proliferation. Such techniques include relaxation, meditation, music, and exercise, among others.

19.6 Gene–Meme Cooperation vs. Gene–Meme Conflict: "Mind" and "Body"

An important aspect of education should be to discuss the "mind–body" problem in memetic terms. The "body" is the manifestation of the genes in action. The "mind" is the activity of the brain processing memes. Since the brain is made of genes and their products, it is geared to be on the side of the genes if there is a conflict between genes and memes. Memes are, of course, concerned only with their own replication even at the expense of genetic interests. Infectious martyrdom is an example of a virulent meme that spreads at the expense of the individual and his/her genes.

Recognition of the potential conflict of interest between genes and memes can result in a rational analysis of the conflict, and thus identify the self-interest of the meme masquerading as altruism or a "holy cause." On the other hand, reason may be on the side of the memes when an impulse generated by genes threatens to take hold of the brain and result in an injudicious action.

A memetic analysis of history will reveal how human beings have been exploited by virulent memes in various epochs, in the forms of oppressive religion, nationalism, racism, and communism, among others, resulting in holy wars, holocausts, and genocides.

Memes arose from genes in the course of evolution. With *Homo sapiens*, memes have evolved exponentially while genes remained stagnant. As memes evolved, i.e., became more sophisticated in replication, they co-opted the gene-based bodies for their own purpose and dictated individuals to obey their bidding. Now memes may have matured enough and developed enough not to require human brains to replicate. This may have a liberating effect on the humans, as those memes that remain in human brains may become more symbiotic rather than virulently parasitic. If memes can live independently and thrive outside of the brain in computers and cyberspace, then they do not have to take over the brain, but could cooperate with the genes of the brain for mutual benefit. The brain may be just a temporary residence for some memes. While memes may no longer need the brain, the brain may still be able to contribute to memes, perhaps by creating novel ones.

References

Brody, B. A. (2002) Freedom and responsibility in genetic testing. *Soc Philos Policy*, **19**, 343–359.

Caspi, A., McClay, J., Moffitt, T. E., et al. (2002) Role of genotype in the cycle of violence in maltreated children. *Science*, **297**, 851–854.

Caspi, A., Sugden, K., Moffitt, T. E., et al. (2003) Influence of life stress on depression: Moderation by a polymorphism in the 5-HTT gene. *Science*, **301**, 386–389.

Chipman, P. (2006) The moral implications of prenatal genetic testing. *Penn Bioeth J*, **2**, 13–16.

Codori, A. M., Petersen, G. M., Boyd, P. A., et al. (1996) Genetic testing for cancer in children. Short-term psychological effect. *Arch Pediatr Adolesc Med*, **150**, 1131–1138.

Codori, A. M., Zawacki, K. L., Petersen, G. M., et al. (2003) Genetic testing for hereditary colorectal cancer in children: Long-term psychological effects. *Am J Med Genet A*, **116A**, 117–128.

Crofford, L. J. (2007) Violence, stress, and somatic syndromes. *Trauma Violence Abuse*, **8**, 299–313.

Ducci, F., Enoch, M. A., Hodgkinson, C., et al. (2008) Interaction between a functional MAOA locus and childhood sexual abuse predicts alcoholism and antisocial personality disorder in adult women. *Mol Psychiatry*, **13**, 334–347.

Eley, T. C. (1999) Behavioral genetics as a tool for developmental psychology: Anxiety and depression in children and adolescents. *Clin Child Fam Psychol Rev*, **2**, 21–36.

Gold, J., Shanks, N. (2002) Mind viruses and the importance of cultural diversity. In *Community, Diversity, and Difference: Implications for Peace* (A. Bailey and P. J. Smithka eds.), pp. 187–199. Rodopi Press, Amsterdam, New York.

Hercher, L., Bruenner, G. (2008) Living with a child at risk for psychotic illness: The experience of parents coping with 22q11 deletion syndrome: An exploratory study. *Am J Med Genet A*, **146A**, 2355–2360.

Kubiak, W. D. (1998) The abhorrence of exotic ideas: Japan's comparative advantage in memetic immunity.

Meyer-Lindenberg, A., Buckholtz, J. W., Kolachana, B., et al. (2006) Neural mechanisms of genetic risk for impulsivity and violence in humans. *Proc Natl Acad Sci USA*, **103**, 6269–6274.

Michie, S., Bobrow, M., Marteau, T. M. (2001) Predictive genetic testing in children and adults: A study of emotional impact. *J Med Genet*, **38**, 519–526.

Pezawas, L., Meyer-Lindenberg, A., Drabant, E. M., et al. (2005) 5-HTTLPR polymorphism impacts human cingulate-amygdala interactions: A genetic susceptibility mechanism for depression. *Nat Neurosci*, **8**, 828–834.

Spriggs, M., Olsson, C. A., Hall, W. (2008) How will information about the genetic risk of mental disorders impact on stigma? *Aust N Z J Psychiatry*, **42**, 214–220.

Suomi, S. J. (2003) Gene-environment interactions and the neurobiology of social conflict. *Ann NY Acad Sci*, **1008**, 132–139.

Suomi, S. J. (2005) Aggression and social behaviour in rhesus monkeys. *Novartis Found Symp*, **268**, 216–222, discussion 222–216, 242–253.

Tercyak, K. P., Peshkin, B. N., Streisand, R., et al. (2001) Psychological issues among children of hereditary breast cancer gene (BRCA1/2) testing participants. *Psychooncology*, **10**, 336–346.

van Ommen, G. J. (2002) The Human Genome Project and the future of diagnostics, treatment and prevention. *J Inherit Metab Dis*, **25**, 183–188.

Wasserman, D., Geijer, T., Sokolowski, M., et al. (2007) Nature and nurture in suicidal behavior, the role of genetics: Some novel findings concerning personality traits and neural conduction. *Physiol Behav*, **92**, 245–249.

Wasserman, D., Sokolowski, M., Rozanov, V., et al. (2008) The CRHR1 gene: A marker for suicidality in depressed males exposed to low stress. *Genes Brain Behav*, **7**, 14–19.

Wasserman, L., Flatt, S. W., Natarajan, L., et al. (2004) Correlates of obesity in postmenopausal women with breast cancer: Comparison of genetic, demographic, disease-related, life history and dietary factors. *Int J Obes Relat Metab Disord*, **28**, 49–56.

Widom, C. S., Brzustowicz, L. M. (2006) MAOA and the "cycle of violence:" childhood abuse and neglect, MAOA genotype, and risk for violent and antisocial behavior. *Biol Psychiatry*, **60**, 684–689.

Part IV
Specific Psychiatric Syndromes

Chapter 20
Overview of Specific Syndromes

Contents

20.1 Introduction

In subsequent chapters in Part IV, we will briefly discuss specific psychiatric syndromes and their treatment. We will here use a model of mental illness that represents a dysregulation of normal brain function as a result of gene × meme × environment interaction through development (Chapter 12, 13, and 14). The diagnostic nomenclature is phenomenological and memetic, and depending on the degree of the dysregulation, gradations of diagnosis could be made, e.g., from anxiety as a symptom to anxiety neurosis to major depression and/or psychosis (Axis I in my scheme, see (Chapter 14).

It should be emphasized that by "genetic," I do not mean just the DNA but also the products of the genes in action, i.e., the organism. By "memes," I mean the information processed by the brain that is or potentially is transmitted (i.e., leave the brain) to the outside.

Thus, an Axis I phenomenological (neurophysiomemetic) classification clustered around presumed brain function/dysfunction may be as follows:

A. Attention-cognition spectrum syndromes (delirium, dementia, impulse control syndromes, ADHD, antisocial personality, obsessive-compulsive personality traits, obsessive-compulsive syndrome);
B. Fear–anxiety–depression spectrum syndromes (anxiety, panic, ASD, PTSD, depression – neurotic and syndromic, borderline syndrome, mania, adjustment disorders, avoidant traits and personality, phobias);
C. Reality perception spectrum syndromes (psychosis, dissociation, conversion, somatoform, misattribution somatization);

H. Leigh, *Genes, Memes, Culture, and Mental Illness*,
DOI 10.1007/978-1-4419-5671-2_20, © Hoyle Leigh, 2010

Early Life   Later Life

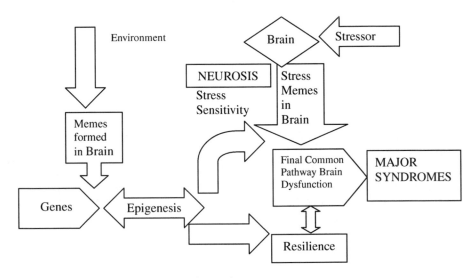

A model of gene–meme–environment interaction

D. Pleasure-motivation spectrum syndromes (substance use/abuse, addictions to substances and beliefs, fanaticism);
E. Primary memetic syndromes (eating disorders, factitious syndromes, malingering, meme-directed irrational acts).

20.2 Gene–Meme Symbiosis and Mental Illness

Memes originally arose to aid the particular genes that either created them or as genes found the incoming meme(s) to be advantageous. Thus there developed a symbiotic relationship between genes and memes. Such symbiotic memes may serve the function of nurturing the organism or primarily serve to facilitate the reproduction and replication of the genes and memes together. With the advent of language and symbols, memes arose that transcend immediate perception. Imagination and fantasy are alternate realities which are created by memes and populated solely by memes. Abstraction is another purely memetic process that brings a memetic order to the universe.

Abstract memes are complex and often recruit and incorporate various memes as they become larger (having more memes in it), more powerful (drive to replicate), and thus more competitive. This is particularly so when the memeplex is competing for whole populations. One can be both a farmer and a carpenter, but one cannot be both a Christian and a Muslim.

Memes that are primarily geared to replication of themselves often at the expense of the genetic needs of the organism may be toxic to the individual. Such memes include most fanaticisms and fanatical religions and superstitions. They are toxic because they suppress, paralyze, and stunt the development of the filtering and sorting function of the brain (ego).

The state of symbiotic relationship between genes and memes in the brain represents the state of mental health or illness (Chapter 12 and 13). When there is a harmonious relationship among the memes in the brain, and their overall function is in the service of the genetic needs of the organism, and when there is a harmonious relationship among the genes in the brain as a result of epigenesis, and they have a harmonious relationship with the goals and plans that the selfplexes are striving for, there is mental health. When there is conflict between the needs of the genes and the memes, or among the memes and genes, then there is distress of varying severity. When the distress reaches a certain threshold, an autonomous syndrome may ensue, which represents a final common pathway brain dysfunction (Chapter 13). Exactly which symptom or syndrome occurs depends on specific gene × meme interaction and vulnerability determined through epigenesis and development of selfplex. Thus, there may be individuals primed to develop anxiety, depression, dissociation, psychosis, etc., due to the genetic trait in interaction with the memetic environment, e.g., Is it more acceptable to express distress with a somatic symptom? By acting crazy? Withdrawing?

20.3 Toward a Dimensional Approach in Identifying and Treating Mental Illness

All the conditions in the five categories of mental illness listed in Section 20.1 may coexist with each other and may overlap as the categories are simply representations of important brain functions. Each of the categories except the primary memetic/imitation conditions can be represented in a continuum using scales and subscales of assessment as below. Scales for many of these items are currently available, others need to be developed.

It should thus be possible to develop treatment strategies geared to improving each dimensional scale representing dysfunction or symptoms. Thus, for a patient who has a severe dysfunction in Af. Obsessiveness scale, Ag. Compulsiveness ccale, Bb. Depression scale, Bf. Neurovegetative symptoms scale, and Cb. Dissociation scale may be best treated with a selective serotonin reuptake inhibitor (SSRI) which is known to reduce both depressive and obsessive-compulsive symptoms. The dissociative symptoms may be treated with meme-oriented therapies to reduce anxiety and to experience the obsessive thoughts as a dysfunction in meme-processing loop, and through self-hypnosis to gain mastery over the dissociative experience and to strengthen a sense of selfplex.

The degree of efficacy of treatment may be monitored through repeated administration of relevant scales.

Diagnostic Scales (Normal—Neurosis/Trait— Major Syndrome)

A. Attention-cognition spectrum conditions

    a. Attention scale
    b. Hyperactivity scale
    c. Cognitive achievement/impairment scale
    d. Rationality scale
    e. Impulsiveness scale
    f. Obsessiveness scale
    g. Compulsiveness scale
    h. Antisociality scale

B. Anxiety-mood spectrum conditions

    a. Anxiety scale
    b. Depression scale
    c. Stress disorder scale
    d. Mania scale
    e. Self-esteem scale
    f. Neurovegetative symptoms scale
        Sleep subscale
        Appetite subscale
        Libido subscale
    g. Avoidant trait scale
    h. Specific phobia scale with specification of phobic object

C. Reality perception spectrum conditions

    a. Selfplex integrity (smoothness of selfplex transition) scale
    b. Dissociation scale
    c. Psychosis scale
        Hallucination subscale
        Delusion subscale
        Association subscale
    d. Eccentricity/unconventionality scale
    e. Misattribution/somatization scale

D. Pleasure-motivation spectrum conditions

    a. Anhedonia (reward deficiency) scale
    b. Substance use scale
    c. Memetic pleasure scale

      Rationality subscale
      Hobby subscale
      Idealism subscale
      Sprituality/religiosity/fanaticism subscale

E. Primary memetic/imitation conditions

   a. Eating disorders
      Body weight perception scale
      Attractiveness perception scale
   b. Suggestibility/Gullibility Scale
   c. Conformity Scale

Chapter 21
Attention-Cognition Spectrum Syndromes: Delirium, Dementia, Impulse Control Syndromes, ADHD, Antisocial Personality, Obsessive-Compulsive Personality Traits, Obsessive-Compulsive Syndrome

Contents

21.1 Gene × Meme Interaction, Evolutionary Adaptation, and Syndromes

Attention is a basic brain function necessary for any action from finding food to fight/flight reaction. Attention to internal physical stimuli such as distended bladder is also important to maintain health. Cognition is essentially the brain's meme-processing function and developed extensively with the growth of the neocortex.

Attention system seems to be separate from the data-processing systems of the brain and involves specific neural networks that carry out specific functions related to attention (Posner and Petersen, 1990). Posner and Peterson (1990) describe the components of the attention system as (1) orienting to sensory stimuli involving the parietal lobes and midbrain structures, (2) detecting signals for processing involving the parietal lobes and their connection to the frontal lobes and the anterior cingulate gyrus, and (3) maintaining an alert, vigilant state, involving the locus ceruleus and the right hemisphere.

There are normal degrees of attention and inattention depending on the nature and amount of external and internal stimuli, physiologic state, and the amount of internal processing of data that may require attention. It is obvious that well-functioning attention system has evolutionarily adaptive value, but the ease of shifts

H. Leigh, *Genes, Memes, Culture, and Mental Illness*,
DOI 10.1007/978-1-4419-5671-2_21, © Hoyle Leigh, 2010

of attention vs. ability to stick to a task without distraction may have differential adaptive value depending on the habitat. When one is in constant threat of being attacked by a predator, easy shift of attention to a footstep may be lifesaving, on the other hand, if one has to concentrate to sharpen a sword before a battle, being able to ignore distractions may be all important. Thus, attention-regulating genes adapted for one environment may prove to be maladaptive for another.

Thinking, or cognition, is mainly a function of the frontal cortex with contributions from the sensory and association cortices. Working memory, associated with the dorsolateral prefrontal cortex and its connections (see Chapter 9) plays an essential part in cognition. The left brain is generally considered to be involved in logical, linear thinking, while the right brain is more involved with global, holistic, and intuitive thinking. Cognition is greatly affected by attention and arousal, as well as by emotions.

With the rapid growth of the neocortex with hominids that parallels the development and multiplication of memes, our brain's activity has become increasingly that of cognition. With ever increasing influx of memes in the form of language and information, the brain is challenged with the need for ever increasing efficiency in meme processing that we call cognition.

Prolongation of human life through technologies developed by memes may be responsible for the prevalence of degenerative dementias. As evolutionary adaptation functions exclusively during the reproductive period, there is no evolutionary disadvantage for diseases of the post-reproductive period in life.

In discussing treatment for syndromes in this section, we will first briefly deal with global dysregulation of meme processing associated with clear physiologic and/or structural aberrations, i.e., delirium and dementia, as it is beyond the scope of this book to discuss this large and important area in detail. Then, we will discuss in some detail the conditions associated with attention-deficit hyperactivity, impulse control problems, obsessions, compulsions, and preoccupations in two separate subsections.

21.1.1 Global Dysregulation of Meme Processing: Delirium and Dementia

Global dysregulation of meme processing occurs when there is a metabolic or toxic dysfunction of the brain as a whole. In delirium, which is characterized by relatively acute fluctuations in global brain function, the memetic content is confused and erratic. Because of the disturbances in neural circuitry and in neural firing and conduction due to electrolyte imbalance, toxins, etc., there are disturbances in the functions they serve, including perception, memory, thinking process, judgment. Hallucinations, delusions, preoccupations, etc., are common as well as emotional lability, agitation, and altered levels of awareness, e.g., sleepiness and stupor.

In dementia, there is often progressive degeneration of brain structures and thus reduction in their meme-processing function. Higher cortical functions necessary for higher level meme processing, such as logical thinking and judgment are often impaired, and often results in disinhibition of normal memetic demands such as following social conventions of dress and behavior. Delirium is often superimposed on dementia resulting in more impairment and confusion.

The memetic diagnosis for delirium and dementia is based on recognizing the global deficits in meme processing, and the treatment should be geared to providing a nonthreatening and easy to comprehend memetic environment. Memetic treatment should be accompanied by drugs as needed. In delirium, the underlying metabolic or toxic cause must be identified and treated. Drug treatment may be geared toward immediate agitation and confusion as well as possible specific dementias.

21.1.2 Dysregulation of Infrastructure for Meme Processing: Attention-Deficit Disorder (ADHD), Impulse and Aggression Dyscontrol, Antisocial Personality

This dysregulation spectrum involves the infrastructures for meme processing, i.e., the tools needed to think and behave normally. This involves being able to shift and maintain attention, recognize and modulate impulses that may arise from gene- or meme-determined needs and to modulate and channel aggression which may also be determined by genes, memes, or both.

Neuropsychological and imaging studies indicate that attention-deficit hyperactivity disorder (ADHD) is associated with alterations in prefrontal cortex (PFC) and its connections to striatum and cerebellum. PFC is critical for utilizing representational knowledge in the regulation of behavior, attention, and affect. PFC is involved in sustaining attention, inhibiting distraction, and dividing attention, while more posterior areas are necessary for perception and allocation of attention. The right PFC seems especially important in behavioral inhibition as its lesions produce distractibility, forgetfulness, impulsivity, poor planning, and motor hyperactivity. PFC is very sensitive to levels of dopamine and norepinephrine. Norepinephrine may enhance signals through postsynaptic alpha-2A receptors in PFC, while dopamine decreases noise through D1 receptor stimulation (Brennan and Arnsten, 2008).

A number of candidate genes for ADHD have been identified, including the dopamine transporter gene (DAT1 or SLC6A3), the dopamine D2, D4, and D5 receptor genes, the serotonin transporter gene (SLC6A4 or 5-HTT), the serotonin 2A receptor gene (5-HT2A), and SNAP25. Other genes that have received significant study include the norepinephrine transporter (NET), catechol-O-methyltransferase (COMT), and the nicotinic acetylcholinereceptor alpha 4 subunit (CHRNA4).

Gene–environment interactions have been studied in ADHD. Interestingly, given childhood abuse, the long allele of the serotonin transporter promoter gene, rather than the short allele which is associated with neuroticism and later depression, was associated with ADHD (see Chapter 1 for further discussion of serotonin transporter promoter gene). It is possible that individuals with the long allele might cope with stress through inattention while those with the short allele might be unable to cope and thus become more fearful and depressed. The short allele was associated with more severe ADHD pathology if the stresses were early in life (Muller et al., 2008). 5-HTTLPR thus may act as a moderator of environmental influences in ADHD (Muller et al., 2008).

Smoking seems to contribute to gene–environment interaction in the risk of ADHD and impulsive behavior (Wallis et al., 2008). Child hyperactivity–impulsivity and oppositional behaviors were associated with a DAT polymorphism but only when the child also had exposure to maternal prenatal smoking. In addition, interaction between DAT1 genotypes and maternal use of alcohol during pregnancy suggests that DAT1 moderates the environmental risk. Prenatal exposure to smoking and variations in the DAT1 and DRD4 loci seem to interact in children with the ADHD combined subtype. CHRNA4 gene polymorphisms interacted with prenatal smoking exposure on risk for severe combined type ADHD. Gene–environment interactions have been reported for DRD2 genotypes as well as COMT polymorphisms for ADHD and conduct disorder.

The short allele of the MAOA (MAOA-uVNTR) has been associated with aggressive behavior, violence, and antisocial behavior (Reif et al., 2007).

Carrying a short allele of the MAOA-uVNTR acted as a true and independent risk factor for later-life aggression, further adding to the risk conveyed by childhood maltreatment. Other behavioral traits such as disruptiveness and cluster B personality traits (dramatic, colorful, histrionic, antisocial, borderline) but not cluster C (shy and fearful) may be contributed to and regulated by the MAOA gene as well.

MAOA short allele has also been associated with hyperreactivity of the amygdala in response to emotional arousal, associated with impaired response of the prefrontal and anterior cingulate cortex in fMRI studies. In fact, stronger coupling between amygdala and the ventromedial prefrontal cortex through the rostral cingulate cortex predicted increased harm avoidance and decreased reward dependence (Buckholtz et al., 2008).

In pathologically aggressive individuals, serotonin transporter concentration was significantly reduced in the anterior cingulate cortex (Frankle et al., 2005). As the short allele of the 5-HTTLPR is associated with decreased levels of serotonin transporter, it may play a role in aggression. Homozygotes for the long allele have been shown to be less likely to develop later-life aggressive behavior, while the short allele homozygotes do. Most interestingly, only heterozygotes were influenced by environmental factors, that is, this polymorphism might have a role in balancing aggressive behaviors in differing societies (Reif et al., 2007).

21.1.3 Dysregulation of Meme-Processing Loop: Preoccupations, Obsessions, Compulsions

An evolutionarily important event was the development of romantic love, which serves as an example of memetic preoccupation, obsession, and compulsion, usually but not always within normal range. Helen Fisher studied romantic love extensively. She states, "The sex drive evolved to motivate individuals to seek a range of mating partners; attraction evolved to motivate individuals to prefer and pursue specific partners; and attachment evolved to motivate individuals to remain together long enough to complete species-specific parenting duties. These three behavioural repertoires appear to be based on brain systems that are largely distinct yet interrelated, and they interact in specific ways to orchestrate reproduction, using both hormones and monoamines. Romantic attraction in humans and its antecedent in other mammalian species play a primary role: this neural mechanism motivates individuals to focus their courtship energy on specific others, thereby conserving valuable time and metabolic energy, and facilitating mate choice" (Fisher et al., 2006).

The neural circuit underlying romantic love involves the right ventral tegmental area of the brain stem and right posterodorsal body of the caudate nucleus. The dopaminergic reward and motivation pathways contribute to aspects of romantic love.

The complex neurotransmitter network of the cortico-striatal-thalamo-cortical (CSTC) circuit involving dopamine, serotonin, glutamate, and gamma-amino butyric acid (GABA) may be dysfunctional in obsessive-compulsive syndrome (Harvey et al., 2001). The dysfunction in this loop may arise from an attenuation of feedback signal indicating reward which results in compulsive lever pressing in rats, which is further enhanced by lesions of the orbitofrontal cortex (Joel et al., 2005). Compulsions may also develop from an operant conditioning (memetic) paradigm as in compulsive gambling, which in turn may result in functional changes in the brain such as impairment of decision-making capacity (Fellows, 2007; Hariri et al., 2006; Kalenscher et al., 2006).

Tourette's syndrome is an example of brain dysfunction that involves dysregulation of both meme processing and motoric function illuminating the role of the basal ganglia in both. In this syndrome, there are simple and complex motor tics, vocal tics, and frequently obsessive-compulsive symptoms. Its onset occurs before the age of 21 and the course is waxing and waning. Tourette's syndrome occurs mainly in boys and is genetically transmitted with variable penetrance but it has also been associated with various infections and immunological conditions such as the PANDAS (pediatric autoimmune neuropsychiatric disorder associated with streptococcal infection). The neuropathology seems to involve a disturbance of the dopaminergic system in the basal ganglia.

Gene–environment interaction involving the serotonin transporter promoter gene (5-HTTLPR) has also been reported in OCD, i.e., those with the s/s allele and childhood trauma were more likely to develop OCD with dissociative experiences (Lochner et al., 2007). Clearly, same gene–environment interaction may lead to multiple vulnerabilities in the CNS, including OCD, dissociation, anxiety, and depression.

In our discussion above, it seems that we are at a threshold of understanding the neurobiological mechanisms of normal functioning such as attention, thinking, aggressivity, and impulse control. Normal thinking process may become abnormal if stuck in a loop, as in preoccupations, obsessions, and compulsions. Structural and metabolic change in the brain may cause temporary or permanent loss of the ability to perceive and process memes in the form of information and memory.

Attention deficit and hyperactivity are behavioral observations, i.e., what do the patients look like and how do they behave? Individuals with these problems may not initially complain of any distress, but their grades may suffer, and family and friends may be frustrated. The memetic content may be those of puzzlement and bewilderment. "Why do I forget so easily? I can't focus" Low self-esteem memes are introduced and proliferate, "I am not good at studying, math, . . ." With hyperactivity and impulse control problems, "badness" memes will be introduced and replicate – "I am a trouble-maker" "I am bad" "Nobody likes me."

With ADHD, however, the individual often fails to store sufficient variety and number of memes in the brain to function well, as well as being distracted by differing memes in the environment vying for attention to get into the brain. Many such memes may be poorly processed in the brain, and thus poorly integrated with existing memes.

With aggression, violence, and antisocial personality, the environment in the gene × meme × environment interaction infuses abuse and neglect memes that cause the epigenetic changes for poor impulse control through attenuation of meme-processing abilities. Furthermore, the abuse and neglect memes take up residence in the brain providing a model for future selfplexes – to be uncaring and abusing.

Preoccupations are excessive memetic replications in the brain. By replication, I do not mean that the neurons are replicating themselves – rather, the intensity of the firing of the neuronal cluster that makes the meme is increased, it recruits other clusters of neurons to fire and develop long-term potentiation like themselves, which is how memes replicate (Chapter 9). The enhanced firing may recruit the motor neurons to fire, thus expressing the meme to the outside, and when this is in the form of language, it is likely to infect the receiver. In other words, if I am preoccupied with love, I may say it aloud, may write an e-mail, and perhaps a poem. All of these will transmit my "love" meme to myself, my beloved, my friends, and the world at large.

Preoccupations, obsessions, and compulsions may occur unwantedly and unexpectedly, depending on the state of the brain and the memetic nature of the thought. In the obsessive-compulsive disorder (OCD), there may be a primary dysfunction of the cortico-striatal-thalamo-cortical network involving dopamine and serotonin discussed above. Symptoms of OCD may also occur because the meme representing the thought may be particularly strong because it is fed by energies from related preexisting memes in the brain. For example, a suicide meme may be introduced by seeing a film to a depressed brain that has many preexisting self-punishment and guilt memes, thus the suicide meme may gain strength, proliferate, and recruit the motor neurons to carry out suicide. Other memes, like earworms which are unwanted melodies or sounds that keep on occurring in the mind, may replicate because of the strength of their vehicles (the rhythm, melody, form of presentation, color, smell, texture, etc.). Some such memes may represent "supernormal stimulus," the kinds of stimuli that are evolutionarily determined to elicit strong preferences, or results of early imprinting (Burkhardt, 2005).

The diagnosis of obsessions, compulsions, and OCD is made on the basis of the severity of the phenomena and the degree of distress. Earworms are nuisances but not necessarily distressing, ego-alien obsessions can be very distressing, and compulsions may be disabling.

21.2 Treatment

Genetic and pharmacologic treatment should be geared to the suspected or demonstrated brain dysfunction, and may include SSRIs, often in high doses, and surgical interventions including deep brain stimulation and capsulotomies have been used successfully in treatment-resistant OCD (Cecconi et al., 2008; Dowling, 2008; Nuttin et al., 2008). Treatment of delirium and dementia involves providing memetic environment that is stable and protective and appropriate medications. For ADHD, stimulants are effective as well as meme-oriented broad spectrum and specific therapies enhancing positive selfplexes.

Several symptom subtypes of obsessive-compulsive disorder (OCD) have been identified on the basis of the predominant obsessions and compulsions. Overt compulsions have been associated with a relatively good response to the exposure and response prevention (ERP) therapy and with poorer response to serotonin reuptake inhibitors (SSRIs). Washing and cleaning and checking compulsions tend to respond well to ERP, but and rather poorly to SSRIs. Patients with symmetry, ordering, and arranging subtype do tend to respond equally well to ERP and SSRIs. Some studies suggest that obsessions might respond to SSRIs somewhat better than to ERP. Hoarding and the subtype characterized by sexual or religious obsessions and absence of overt compulsions have been associated with poor response to ERP and SSRIs (Starcevic and Brakoulias, 2008).

Cognitive–behavioral therapy and antipsychotic medications have also been used effectively in OCD.

The memetic approach to preoccupations, obsessions, and compulsions should involve an analysis of the memetic content of the thoughts, and their memetic connections (and vehicles) such as the visual, auditory, olfactory, gustatory, and tactile associations. One might find that the energy for replication of the obsessive meme may indeed come from a conflict with a nondominant (repressed) meme that is associated with it.

Treatment should then include, in addition to cognitive behavioral and exposure and response techniques, direct memetic neutralization of the replicating thought (obsession) through infusion of new memes and/or strengthening of existing ones as with repetition of a word or phrase, visualization, and music therapy. Such specific treatments may be in conjunction with broad-spectrum anti-meme therapy (see Chapter 17) to reduce the unchecked proliferation of memes seen in OCD.

References

Brennan, A. R., Arnsten, A. F. (2008) Neuronal mechanisms underlying attention deficit hyperactivity disorder: The influence of arousal on prefrontal cortical function. *Ann N Y Acad Sci*, **1129**, 236–245.

Buckholtz, J. W., Callicott, J. H., Kolachana, B., et al. (2008) Genetic variation in MAOA modulates ventromedial prefrontal circuitry mediating individual differences in human personality. *Mol Psychiatry*, **13**, 313–324.

Burkhardt, R. W., Jr. (2005) *Patterns of Behavior: Konrad Lorenz, Niko Tinbergen, and the Founding of Ethology.* University of Chicago Press, Chicago.

Cecconi, J. P., Lopes, A. C., Duran, F. L., et al. (2008) Gamma ventral capsulotomy for treatment of resistant obsessive-compulsive disorder: A structural MRI pilot prospective study. *Neurosci Lett*, **447**, 138–142.

Dowling, J. (2008) Deep brain stimulation: Current and emerging indications. *Mo Med*, **105**, 424–428.

Fellows, L. K. (2007) The role of orbitofrontal cortex in decision making: A component process account. *Ann N Y Acad Sci*, **1121**, 421–430.

Fisher, H. E., Aron, A., Brown, L. L. (2006) Romantic love: A mammalian brain system for mate choice. *Philos Trans R Soc Lond B Biol Sci*, **361**, 2173–2186.

Frankle, W. G., Lombardo, I., New, A. S., et al. (2005) Brain serotonin transporter distribution in subjects with impulsive aggressivity: A positron emission study with [11C]McN 5652. *Am J Psychiatry*, **162**, 915–923.

Hariri, A. R., Brown, S. M., Williamson, D. E., et al. (2006) Preference for immediate over delayed rewards is associated with magnitude of ventral striatal activity. *J Neurosci*, **26**, 13213–13217.

Harvey, B. H., Scheepers, A., Brand, L., et al. (2001) Chronic inositol increases striatal D(2) receptors but does not modify dexamphetamine-induced motor behavior. Relevance to obsessive-compulsive disorder. *Pharmacol Biochem Behav*, **68**, 245–253.

Joel, D., Doljansky, J., Schiller, D. (2005) 'Compulsive' lever pressing in rats is enhanced following lesions to the orbital cortex, but not to the basolateral nucleus of the amygdala or to the dorsal medial prefrontal cortex. *Eur J Neurosci*, **21**, 2252–2262.

Kalenscher, T., Ohmann, T., Gunturkun, O. (2006) The neuroscience of impulsive and self-controlled decisions. *Int J Psychophysiol*, **62**, 203–211.

Lochner, C., Seedat, S., Hemmings, S. M., et al. (2007) Investigating the possible effects of trauma experiences and 5-HTT on the dissociative experiences of patients with OCD using path analysis and multiple regression. *Neuropsychobiology*, **56**, 6–13.

Muller, D. J., Mandelli, L., Serretti, A., et al. (2008) Serotonin transporter gene and adverse life events in adult ADHD. *Am J Med Genet B Neuropsychiatr Genet*, **147B**, 1461–1469.

Nuttin, B. J., Gabriels, L. A., Cosyns, P. R., et al. (2008) Long-term electrical capsular stimulation in patients with obsessive-compulsive disorder. *Neurosurgery*, **62**, 966–977.

Posner, M. I., Petersen, S. E. (1990) The attention system of the human brain. *Annu Rev Neurosci*, **13**, 25–42.

Reif, A., Rosler, M., Freitag, C. M., et al. (2007) Nature and nurture predispose to violent behavior: Serotonergic genes and adverse childhood environment. *Neuropsychopharmacology*, **32**, 2375–2383.

Starcevic, V., Brakoulias, V. (2008) Symptom subtypes of obsessive-compulsive disorder: Are they relevant for treatment? *Aust NZ J Psychiatry*, **42**, 651–661.

Wallis, D., Russell, H. F., Muenke, M. (2008) Review: Genetics of attention deficit/hyperactivity disorder. *J Pediatr Psychol*, **33**, 1085–1099.

Chapter 22
Anxiety-Mood Spectrum Syndromes: Anxiety, Panic, Phobias, ASD, PTSD, Borderline Syndrome, Dependent and Avoidant Personalities, Social Phobia, Bipolarity and Mania, Depression – Neurotic and Syndromic, Adjustment Disorders

Contents

22.1 Gene × Meme Interaction, Evolutionary Adaptation, and Syndromes

Anxiety is ubiquitous and is a natural function of the brain structure, conserved and evolved over time in animals to be aware of danger situations. The limbic system, particularly the amygdala, hippocampus, and the cingulate gyrus, is involved in anxiety and depression (see Chapters 1 and 2). Like a smoke detector, the generation of anxiety allows an animal to prepare for fight or flight, conferring survival and thus reproductive advantage. Sad expression and withdrawal behavior in depression draw attention and support from others and thus may confer survival value.

H. Leigh, *Genes, Memes, Culture, and Mental Illness*,
DOI 10.1007/978-1-4419-5671-2_22, © Hoyle Leigh, 2010

We examined at some length in Chapters 1 and 2 how stress may affect certain genes, which may in turn affect the morphology and function of brain structures such as the connection between the amygdala and the cingulate gyrus. Anxiety is the experience of stress within the brain – how the sensory input is processed within the brain as a danger signal. When a sensory input, which may be either physical (e.g., cold weather) or memetic (e.g., words), enters the sensory cortex, it is presented to the amygdala, to the hippocampus, and to the association cortex where the sensory input is compared with memory (existing memes), then an interpretation is made as to whether it is dangerous or not, and this information is fed back to the amygdala. Many sensations turn out to be not very dangerous, and the feedback will tune down the amygdala in most persons. In individuals with the short allele of the serotonin transporter promoter gene (5-HTTLPR), especially in those who had been exposed to abuse as a child, there is a reduction in this feedback loop back to amygdala. Thus, such individuals tend to have heightened and more frequent anxiety responses to stress in adult life and eventually an increased risk of depression and suicidal behavior (Caspi et al., 2003; Pezawas et al., 2005; Ribases et al., 2008; Stein et al., 2008). It appears that repeated and unabated activation of the anxiety-fear circuit eventually results in depression.

Abuse in childhood represents not only physical stress from trauma, but also the infusion of memes into the immature brain. The memes associated with childhood abuse are exactly the kinds of memes that are associated with fear, anxiety, and depression – "The world is a dangerous and hostile place" "I am not worthwhile" "I deserve to be punished," etc. Stress in adult life, with infusion of similar memes, may result in an unchecked proliferation of anxiety and depressive memes.

In rhesus monkeys, animals heterozygous for the *s* allele were shown to exhibit exaggerated stress responses only in already stressful situations, such as being in a new cage, while in their home cages, they exhibited similar responses as the *l/l* allele monkeys (Kalin et al., 2008).

Recent studies have shown that fear conditioning and extinction involve two different sets of neurons in the amygdala with connections to the medial prefrontal cortex and the hippocampus (Herry et al., 2008). The fear neurons received input from the hippocampus and projected to the medial prefrontal cortex, while the extinction neurons had bidirectional connections to medial prefrontal cortex. During extinction of fear response, the extinction neurons were active even when the fear neurons were not. In effect, extinction occurs through the creation of memory, i.e., a meme. The introduction of a meme could thus extinguish fear.

22.1.1 Anxiety

Anxiety is identifiable through the transmission of memes indicating its presence, which may be in words, facial expression, or behavior. It may be experienced as pure emotion, a subjective sense of anxiety which is not expressed, or it may be feigned or mimicked, as in playacting. Even when anxiety is not communicated, the pure experience may replicate inside the brain as a meme, eventually building up pressure to be expressed.

While anxiety is usually experienced as a negative emotion, it is necessary and desirable as a warning signal of an impending danger (both external and internal, which may be a result of a memetic conflict). As anxiety involves arousal and attention, it facilitates performance in moderate amounts. When anxiety is excessive, however, there is a decline of performance, sometimes to the point of paralysis or extreme purposeless agitation.

Locus ceruleus, the nucleus of a majority of noradrenergic neurons in the brain, plays an important role in anxiety. Activation of the locus ceruleus is an important aspect of the physiologic activation associated with anxiety. This response may be explosive and if unchecked, results in the panic syndrome. Panic may be precipitated by a memetic stimulus, such as a thought or perception of an open space in an agoraphobic patient.

Phobias represent severe anxiety and fear associated with memes and memetic stimuli.

22.1.2 Panic Syndrome and Agoraphobia

In panic syndrome, there is unexpected and repeated episodes of intense fear accompanied by physical symptoms that may include chest pain, heart palpitations, shortness of breath, dizziness, or abdominal distress. The symptoms usually last minutes, peaking in about 10 min, though sometimes longer. This may be accompanied in about a third of cases by agoraphobia, the fear of public or unfamiliar places, or even going out of the house lest a panic attack might occur. Various genes have been identified that might contribute to anxiety proneness in general and panic syndrome and agoraphobia in particular (Domschke et al., 2008a, b; Hettema et al., 2008; Strug et al., 2008). It appears that panic syndrome with agoraphobia may have a stronger genetic component.

Panic syndrome clearly represents a severe and episodic dysregulation of the fear-anxiety apparatus, probably determined by an unstable regulatory mechanism. Memetic stimulus such as being in an unfamiliar place might provide the initial ignition of anxiety that results in a full blown panic attack.

22.1.3 Specific Phobias

Phobias to specific objects, such as acrophobia, misophobia, arachnophobia, and ailurophobia probably represent conditioned anxiety to memetic stimuli. The phobic object may be symbolic of a meme that one fears, such as a feared person. Phobic memes are common in most cultures and some may be even inherent, such as the fear of spiders and snakes. Others, such as the fear of germs and contamination (misophobia) are results of modern civilization.

Phobic symptoms are more likely to develop in individuals with genetic predisposition for anxiety, and who also had exposure to the phobic memes. Most phobic objects can be avoided and thus not a source of great distress, but when a person is unexpectedly exposed to a phobic object, panic may ensue. Such exposure may be traumatic enough to leave lasting consequences.

22.1.4 Acute Stress and Posttraumatic Stress Syndromes

These represent the effects of overwhelming stress on the brain, i.e., overwhelming infusion or activation of stress memes that take over the function of the brain. The stress reaction involves the activation of the hypothalamo-pituitary-adrenocortical axis and massive production of glucocorticoids which are neurotoxic to the hippocampus, and may result in a smaller volume and difficulty in processing memory (see Chapter 2).

With PTSD, there may be a permanent damage to the meme-processing ability of the brain, setting the stage for a labile equilibrium among conflicting memes and susceptibility to be overwhelmed with new incoming memes or an inability to process new and useful memes. The stress memes that overwhelmed the brain are likely to reside in the brain and proliferate at every opportunity. Note that strong emotions may enhance long-term potentiation and thus memory formation through dopaminergic and serotonergic mechanisms ("flashbulb memory"; see Chapter 9).

Persons who have no memory of a traumatic event in 24 h were shown to be less likely to develop PTSD in 6 months than those who had memories of the trauma (Gil et al., 2005). This finding supports the notion that the ability to inhibit the traumatic meme proliferation (memory) prevents PTSD.

Once PTSD has been established, reservoirs of traumatic memes may proliferate unpredictably and uncontrollably as in flashbacks and nightmares. EMDR (eye movement desensitization and reprocessing therapy) might be effective as it simulates the saccadic eye movements of the REM (rapid eye movement) sleep during which traumatic memes may be processed in the cortex (Stickgold, 2002).

22.1.5 Borderline Syndrome and Traits

Characterized by emotional instability, stormy relationships, and tendency for dissociation, this syndrome overlaps considerably with the symptoms and neurophysiology of PTSD and depression, and may indeed represent the sequelae of childhood traumas interacting with genetic vulnerability (Hunt, 2007; Minzenberg et al., 2008). Nightmares and dream anxiety are quite common in borderline syndrome and may represent intense replication of trauma memes as in PTSD (Semiz et al., 2008).

Borderline syndrome patients often have identity diffusion, or a fragmented sense of self (Brenner, 1996; Charry, 1983; Fuchs, 2007; Jorgensen, 2006). This may represent a failure to develop harmonious relationships among several competing selfplexes (the memes that constitute the sense of self, see Chapter 12). Thus, there may be no consistent selfplex that presides over other selfplexes and use them as the occasion demands, and the contradictory selfplexes may alternate or shift unpredictably instigated by otherwise insignificant stress memes. Depending on which selfplex is dominant at the moment, the individual may feel different emotions and exhibit different behavioral traits.

22.1.6 Dependent Personality Traits and Syndrome

This is characterized by degrees of psychological dependence on others for decision making and submissive and clinging behavior and a lack of initiative.

Everyone has some dependency needs – in fact, all mammals are dependent on their mothers in the early stages of life. There are, however, genetic polymorphisms that may predispose an individual to various personality traits including extraversion, novelty seeking, withdrawal from angry faces, tendency for drug use (Han et al., 2008; Luo et al., 2008; Perlis et al., 2008). As in borderline personality, there may be specific gene × meme interactions in the development of dependent personality traits and syndrome.

Early memetic environment that discouraged independence and fostered dependence would strongly contribute to the development of dependent personality. This would be particularly so if dependence was expected because of the gender, race, or social class of the child, and there were numerous memetic models (identification figures) for this.

22.1.7 Avoidant Personality Traits and Syndrome, Social Phobia

Avoidant persons show pervasive social inhibition, feelings of inadequacy, extreme sensitivity to negative evaluation and avoidance of social interaction. They often consider themselves to be socially inept, and avoid social interactions for fear of being rejected. They often consider themselves to be loners and feel alienated. In Social Phobia, there is excessive anxiety in social situations for fear of being humiliated or ridiculed. Such persons may show physiologic signs of anxiety such as blushing and sweating, which may further cause embarrassment and anxiety. Avoidant personality may be a more pervasive type of social phobia (Chambless et al., 2008). Like any other anxiety conditions, these traits develop over development through interaction between genetic disposition and memes introduced from the environment. Repeated exposure in childhood to critical memes in social situations, or the stress of having to repeatedly adapt to new and strange environments in an anxiety-prone person would set the stage for social phobia and avoidant personality.

22.1.8 Bipolarity and Mania

Bipolar disorder in current terminology means one or more episodes of abnormally elevated mood, either hypomania or the more severe form, mania. Hypomania or mania often occurs in persons who also have episodes of depression, thus the original term, bipolar. There may also be mixed episodes of both depression and mania/hypomania. These episodes are usually separated by periods of euthymia, but in some individuals, depression and mania may rapidly alternate. During manic states, the person may be very speeded up, with rapid thoughts, pressured speech, and the mood may be irritable rather than euphoric, sometimes with grandiose delusions and hallucinations.

There is considerable overlap between borderline personality and bipolar disorder (Hunt, 2007; Smith et al., 2004). Seventeen percent of first degree relatives of borderline personality had bipolar disorder according to one study (Akiskal, 1981). The rate of bipolar disorder among first degree relatives of unipolar depression was 3.5% (Andreasen et al., 1987).

Affective instability may be seen to be an underlying mechanism for both (Mackinnon and Pies, 2006). The mechanism of switch between depression and mania is unclear. In one study, 9 of 11 patients with bipolar depression switched to an elevated mood state with the administration of S-adenosyl methionine (SAM), indicating the involvement of dopamine and serotonin (Carney et al., 1989).

While mania may be considered to be a dysregulation of mood, it has also been proposed that mania may represent a dysfunction of *reentry* described by Edelman (see Chapter 9), the process of ongoing parallel and recursive signaling between separate neuronal groups along parallel reciprocal fibers that link these groups anatomically. According to this view, reentry is speeded up through some biochemical mechanism, resulting in rapid recursive signaling and thought (Mellerup and Kristensen, 2004). As reentry is the process through which memes are consolidated and replicate, there would be a rapid proliferation of memes under those conditions. The kinds of memes that would proliferate would depend on the mood state, which is elevated in manic states. Thus, there is proliferation of euphoric, high self-esteem, and grandiose memes, at times to the point of delusions and hallucinations when a psychotic process is activated when the manic state reaches a threshold.

22.1.9 Depression – Neurotic and Major Depressive Syndrome

How do you know a person is depressed? By simply looking at a person, then, by talking with the person. Depression is perhaps one of the states that illustrates the meme as something imitatable. We know how to look depressed and feel depressed, and when we imitate someone's depressed expression, we feel depressed. This empathy, feeling what another feels by imitation, is in fact the first mode of communication between a preverbal child and caregiver and involves the activation of the mirror neurons, prefrontal cortex, and the limbic system through the insula (Carr et al., 2003; Lenzi et al., 2008).

The verbal communication of a depressed person is, of course, full of depressive memes and represents a state of unchecked proliferation of such memes. In other words, the neurobiology of depression permits explosive replication of depressive memes. It is important, however, to recognize that in very severe depression, there may be sufficient psychomotor retardation such that the depressive memes are predominantly nonverbal.

Common memes replicated in depressive states are sad, crying, helpless, hopeless, pessimistic, self-reproach, self-punitive, uncaring, apathetic, self-destructive, and suicidal memes.

With severe depression or depressive syndrome, there is often physiologic signs such as insomnia, fatigue, anhedonia, and anorexia. Anhedonia is also associated with a dampening of feedback information, such as reward for an action. This is associated with functional changes in the brain, such as activation of ventral striatum that indicates a reward stimulus (Steele et al., 2007). There may also be psychotic symptoms, such as depressive delusions and hallucinations.

Sadness is often a consequence of an event about which one had felt anxious – inability to master a threat may result in sadness and helplessness and may trigger the depressive syndrome in vulnerable individuals. Depression may occur purely from memetic processes, such as the recognition of an inability to meet the demands of a memeplex (ego ideal) (Busch et al., 2004).

Depressed mood, cognition, and behavior are memes that can be imitated and feigned, and serve a communicative purpose. They draw attention to the helplessness of the individual and may elicit support and protection by others. Depressed memes may also represent submissiveness, as displayed by some animals toward a higher ranking one, thus avoiding confrontation and harm. "Learned helplessness" to unavoidable danger situations may protect the organism from futile expenditure of energy and effort. Such "learning," however, may be maladaptive as the situation may have changed, and there may indeed be ways of mastering the current situation. There is evidence that the experience of learned helplessness may lead to specific activation of the amygdala and the mammillary bodies (Schneider et al., 1996; Seligman, 1972).

Depression may vary in severity from sad affect to *depressive neurosis* to major depressive syndrome. Sad affect is generally associated with an identifiable loss or an anniversary of a loss and is temporary. Depressive neurosis represents a depressive trait – a tendency to experience mild to moderate depressed mood with minor stresses. They may have a pessimistic outlook, and may feel helpless in warding off depressogenic stresses.

In *major depression*, which often arises in persons with depressive neurosis, there are several categories of symptoms and signs – (1) affective (sad, blue, apathetic, crying), (2) cognitive (pessimistic, helpless, hopeless, low self-esteem, self-reproach, guilt, suicidal ideation and plans), (3) neurovegetative and physiologic (anhedonia, insomnia, hypersomnia, psychomotor agitation/retardation, constipation, fatigue, vague pains and discomfort), (4) Behavioral (self neglect,

neglect of hygiene, social withdrawal, substance use/abuse, suicidal behavior). Once major depressive syndrome develops, it usually has an autonomous course lasting on the average 6–12 months without specific treatment and suicide is a serious risk. Major depressive syndrome is a final common pathway brain dysfunction requiring coordinated psychiatric treatment.

22.1.10 Adjustment Disorders

In a sense, all psychiatric syndromes may be considered to be adjustment disorders, but the term is generally reserved for relatively mild and transient symptoms of distress to stressful situations that do not reach the threshold for diagnosing a more serious and persistent conditions such as neurosis or major psychiatric syndromes (e.g., major depression, psychosis).

In adjustment disorders, the symptoms, while distressing, is usually within the boundaries of normality and the autonomous course of a final common pathway syndromes has not been triggered.

Adjustment disorders may be characterized with prominent anxiety and/or depressed mood and/or behavioral problems including acting out, substance use, which may be a maladaptive way of coping with the stress.

There is a proliferation of stress and distress memes in adjustment disorders which may threaten to trigger a proliferation of depressive and/or psychotic memes if these are already present in the brain in relatively large quantities. The stress memes may also induce certain physiologic symptoms such as insomnia and other manifestations of anxiety.

22.2 Treatment

22.2.1 Prevention

There has been little genetic evolution in humans during the eyeblink of time between the stone age and the modern age, though the memes have evolved at an exponential rate. It is no wonder, then, that the genetic machinery of our brain is often mismatched for the memetic onslaught through our perceptual apparatus. Thus, brains well adapted to generate anxiety at the slightest sensation indicating the presence of a predatory animal may find itself generating anxiety signals at various sensations arising from memetic (e.g., images, voice, words) and physical (e.g., speeding vehicles, being in tall buildings) stimuli that are commonplace and benign.

The anxiety-prone genes may have been adaptive in the stone age, but may cause vulnerability to anxiety in modern age. Identification of children with highly threat-sensitive genes and providing them with training on stress management and coping skills may prevent future development of symptoms and syndromes.

22.2.2 Mild Symptoms (Problems of Living and Adjustment Reactions)

Mild anxiety and depressive symptoms may arise as a function of the individual vulnerability interacting with perceived stress. Intervention should be geared toward reduction of perceived stress through reframing if the perception of danger is excessive, or through more effective coping. Broad-spectrum meme-oriented therapy, such as relaxation, meditation, and massage therapy may be particularly useful (Chapter 17), as well as certain specific meme-oriented therapies (Chapter 18). Enhancing coping ability and thus reducing helpless feelings may be particularly useful for mild depressive symptoms.

22.2.3 Neurosis

Neurosis indicates the presence of a pattern of behavior and emotional arousal that is distressing and that is often the patient's own making. Such patients are often self-defeating and pessimistic. Neurosis may be truly memetic, i.e., learned (imitated) way of living patterned after a parent or surrogate, or arise out of repeated adjustment reactions with failure to cope.

Specific meme-oriented therapies should be used for neurosis, augmented with broad-spectrum therapies and medications as needed. The medications may be antianxiety agents when the patients find themselves in an excessively anxiety-provoking situation, even if it is of their own making, or antidepressants or hypnotics as the occasion demands.

Therapy for neurosis should be geared toward the memes that constitute the pattern of behavior and emotional arousal by modifying and replacing them with more effective memes and thus creating a healthier selfplex.

22.2.4 Major Syndromes

Major syndromes of the fear–anxiety–depression spectrum syndromes include panic syndrome, phobias, acute stress disorder (ASD), posttraumatic stress disorder (PTSD), borderline syndrome, mania, and major depressive syndrome.

Gene-oriented treatment should be ideally geared to turning off the expressed genes that may cause the dysfunction of the brain structures. This may be possible through drugs that might be developed for specific genes or choice of drugs in a pharmacogenetically informed way. For example, SSRIs may be more effective for specific genomic groups, while alpha II agonists such as clonidine might be more effective for others whose locus ceruleus may be hypersensitive.

Current gene-oriented therapy, unfortunately, remains at the level of trial and error of drugs that have been shown to be effective for a significant but less than satisfactory percentage of patients with overlapping symptoms and that are associated with often highly undesirable and dangerous side effects. They include antidepressants (tricyclics, SSRIs), serotonergic-noradrenergic drugs (SNRIs, mirtazapine), mood stabilizers (lithium, anticonvulsants, antipsychotics), and benzodiazepines. All of these drugs except lithium (which is used more specifically for bipolar and recurrent depression) have been used for any of the above syndromes largely on a trial and error basis.

There is clearly a need to develop more specific gene- and genome-oriented drugs. Gene-oriented therapy is not confined to pharmacotherapy. As has been shown in rhesus monkeys (Suomi, 2003, 2005), good nurturance can reverse the adverse effects of genes such as the short allele of 5-HTTLPR. Long-term psychotherapy and/or nurturing environment in adulthood may also affect genes.

General meme-oriented therapy for anxiety and depression would include all broad-spectrum therapies outlined in Chapter 17. Meme-oriented therapy includes all of the specific therapies discussed in Chapter 18. Specific therapies such as cognitive–behavioral therapy (CBT) and interpersonal therapy (IPT) for anxiety and depression should be used, as well as dialectical behavioral therapy (DBT) for borderline syndrome.

Memetically, anxiety symptoms may represent a tension among existing memes in the brain or between an incoming meme and existing memes. Specific techniques could be developed to examine recently introduced memes and their relationship to existing ones, so as to achieve a reconciliation if a conflict is found. Note that the newly introduced meme may have arrived unconsciously or semiconsciously, sometimes as a part of a complex meme such as a song or other works of art. Resident memes that may tend to generate anxiety easily, such as rigid and punitive moral codes, may be reexamined and reprocessed rationally if they are identified.

When anxiety remains unabated, or the stressful situation is perceived to be hopeless, hopeless and helpless memes replicate and predominate and depressive syndrome ensues. Depressive syndrome may also be the result of new infusion of depressive memes or the replication of existing depressive memes because of a change in the brain environment (e.g., cytokines associated with a viral infection) or triggered by incoming depressive memes.

Specific antianxiety and/or antidepressive memes could be infused through words (e.g., mantra, self-suggestion), song, visual imagery, or physical activity (e.g., flexing and relaxing muscles).

Combined gene- and meme-oriented therapy may be used. For example, desensitization to an anxiety-provoking meme may be conducted through exposure after medication with an anxiolytic drug. Antidepressive memes could be infused after medication with a stimulant drug. In ASD and PTSD, neuroprotective drugs should be used as well as treating the proliferation of unintegrated trauma memes through broad-spectrum therapies as well as specific meme-oriented therapies that may include reexperiencing trauma with beta blockade or controlled exposure therapy.

Virtual reality therapy can be used effectively to treat situational anxieties including social anxiety and phobias through desensitization. Avatars may also be used to introduce new memes, such as mastery of fear and assertiveness in social situations. An avatar is a virtual image of oneself, and there is nothing more effective than watching and imitating oneself actually doing the things one wished one could do. Avatars could show the patient how he/she can interact with people confidently, become physically fit, and enjoy life. A new selfplex could be built.

References

Akiskal, H. S. (1981) Subaffective disorders: Dysthymic, cyclothymic and bipolar II disorders in the "borderline" realm. *Psychiatr Clin North Am*, **4**, 25–46.

Andreasen, N. C., Rice, J., Endicott, J., et al. (1987) Familial rates of affective disorder. A report from the National Institute of Mental Health Collaborative Study. *Arch Gen Psychiatry*, **44**, 461–469.

Brenner, I. (1996) The characterological basis of multiple personality. *Am J Psychother*, **50**, 154–166.

Busch, F., Rudden, M., Shapiro, T. (2004) *Psychodynamic Treatment of Depression*. American Psychiatric Pub, Washington, DC.

Carney, M. W., Chary, T. K., Bottiglieri, T., et al. (1989) The switch mechanism and the bipolar/unipolar dichotomy. *Br J Psychiatry*, **154**, 48–51.

Carr, L., Iacoboni, M., Dubeau, M. C., et al. (2003) Neural mechanisms of empathy in humans: A relay from neural systems for imitation to limbic areas. *Proc Natl Acad Sci USA*, **100**, 5497–5502.

Caspi, A., Sugden, K., Moffitt, T. E., et al. (2003) Influence of life stress on depression: Moderation by a polymorphism in the 5-HTT gene. *Science*, **301**, 386–389.

Chambless, D. L., Fydrich, T., Rodebaugh, T. L. (2008) Generalized social phobia and avoidant personality disorder: Meaningful distinction or useless duplication? *Depress Anxiety*, **25**, 8–19.

Charry, D. (1983) The borderline personality. *Am Fam Physician*, **27**, 195–202.

Domschke, K., Hohoff, C., Jacob, C., et al. (2008) Chromosome 4q31–34 panic disorder risk locus: Association of neuropeptide Y Y5 receptor variants. *Am J Med Genet B Neuropsychiatr Genet*, **147B**, 510–516.

Domschke, K., Ohrmann, P., Braun, M., et al. (2008) Influence of the catechol-O-methyltransferase val158met genotype on amygdala and prefrontal cortex emotional processing in panic disorder. *Psychiatry Res*, **163**, 13–20.

Fuchs, T. (2007) Fragmented selves: Temporality and identity in borderline personality disorder. *Psychopathology*, **40**, 379–387.

Gil, S., Caspi, Y., Ben-Ari, I. Z., et al. (2005) Does memory of a traumatic event increase the risk for posttraumatic stress disorder in patients with traumatic brain injury? A prospective study. *Am J Psychiatry*, **162**, 963–969.

Han, D. H., Yoon, S. J., Sung, Y. H., et al. (2008) A preliminary study: Novelty seeking, frontal executive function, and dopamine receptor (D2) TaqI A gene polymorphism in patients with methamphetamine dependence. *Compr Psychiatry*, **49**, 387–392.

Herry, C., Ciocchi, S., Senn, V., et al. (2008) Switching on and off fear by distinct neuronal circuits. *Nature*, **454**, 600–606.

Hettema, J. M., An, S. S., Bukszar, J., et al. (2008) Catechol-O-methyltransferase contributes to genetic susceptibility shared among anxiety spectrum phenotypes. *Biol Psychiatry*, **64**, 302–310.

Hunt, M. (2007) Borderline personality disorder across the lifespan. *J Women Aging*, **19**, 173–191.

Jorgensen, C. R. (2006) Disturbed sense of identity in borderline personality disorder. *J Personal Disord*, **20**, 618–644.

Kalin, N. H., Shelton, S. E., Fox, A. S., et al. (2008) The serotonin transporter genotype is associated with intermediate brain phenotypes that depend on the context of eliciting stressor. *Mol Psychiatry*, **13**, 1021–1027.

Lenzi, D., Trentini, C., Pantano, P., et al (2008) Neural basis of maternal communication and emotional expression processing during infant preverbal stage. *Cereb Cortex*, **19**, 1124–1133.

Luo, X., Kranzler, H. R., Zuo, L., et al. (2008) ADH7 variation modulates extraversion and consci-entiousness in substance-dependent subjects. *Am J Med Genet B Neuropsychiatr Genet*, **147B**, 179–186.

Mackinnon, D. F., Pies, R. (2006) Affective instability as rapid cycling: Theoretical and clinical implications for borderline personality and bipolar spectrum disorders. *Bipolar Disord*, **8**, 1–14.

Mellerup, E., Kristensen, F. (2004) Mania as a dysfunction of reentry: Application of Edelman's and Tononi's hypothesis for consciousness in relation to a psychiatric disorder. *Med Hypotheses*, **63**, 464–466.

Minzenberg, M. J., Fan, J., New, A. S., et al. (2008) Frontolimbic structural changes in borderline personality disorder. *J Psychiatr Res*, **42**, 727–733.

Perlis, R. H., Holt, D. J., Smoller, J. W., et al. (2008) Association of a polymorphism near CREB1 with differential aversion processing in the insula of healthy participants. *Arch Gen Psychiatry*, **65**, 882–892.

Pezawas, L., Meyer-Lindenberg, A., Drabant, E. M., et al. (2005) 5-HTTLPR polymorphism impacts human cingulated–amygdala interactions: A genetic susceptibility mechanism for depression. *Nat Neurosci*, **8**, 828–834.

Ribases, M., Fernandez-Aranda, F., Gratacos, M., et al. (2008) Contribution of the serotoninergic system to anxious and depressive traits that may be partially responsible for the phenotypical variability of bulimia nervosa. *J Psychiatr Res*, **42**, 50–57.

Schneider, F., Gur, R. E., Alavi, A., et al. (1996) Cerebral blood flow changes in limbic regions induced by unsolvable anagram tasks. *Am J Psychiatry*, **153**, 206–212.

Seligman, M. E. (1972) Learned helplessness. *Annu Rev Med*, **23**, 407–412.

Semiz, U. B., Basoglu, C., Ebrinc, S., et al. (2008) Nightmare disorder, dream anxiety, and sub-jective sleep quality in patients with borderline personality disorder. *Psychiatry Clin Neurosci*, **62**, 48–55.

Smith, D. J., Muir, W. J., Blackwood, D. H. (2004) Is borderline personality disorder part of the bipolar spectrum? *Harv Rev Psychiatry*, **12**, 133–139.

Steele, J. D., Kumar, P., Ebmeier, K. P. (2007) Blunted response to feedback information in depressive illness. *Brain*, **130**, 2367–2374.

Stein, M. B., Schork, N. J., Gelernter, J. (2008) Gene-by-environment (serotonin transporter and childhood maltreatment) interaction for anxiety sensitivity, an intermediate phenotype for anxiety disorders. *Neuropsychopharmacology*, **33**, 312–319.

Stickgold, R. (2002) EMDR: A putative neurobiological mechanism of action. *J Clin Psychol*, **58**, 61–75.

Strug, L. J., Suresh, R., Fyer, A. J., et al. (2008) Panic disorder is associated with the serotonin transporter gene (SLC6A4) but not the promoter region (5-HTTLPR). *Mol Psychiatry*.

Suomi, S. J. (2003) Gene–environment interactions and the neurobiology of social conflict. *Ann NY Acad Sci*, **1008**, 132–139.

Suomi, S. J. (2005) Aggression and social behaviour in rhesus monkeys. *Novartis Found Symp*, **268**, 216–222; discussion 222–216, 242–253.

Chapter 23
Reality Perception Spectrum Syndromes (Imagination, Dissociation, Conversion, Somatoform, Misattribution Somatization, Psychosis)

Contents

23.1 Gene × Meme Interaction and Evolutionary Adaptation

What is reality? In humans, reality is a representation, integration in the brain of complex perceptions. Once perception is encoded in memory as a percept, it is a meme, i.e., it is capable of reproduction and multiplication. Imagination is also a representation – a creation or reassembly of percepts within the brain. Imagination may be directed (e.g., imagine a smiling face) or nondirected. There is evidence that similar areas of the brain are activated in actual perception and in imagination (Iseki et al., 2008; Kim et al., 2007; Qiu et al., 2008).

Reality is a complex memeplex, i.e., it consists of sets of memes or percepts that have been accepted by the selfplex as "real," as opposed to other sets of percepts that the selfplex has either ignored or adjudged to be "unreal" or illusory.

H. Leigh, *Genes, Memes, Culture, and Mental Illness*,
DOI 10.1007/978-1-4419-5671-2_23, © Hoyle Leigh, 2010

Existing perceptual memes replicate and gain force when attention is paid to them internally and when they are reassembled as imagination. When this process is intense as in fantasy, the perceptual memes being manipulated or processed by the brain may replicate to the extent that their intensity may equal those of "real" perception.

23.1.1 Imagination and Dreaming

Normal persons can differentiate between imagination and reality in spite of similar activation of brain areas, but in the dreaming state, normal persons actually experience hallucinations and delusions as reality. The REM state during which dreaming usually occurs is phylogenetically ancient and probably serves important physiologic function. Dreaming is significantly influenced by the activity of the frontal cortex (Solms, 2000) and may serve the function of rehearsing coping with threatening stimuli (Revonsuo, 2000).

Imagination and dreaming are necessary (see Chapter 2 for more about dreaming) for problem solving and creativity. Being unable to distinguish between imagination, dreaming, and reality and being unable to return to reality result in distress and thus mental illness. The inability to distinguish may arise from either reduction in the evaluative aspect of meme processing, attenuation of reality perception, or excessive attention to the internal processing of memes at the expense of the patency of the perceptual apparatus as in dreaming.

23.1.2 Dissociation

Dissociation, and the associated phenomena of depersonalization and derealization are not uncommonly experienced in normal persons when absorbed in a task or under stress. Dissociation may be adaptive and may be hardwired as an adaptive mechanism (Berrios and Sierra, 1997; Sierra and Berrios, 1998). In the face of acute stress situations where the individual lacks control over the environment and cannot localize the source of threat, the inhibition of nonfunctional emotional response may serve an adaptive function, i.e., not engage in useless fight/flight but heightening alertness for the environment. Such inhibition of emotional responses and suppression of autonomic arousal creates a feeling of unreality – depersonalization seen in dissociative states (Seligman and Kirmayer, 2008). In both trauma-related dissociation and hysterical conversion, there seems to be a sense of distancing or disconnection from self and the world that characterizes depersonalization and derealization, related to cortical inhibition of emotional processing. The experience of subjective loss of voluntary control over parts of the body appears tied to cortical inhibition of attention and awareness as well as disruption of the link between volition and execution. This is consistent with studies of hypnosis which show that, in highly hypnotizable individuals, specific suggestions can reduce conflict between ordinarily competing attentional processes (Raz et al., 2005). Functional brain imaging in this situation shows an effective disconnection between anterior cingulate cortex, thought to be involved in monitoring cognitive conflicts, and other cortical regions involved in the cognitive or perceptual task.

Through these mechanisms, hypnotic suggestion can cause a functional dissociation that reduces conflict between otherwise incompatible cognitive processes (i.e., conflicting memes), allowing potentially contradictory streams of information processing to coexist.

Under circumstances that increase suggestibility, and in susceptible individuals, misattribution of distress to parts of the body rather than to a memetic stress may occur as in conversion and somatization syndromes, as well as misattribution of percepts from within the brain (imagination) to outside of the brain (hallucination). Hallucinations and delusions occur regularly in "normal" individuals in hypnotic trance or religious frenzy.

Memetic environment often determines the content of dissociative and misattribution experiences, e.g., "possession" by spirits, fibromyalgia.

23.1.3 Dissociative Identity Disorder (DID, Multiple Personality)

In one study, some 18% of women in the general population had some dissociative disorder, while about 1% had a diagnosis of dissociative identity disorder (Sar et al., 2007).

In Chapter 11, I argued that we are all multiple personalities, that our brain contains a number of different selfplexes that are hopefully coexisting in a democracy. In such a state, each selfplex is experienced as a part of *me*. So, I sometimes say, "A part of me agrees with your idea, but another part of me is in violent disagreement." This is akin to a country in which there are strongly opposing forces toward an issue, for example, a war. Problems arise when authoritarian governments take over in succession and forcibly suppress other points of view, often even suppressing historical memory. Such is the state in dissociative identity disorder when there is a disturbance in the formation of a coherent set of mutually recognized selfplexes. At times of stress or vulnerability, a suppressed, unrecognized selfplex may take over and suppress other selfplexes. The newly dominant selfplex may not be connected to the memory memes of previous selfplexes, thus may suffer from global amnesia. More often, there is a mostly dominant selfplex which is from time to time overwhelmed by one or more selfplexes that incorporate memes disavowed by the mostly dominant selfplex.

Why does tolerant democracy of selfplexes fail to develop in certain brains? Childhood physical and sexual trauma is usually considered to be associated with DID. With severe trauma, there may be a degeneration of the hippocampus which in turn reduces the meme-processing ability of the brain (Ehling et al., 2008; Kihlstrom, 2005). There may also be a developmental arrest of the orbitofrontal cortex involved with the sense of self (Forrest, 2001). The ventromedial cortex including the orbitofrontal cortex, the cingulate gyrus, and areas of temporoparietal cortex seem to be intimately involved in the sense of self (David et al., 2006; Devinsky et al., 1995; Lou et al., 2005). Thus, normal, integrated sense of self with different personality aspects may represent a democracy of selfplexes that control the ventromedial cortex and associated brain areas.

In DID, competing and contradictory selfplexes may take over the brain areas, often incompletely. As selfplexes are clusters of meme-representing neurons, "taking control" means that the meme-containing neural clusters strengthen their connection to the sense of self areas of the brain.

In certain meme pools such as the Afro-Brazilians with the Candomblé religion, the religious memes provide a normalizing explanation for dissociative identity disorder and the stress that precipitates it. The Candomblé belief system involves the idea that a pantheon of deities, called the Orixas, control human destinies and human bodies. Orixas may choose to possess particular individuals. Hence, individuals experiencing acute psychosocial stress and dissociation may interpret these experiences as products of a spiritual disturbance caused by the Candomblé deities. By facilitating such interpretations, Candomblé encourages the belief that individuals may experience discontinuity among aspects of the self, including body, memory, responsibility, and personal identity. Such attributions allow individuals to understand their stressful experiences as non-self-implicating, thus alleviating the need to face the trauma directly. Belief in possession also allows them to embrace their dissociative experiences as spiritually productive, as such alterations in consciousness represent the replacement of their own self with that of a possessing deity. In fact, individuals learn how to induce such states of awareness in ritual contexts (Seligman and Kirmayer, 2008).

23.1.4 Misattribution Syndromes: Conversion, Somatization, Hypochondriasis, Chronic Pain (Somatoform Disorders)

Bodily symptoms without obvious physiological explanation are considered to be *somatoform* disorders. They presumably have psychological explanations.

Conversion disorder, or hysteria, is an age-old entity, first attributed to wandering uterus by Hippocrates. Conversion symptoms are such physical symptoms as anesthesia, paralysis, syncope, ataxia, globus hystericus, and seizures. Somatization disorder or Briquet's syndrome consists of physical symptoms in various parts of the body without demonstrable underlying pathophysiology. Chronic pain syndrome, or psychogenic pain, is pain without organic pathology or in excess of what is expected from organic pathology. Hypochondriasis is a preoccupation that one has the symptoms of a serious disease. There are other somatic symptoms such as chemical intolerance, fibromyalgia, chronic fatigue.

Some of the disorders arise relatively early in life, often in families, and associated with stress. Freud considered hysteria to be a result of unconscious psychological conflicts: the symptom represents a compromise resolution of the unconscious conflict between an unacceptable wish (such as a gene-driven aggressive wish toward an authority figure) and a meme-driven inhibition (conscience), which compromise allows the conflict to be unconscious and thus avoid experiencing the anxiety had it become conscious, but also drawing attention to the prohibited wish by the symptom itself, such as the paralysis of an arm that would have struck at the authority figure.

Conversion symptoms tend to occur more easily in patients with brain injury, and conversion seizures often coexist with electrical seizures. There may be specific cortical inhibition in certain conversion symptoms (Aybek et al., 2008).

In somatization, hypochondriasis, and chronic pain, there may be an amplification of mild discomfort into more severe one in the brain (Barsky and Borus, 1999; Barsky et al., 1988; Barsky and Wyshak, 1990).

Early-life stress and negative parental relationships have been associated with chemical intolerance syndrome in women (Bell et al., 1998). It is well known that fibromyalgia, chemical sensitivity, and hypoglycemia achieved epidemic proportions in recent time (Ross, 1999).

In general, the symptoms may arise through a process of brain's misattribution of distress to somatic (sensory and visceral) sources when they are central and often memetic in origin. This distress misattribution process may be facilitated in certain individuals through epigenetic factors, early memetic infection from another person who somatizes or is in the sick role, or both, and current stress that both causes the distress and reawakens the sick role memes.

23.1.5 Psychosis

Psychosis is an alternative mode of experiencing reality, often occasioned by an inability to distinguish fantasy and dreaming from reality. Drugs such as LSD as well as prolonged sensory deprivation can produce symptoms of psychosis. Susceptibility to psychosis may arise from genetic and epigenetic factors during the maturation of the brain. Auditory hallucinations may be a misattribution of the source of memes to the outside when it is actually a perception of memetic proliferation within the brain, particularly in the nondominant hemisphere. The "inner voice" may be actually heard as auditory hallucination in affected individuals. Crow proposed that such hallucination may be a result of failure of the left brain to exert complete dominance in language production and thus an inability to differentiate between self-generated thoughts and voices coming from outside (Crow, 2000).

The memetic content of psychosis is clearly dependent on the meme pool to which the individual has been exposed. Thus, delusions and hallucinations may be religious in religious societies, paranoid in secular societies, etc. (see Chapter 4).

23.1.6 Schizophrenia

Schizophrenia is a group of chronic psychotic syndromes characterized by a relatively early age of onset and a general decline in function without treatment. The risk of developing schizophrenia in the general population is somewhat less than 1%, while the prevalence for parents of children who are known schizophrenics is 12%. The morbidity risk for schizophrenia for full siblings of schizophrenic patients is 13–14%. The risk for children with one schizophrenic parent is 8–18%. If both parents are schizophrenic, the morbidity risk for their children may be as high as 50%. In the case of twins, heterozygous twins have the same risk as other siblings, while homozygous (identical) twins have a concordance rate for schizophrenia of approximately 50%. (However, there is much variability in the concordance rate depending on the study, from practically 0 to 86%.)

In spite of the demise of the term *dementia praecox*, cognitive disturbance has recently become a cornerstone of understanding schizophrenia. Schizophrenia is conceptualized as a neurodevelopmental disorder resulting in a reduction in cortical volume and dysfunctions in glutamatergic, GABA (γ-aminobutyric acid)ergic, and dopaminergic transmission. There seems to be a hyperfunction of the mesolimbic and a hypofunction of the mesocortical dopaminergic transmission.

Mesocortical dopaminergic transmission is stimulated by glutamatergic transmission and reduced by GABAergic transmission, and it plays an important role in working memory often disturbed in schizophrenia (Romanides et al., 1999). There is evidence of dysfunction in schizophrenia of the GABAergic cortical chandelier cells that synchronize the firing of the glutamatergic pyramidal cells, which are necessary for proper functioning of the working memory (Lewis et al., 2004). A fundamental disturbance in schizophrenia seems to be an inefficiency of the prefrontal cortex, particularly the dorsolateral area, in processing information, and increased "noise" in the local microcircuit function (Meyer-Lindenberg et al., 2005; Weinberger, 2005).

A number of genes have been identified as candidate genes for the susceptibility to schizophrenia: catechol-*O*-methyltransferase *(COMT)* (chromosome 22q), *dysbindin-1* (chromosome 6p), *neuregulin-1* (chromosome 8p), metabotropic glutamate receptor 3 *(GRM-3)* (chromosome 7q), glutamate decarboxylase 1 (chromosome 2q), and disrupted-in-schizophrenia 1 *(DISC1)* (chromosome 1q).

The *COMT* gene affects prefrontal cortical function by changing dopamine signaling in the prefrontal cortex and brainstem. *GRM-3* shows similar results on prefrontal function and has an effect on expression of various glutamate synaptic markers. *DISC1* affects hippocampal anatomy and function. *Dysbindin-1* seems to be a general cognitive capacity gene that is underexpressed in the cortex of schizophrenic patients.

As should be obvious from this discussion, schizophrenia is not a simple genetic disease; rather, it is a syndrome contributed to by susceptibility genes that have functions other than conveying susceptibility to schizophrenia. Such susceptibility may include susceptibility to psychosis in general including psychosis in bipolar disorder (Goes et al., 2008; Nickl-Jockschat et al., 2008; Prasad et al., 2008; Sullivan, 2008; van Haren et al., 2008).

Intrauterine infections may also play a role in the development of schizophrenia as well as early memetic environment and stress.

Schizophrenia has conferred a reproductive disadvantage on the afflicted. Why, then, is schizophrenia extant at more or less a constant rate across human populations? An obvious explanation is that the alleles that, in certain combinations, may predispose one to schizophrenia may be involved in other functions that are adaptive. Some of these may be involved in creativity and eccentricity.

In addition, the susceptibility genes may represent variations of ubiquitous genes subserving basic functions of the human brain. Crow proposed that schizophrenia may represent an extreme of normal genetic variation in the communication between the two hemispheres that is critical in language, a uniquely human acquisition. He postulates that Schneiderian first-rank symptoms such as thought insertion and withdrawal may represent a dysfunction of the coordinated hemispheric communication – a right hemispheric intrusion into left hemispheric linear thinking (Crow, 1997, 2007). Schizophrenia may represent an extreme of variations in the interconnectivity of various structures of the brain, particularly those involved in social cognition and the working memory.

In sum, certain individuals with problems in the normal development of the brain functions involved in meme processing may be susceptible to difficulty in distinguishing between internal and external sources of meme presentation, such that internal memes are perceived as external perception (hallucinations).

Psychotic symptoms, therefore, may represent an intrusion into consciousness of internal existing memes that are ordinarily unconscious but are available in adaptive processes such as fantasy and creativity. In some individuals, psychosis may also be a result of disorganization of the meme-processing functions of the brain due to severe internal or external stress. In such states, certain memes that are in conflict with the dominant selfplex may proliferate, having gained strength by recruiting the perceptual apparatus in the form of hallucination. It is one thing to hear your own conscience, quite another to hear God admonishing you.

Delusions may occur when the meme-processing ability is impaired such that irrational memes are reinforced and become convictions, beyond the control of the meme filter for unreasonable memes. Delusions are irrational memes that have either severed themselves from the rational meme-processing apparatus or overwhelmed it, and have taken up residence as a part of the dominant selfplex. No contradictory memes will then be able to enter the brain and take hold.

The meme pool of the environment may then determine the *presentation* of the psychosis, i.e., what is the "normal" way to become psychotic in that culture? Thus, in some cultures, presenting with acute agitation and uncontrolled behavior may be the accepted way of "being crazy," while in another culture, it may be becoming hypervigilant and paranoid. See Chapter 3 for further discussion of the interplay among culture, stress of migration, and psychiatric symptoms.

The confusing hallucinations and/or delusions arising from faulty meme processing may force the patient to assume the "crazy meme" in the culture, which may in turn serve to reduce the distress, being labeled "crazy" and thus accepted in that role.

The clinical course of schizophrenia is clearly influenced by memetic stress. Memes in the form of expressed emotions, particularly negative ones, have been associated with exacerbations and hospitalizations both on a short-term and long-term basis (Kymalainen and Weisman de Mamani, 2008; Marom et al., 2005).

23.2 Treatment

23.2.1 Mild Dissociative Symptoms, Dissociation in Borderline Syndrome, PTSD

Generally, no treatment is necessary for mild dissociative symptoms including depersonalization and derealization as they tend to be time-limited and do not cause serious distress.

Severe, uncontrolled, and distressing dissociation may occur concomitant to strong emotional arousal with associated autonomic and endocrine arousal, often in the borderline syndrome and PTSD. Management and prevention of strong emotional arousal, especially anxiety, is through broad-spectrum anti-meme therapy and medications when indicated.

Memetic reinforcement of the selfplex may be helpful for the relatively transient dissociative symptoms, in the form of repetition of words or phrases asserting the identity or attributes of the selfplex, e.g., "I am Helen Stein, I am an internist, I am competent and respected." Such repetition will enhance replication of the desired selfplexes in the brain, and facilitate their regaining control over the sense of self brain areas. Memetic reinforcements in the environment, such as comforting photos and mementos may be also helpful.

Learning self-hypnosis may also provide a sense of mastery over the dissociation susceptibility.

23.2.2 Dissociative Identity Disorder (DID, Multiple Personality Syndrome)

Recognition that we are all multiple personalities at some level may provide the basis for acceptance of the multiple personality aspects within one's brain and pave the way toward a more cooperative selfplexes (see Chapter 11). The task is how to change a culture of successive oppressive authoritarian regimes to one of tolerance for differing and contradictory ideas and democratic power sharing and peaceful regime change in the brain.

Rational discussions concerning the existence of multiple selfplexes and the phenomenon of dissociation, and the need to accept their existence as one's own may lead to a strategy of treatment. Various psychotherapeutic techniques have been used successfully in treating DID – all the successful techniques eventually result in an "integration" of the personalities, or an acceptance of different selfplexes to reside in the brain in a more harmonious way.

Hypnosis is a useful tool in inducing a dissociative state in which tolerance for coexistence of contradictory memes might be achieved as well as in investigating the presence of selfplexes that may be latent.

Some have argued that DID is an iatrogenic disorder that develops in the course of psychotherapy by therapists who are interested in the multiple personalities (Piper and Merskey, 2004; Reinders, 2008). As we are all "multiple personalities" as discussed previously in this chapter, it stands to reason that an emphasis on the differences of the selfplexes can lead to a diagnosis of DID in many "normal" people. Nevertheless, DID patients who seek help indeed suffer from the lack of communication among the different selfplexes, and treatment is often effective. DID may also be accompanied by a more serious syndrome such as PTSD and borderline syndrome – the treatment of the more serious syndrome may also reduce the symptoms of DID.

As proneness to dissociation is associated with childhood abuse and trauma, prevention should play an important role.

23.2.3 Misattribution Syndromes: Conversion, Somatization, Hypochondriasis, Chronic Pain, Fibromyalgia, etc.

A rational discussion concerning how stress, both external and internal memetic, can cause a dysequilibrium in the brain, which may in turn result in a misattribution of the source to a body part, can help the patient to recognize the presence of stress. This can also result in a discussion concerning the physiologic arousal accompanying stress which may further contribute to the distressing symptoms. The role of helplessness and depression should also be explored and discussed.

A careful history will usually reveal the original model for misattribution – e.g., a family member who always had a headache when stressed.

Through this process, the fear that the patient has a serious medical disease can be alleviated, at the same time recognizing that the patient has "real" physically experienced distress because of the brain's processing problems. Then methods can be developed to alleviate the distress through stress management, relaxation, and other broad-spectrum anti-meme therapies (see Chapter 17) as well as specific therapies such as cognitive–behavioral therapy as indicated. Pharmacotherapy may be indicated targeting anxiety and/or depression as well as pain.

23.2.4 Psychosis and Schizophrenia

Persistent psychosis and schizophrenia are major final common pathway syndromes that require both gene- and meme-oriented therapies. Pharmacotherapy is often critical in treating the symptoms of psychosis and standard textbooks of psychiatry should be consulted for details. Broad-spectrum meme-oriented therapies include music, art, exercise, and dance therapies. Also useful are specific therapies geared to enhance positive selfplexes as well as specific problem-solving and coping skill enhancing therapies.

Acutely psychotic patients are hypervigilant and their meme-processing apparatus is flooded with threatening and confusing memes.

In acute psychosis or acute exacerbations of schizophrenia, temporary removal from the stressful memetic environment through hospitalization may be necessary.

Psychoeducation of the patient and family concerning the nature and symptoms of schizophrenia, need for reducing stress, adherence to medications, and follow-up visits is also important.

References

Aybek, S., Kanaan, R. A., David, A. S. (2008) The neuropsychiatry of conversion disorder. *Curr Opin Psychiatry*, **21**, 275–280.

Barsky, A. J., Borus, J. F. (1999) Functional somatic syndromes. *Ann Intern Med*, **130**, 910–921.

Barsky, A. J., Goodson, J. D., Lane, R. S., et al. (1988) The amplification of somatic symptoms. *Psychosom Med*, **50**, 510–519.

Barsky, A. J., Wyshak, G. (1990) Hypochondriasis and somatosensory amplification. *Br J Psychiatry*, **157**, 404–409.

Bell, I. R., Baldwin, C. M., Russek, L. G., et al. (1998) Early life stress, negative paternal relationships, and chemical intolerance in middle-aged women: support for a neural sensitization model. *J Womens Health*, **7**, 1135–1147.

Berrios, G. E., Sierra, M. (1997) Depersonalization: a conceptual history. *Hist Psychiatry*, **8**, 213–229.

Crow, T. J. (1997) Is schizophrenia the price that Homo sapiens pays for language? *Schizophr Res*, **28**, 127–141.

Crow, T. J. (2000) Schizophrenia as the price that homo sapiens pays for language: a resolution of the central paradox in the origin of the species. *Brain Res Brain Res Rev*, **31**, 118–129.

Crow, T. J. (2007) How and why genetic linkage has not solved the problem of psychosis: review and hypothesis. *Am J Psychiatry*, **164**, 13–21.

David, N., Bewernick, B. H., Cohen, M. X., et al. (2006) Neural representations of self versus other: visual-spatial perspective taking and agency in a virtual ball-tossing game. *J Cogn Neurosci*, **18**, 898–910.

Devinsky, O., Morrell, M. J., Vogt, B. A. (1995) Contributions of anterior cingulate cortex to behaviour. *Brain*, **118**(Pt 1), 279–306.

Ehling, T., Nijenhuis, E. R., Krikke, A. P. (2008) Volume of discrete brain structures in complex dissociative disorders: preliminary findings. *Prog Brain Res*, **167**, 307–310.

Forrest, K. A. (2001) Toward an etiology of dissociative identity disorder: a neurodevelopmental approach. *Conscious Cogn*, **10**, 259–293.

Goes, F. S., Sanders, L. L., Potash, J. B. (2008) The genetics of psychotic bipolar disorder. *Curr Psychiatry Rep*, **10**, 178–189.

Iseki, K., Hanakawa, T., Shinozaki, J., et al. (2008) Neural mechanisms involved in mental imagery and observation of gait. *Neuroimage*, **41**, 1021–1031.

Kihlstrom, J. F. (2005) Dissociative disorders. *Annu Rev Clin Psychol*, **1**, 227–253.

Kim, S. E., Kim, J. W., Kim, J. J., et al. (2007) The neural mechanism of imagining facial affective expression. *Brain Res*, **1145**, 128–137.

Kymalainen, J. A., Weisman de Mamani, A. G. (2008) Expressed emotion, communication deviance, and culture in families of patients with schizophrenia: a review of the literature. *Cultur Divers Ethnic Minor Psychol*, **14**, 85–91.

Lewis, D. A., Volk, D. W., Hashimoto, T. (2004) Selective alterations in prefrontal cortical GABA neurotransmission in schizophrenia: a novel target for the treatment of working memory dysfunction. *Psychopharmacology (Berl)*, **174**, 143–150.

Lou, H. C., Nowak, M., Kjaer, T. W. (2005) The mental self. *Prog Brain Res*, **150**, 197–204.

Marom, S., Munitz, H., Jones, P. B., et al. (2005) Expressed emotion: relevance to rehospitalization in schizophrenia over 7 years. *Schizophr Bull*, **31**, 751–758.

Meyer-Lindenberg, A. S., Olsen, R. K., Kohn, P. D., et al. (2005) Regionally specific disturbance of dorsolateral prefrontal-hippocampal functional connectivity in schizophrenia. *Arch Gen Psychiatry*, **62**, 379–386.

Nickl-Jockschat, T., Rietschel, M., Kircher, T. (2008) [Correlations between risk gene variants for schizophrenia and brain structure anomalies.]. *Nervenarzt*, **80**(1), 40–42.

Piper, A., Merskey, H. (2004) The persistence of folly: critical examination of dissociative identity disorder. Part II. The defence and decline of multiple personality or dissociative identity disorder. *Can J Psychiatry*, **49**, 678–683.

Prasad, S. E., Howley, S., Murphy, K. C. (2008) Candidate genes and the behavioral phenotype in 22q11.2 deletion syndrome. *Dev Disabil Res Rev*, **14**, 26–34.

Qiu, J., Li, H., Liu, Q., et al. (2008) Brain mechanism of response execution and inhibition: an event-related potential study. *Neuroreport*, **19**, 121–125.

Raz, A., Fan, J., Posner, M. I. (2005) Hypnotic suggestion reduces conflict in the human brain. *Proc Natl Acad Sci USA*, **102**, 9978–9983.

Reinders, A. A. (2008) Cross-examining dissociative identity disorder: neuroimaging and etiology on trial. *Neurocase*, **14**, 44–53.

Revonsuo, A. (2000) The reinterpretation of dreams: an evolutionary hypothesis of the function of dreaming. *Behav Brain Sci*, **23**, 877–901, discussion 904–1121.

Romanides, A. J., Duffy, P., Kalivas, P. W. (1999) Glutamatergic and dopaminergic afferents to the prefrontal cortex regulate spatial working memory in rats. *Neuroscience*, **92**, 97–106.

Ross, S. E. (1999) "Memes" as infectious agents in psychosomatic illness. *Ann Intern Med*, **131**, 867–871.

Sar, V., Akyuz, G., Dogan, O. (2007) Prevalence of dissociative disorders among women in the general population. *Psychiatry Res*, **149**, 169–176.

Seligman, R., Kirmayer, L. J. (2008) Dissociative experience and cultural neuroscience: narrative, metaphor and mechanism. *Cult Med Psychiatry*, **32**, 31–64.

Sierra, M., Berrios, G. E. (1998) Depersonalization: neurobiological perspectives. *Biol Psychiatry*, **44**, 898–908.

Solms, M. (2000) Dreaming and REM sleep are controlled by different brain mechanisms. *Behav Brain Sci*, **23**, 843–850, discussion 904–1121.

Sullivan, P. F. (2008) Schizophrenia genetics: the search for a hard lead. *Curr Opin Psychiatry*, **21**, 157–160.

van Haren, N. E., Bakker, S. C., Kahn, R. S. (2008) Genes and structural brain imaging in schizophrenia. *Curr Opin Psychiatry*, **21**, 161–167.

Weinberger, D. R. (2005) Genetic mechanisms of psychosis: in vivo and postmortem genomics. *Clin Ther*, **27 Suppl A**, S8–S15.

Chapter 24
Pleasure Spectrum Syndromes (Substance Use/Abuse, Addictions to Substances and Beliefs, Fanaticism)

Contents

24.1 Gene × Meme Interaction, Evolutionary Adaptation, and Syndromes

Pleasure is the motivation for all living activity. Volitional action actively seeks pleasure and avoids unpleasure; nonvolitional autonomic dysfunction may cause unpleasure, which then stimulates the organism to correct the dysfunction.

For humans, there are certain activities that predictably produce pleasure, e.g., a good meal, good company, love, sex, good exercise, engaging in favorite hobbies. The emotion of pleasure seems associated with the dopaminergic activation of the medial forebrain bundle, the ascending mesolimbic ventral tegmental pathway and nucleus accumbens (see Chapter 12).

The dopaminergic and endorphinergic reward pathways of the brain are critical for survival since they provide the pleasure drives for eating, love, and reproduction; these are called "natural rewards" and involve the release of dopamine in the nucleus accumbens and frontal lobes (Comings and Blum, 2000).

Dopamine D2 receptor especially has been implicated in pleasure and reward mechanisms. Pleasure seems to be the net effect of neurotransmitter interaction at the mesolimbic brain region when dopamine is released from the neuron at the nucleus accumbens and interacts with a dopamine D2 receptor. "The reward cascade" involves the release of serotonin, which in turn at the hypothalamus stimulates enkephalin, which in turn inhibits GABA at the substantia nigra, which in turn fine tunes the amount of dopamine released at the nucleus accumbens ("reward site"). This normal mechanism of pleasure works well in most of us.

H. Leigh, *Genes, Memes, Culture, and Mental Illness*,
DOI 10.1007/978-1-4419-5671-2_24, © Hoyle Leigh, 2010

When dopamine is released into the synapse, it stimulates a number of dopamine receptors (D1–D5) which results in increased feelings of well-being and reduced stress.

Release of dopamine and the sensations of pleasure can be produced by "unnatural rewards" such as alcohol, cocaine, methamphetamine, heroin, nicotine, marijuana, and other drugs, and by compulsive activities such as gambling, eating, and sex, and by risk taking behaviors. Since only a minority of individuals become addicted to these substances or behaviors, genetic and epigenetic factors play an important role in such vulnerabilities (Margaron, 2004).

When there is a dysfunction of the brain reward cascade often as a result of genetically influenced hypodopaminergic state, the brain may compensate for the lack of pleasure by seeking an external source of dopaminergic stimulation – e.g., drugs. This may result in multiple drug-seeking behavior as alcohol, cocaine, heroin, marijuana, nicotine, and glucose all cause activation and neuronal release of brain dopamine. Carriers of the DRD2 receptor gene Taq I A1 allele have compromised dopamine D2 receptors and a high risk for multiple addictive, impulsive, and compulsive behavioral propensities, such as severe alcoholism, cocaine, heroin, marijuana and nicotine use, glucose bingeing, pathological gambling, sex addiction, ADHD, Tourette's syndrome, autism, chronic violence, posttraumatic stress disorder, schizoid/avoidant cluster, conduct disorder and antisocial behavior. Blum proposed the term, "reward-deficiency syndrome," to describe the hypodopaminergic trait resulting in the breakdown of the reward cascade due to both multiple genes and environmental stimuli and resultant aberrant behaviors (Blum et al., 2000; Comings and Blum, 2000).

The pursuit of pleasure has obvious value to the organism, i.e., genes. When memes arose, they provided a shortcut for pleasure as imitation of successful behaviors, such as cracking open a shell, was more efficient than trial and error. As memes evolved, they tended to attach themselves to the pleasure-reward mechanism as this is a sure way of ensuring replication. For example, one tends to dwell on pleasant thoughts and memories, and tends to communicate (replicate and spread) them. Eventually, some memes co-opted the pleasure mechanism for their own propagation regardless of the welfare of the genes.

As memes in the brain are sophisticated neuronal connections, they are capable of eliciting subtly different pleasures as in sophisticated cooking. Thus, certain types of meditation or asceticism may produce a different kind of "high" while disavowing ordinary pleasures of life.

Some memes became experts in creating dopamine "high's" to the point of addiction, often at the expense of the genetic needs of the individual, as in gambling and in religious experiences (Comings et al., 2000; Previc, 2006). This may be particularly facilitated in conditions of dissociation (see Chapter 23). In religious fanaticism, the search for this dopamine high may result in killing of the self and/or others (e.g., suicide bombing). Religious memes also attached themselves to the fear-anxiety system of the brain – fear of eternal damnation and suffering. Thus armed with the brain mechanisms of ecstasy and terror, religions suppressed the memes geared to the interests of genes, such as reasoning, and engaged in religious wars for centuries.

Inability to feel pleasure, anhedonia, is often seen in depression and schizophrenia and represents a hypodopaminergic state, usually a result of gene × meme interaction. Memes of painful experiences, fear and anxiety, hopelessness, etc., may all contribute to the blockage of the reward-pleasure system.

In summary, pleasure spectrum disorders represent a dopamine system dysregulation caused by gene × meme interaction. Addictions may occur in individuals with a hypodopaminergic reward-deficiency syndrome. Imitating others getting high with drugs (meme) may be an important component in addictions as well as in religious fanaticism.

Syndromes. Why does the pursuit of pleasure (and reward) become problematic? Is not *everything* we do for pursuit of pleasure?

We may say that if the pleasurable activity does not serve the long-term well-being of the organism or of the society, then it is a problem. Obviously, this statement is meme-driven. From the genetic point of view, any pleasurable activity is evolutionarily driven to be adaptive. Considering whether an activity is good or bad in the long run is a product of memetic processing as are considerations of whether it is good or bad for the society. What I am saying here is that, unlike anxiety-mood spectrum syndromes and attention-cognition spectrum syndromes, pleasure spectrum disorders, with the exception of anhedonia, do not involve immediate gene-mediated suffering but are defined as problematic memetically, i.e., meme-defined disorders. We have seen, nevertheless, that gene × meme interaction is important in causing the hypodopaminergic state that probably underlies many serious addictions.

24.1.1 Substance Use/Abuse

We rely on substances for living – food, water, air. Substances derived from plants and animals have been used since time immemorial in the hopes of relieving pain, obtaining an energy boost, as an aphrodisiac, etc. Some of the substances used in herbal medicine are poisonous in large quantities, but then all prescription drugs we use are poisonous in large quantities. Indians in Peru have chewed on coca leaves for centuries without any ill effects or social taboo, and smoking or ingesting marijuana (bhang) has been widely accepted in India and other parts of Southeast Asia since at least 2000 BCE.

Of course, cocaine and marijuana are illegal substances in the United States, and thus their use is considered problematic though there is no evidence that moderate use causes any harm to the adult organism. Alcohol and tobacco, on the other hand, are legal, but they can be quite addicting, and tobacco in particular is not only highly addicting but is known to be detrimental to physical health in a dose dependent fashion. Caffeine is, of course, legal and widely used for its stimulant effect, but can cause anxiety symptoms, insomnia, and sympathetic hyperarousal if used excessively.

Psychotomemetic substances such as LSD and peyote, and designer drugs such as MDMA (3,4-methylenedioxy-*N*-methylamphetamine, "ecstasy") are illegal substances and thus a problem even if used moderately. On the other hand, the "date rape" drug GHB (gamma-hydroxybutyric acid, "liquid ecstasy," "liquid G") is illegal (schedule I) except when prescribed for cataplexy and narcolepsy as xyrem (schedule III). Prescription drugs are legal unless used illegally, i.e., without prescription for the individual using it. All these substances have in common the fact that they are defined as problems by the society memetically rather than because they are inherently problematic.

24.1.2 Addictions to Substances and Beliefs, Fanaticism

Addiction can be to substances (e.g., alcohol, narcotics, stimulants) or memeplexes that may combine belief and behavior, including rituals (e.g., artistic endeavor, gambling, religion, fanaticism). Addiction represents an extreme of pleasure seeking behavior where the degree of pleasure achieved through the substance or activity (or the unpleasure without it) far outweighs considerations for other genetic and memetic needs of the organism. If an addicted individual is deprived of the addictive substance or activity, there results a state of severe unpleasure representing sudden dopamine withdrawal in the pleasure areas of the CNS discussed above. This may be further augmented by the physiologic withdrawal reactions to the addictive substances themselves, such as alcohol withdrawal and cocaine withdrawal.

As discussed earlier in the chapter, genetic polymorphisms interacting with early environment may contribute to a hypodopaminergic CNS thus resulting in a tendency to seek external augmentation of dopaminergic stimulation through substances or activities. Repeated exposure to addictive agents including substances and belief systems provides the opportunity for the commencement of the self-perpetuating addictive process.

Once established, addiction becomes a compulsion, and blends into obsessive–compulsive disorder (OCD). As with OCD, the obsession and compulsion associated with addiction may be ego-alien and the individual may wish to "get over" them, but find it impossible to do so. Environmental cues such as drinking buddies, drug paraphernalia, and religious symbols and rituals are strong memeplexes supporting and maintaining the addiction.

Are all addictions mental illness? Not necessarily. Some hobbies and even work (workaholism) may be addicting but are hardly illnesses. As with other pleasure spectrum conditions, addiction should be memetically considered a problem when it results in a severe conflict between the genetic needs of the organism and the addictive meme.

24.2 Treatment

Detailed descriptions of detoxification and treatment of specific substances including alcohol, narcotics, stimulants, and other substances are available in appropriate textbooks and are beyond the scope of this book. We will discuss here briefly how distortions of the pursuit of pleasure might be approached.

Memes first arose as they provided a shortcut from trial and error in attaining pleasure first by forming memories of the location of food and the activities that resulted in mating, and then by learning to imitate the behavior and/or appearance of the successful ones. As memes evolved as information, and components of culture, certain memes attached themselves to the pleasure apparatus of the brain *regardless* of the welfare of the organism as a whole. Such memes, in the form of tradition and religion, co-opted the brains to spread and perpetuate themselves often at the expense of individual pursuit of pleasure.

In the meanwhile, for those with genetically influenced hypodopaminergic brain, exogenous substances provided the needed "fix," and drug use also spread as memes.

Mild cases of both instances, such as coffee drinking and "spirituality", are instances of normal pursuit of pleasure.

We discussed that drug use per se is not an illness, but defined to be a problem by society arbitrarily only for certain substances. There are powerful irrational memes that compete with substances for pleasure-giving potential, such as religions and other ideologies and they actively seek to suppress the substances for the sake of their own expansion of power and thus replication. It is such puritanical memes that frown upon and criminalize most pleasure-giving activities including drugs. As with the case of the Prohibition in the United States, crime syndicates prosper and countless violent and nonviolent crimes are committed because drugs are illegal.

Education provides an individual with the ability to analyze and process memes concerned with obtaining pleasure, which includes substances, behaviors, activities, and ideals. An informed populace will choose not to use harmful substances even if they are legal and even marketed. Such a populace will also not become addicted to fanaticisms.

Addictions that are ego-alien and compulsive should properly be considered to be an illness as the individual loses control over the activity even when it is obviously detrimental to his/her immediate health and well-being. The treatment for such illness should be individualized, taking into account the genetic and memetic constitution. It may involve detoxification and rehabilitation, controlled and regulated maintenance of the addiction to avoid withdrawal, or substitutive substances or activity to overcome the hypodopaminergic trait. In all these treatment strategies, broad-spectrum anti-meme therapy and specific meme-oriented therapies may be used to neutralize the strong addictive meme (see Chapters 17 and 18).

References

Blum, K., Braverman, E. R., Holder, J. M., et al. (2000) Reward deficiency syndrome: A biogenetic model for the diagnosis and treatment of impulsive, addictive, and compulsive behaviors. *J Psychoactive Drugs*, **32 Suppl**(i–iv), 1–112.

Comings, D. E., Blum, K. (2000) Reward deficiency syndrome: Genetic aspects of behavioral disorders. *Prog Brain Res*, **126**, 325–341.

Comings, D. E., Gonzales, N., Saucier, G., et al. (2000) The DRD4 gene and the spiritual transcendence scale of the character temperament index, *Psychiatr Genet*, **10**, 185 189.

Margaron, H. (2004) Pleasure: From onthogenesis to addiction. *Subst Use Misuse*, **39**, 1423–1434.

Previc, F. H. (2006) The role of the extrapersonal brain systems in religious activity. *Conscious Cogn*, **15**, 500–539.

Chapter 25
Primary Memetic Syndromes: Eating Disorders, Factitious Disorders, Malingering, Meme-Directed Destructive Behaviors

Contents

25.1 Gene × Meme Interaction, Evolutionary Adaptation, and Syndromes

The conditions in this category are characterized by a strong meme-driven quality. As with any other human behavior and experience, early gene × meme interaction determines the brain state that may be more or less receptive to infusion of destructive memes and more or less vulnerable to a takeover by such memes.

Memetic infection is a normal physiologic process for which the human brain is adapted, just as normal microbial flora take up residence in the human gut and serve an essential function. It is only when there is a conflict between the gene-driven needs of the human organism and the demands of the memes that problems arise. Both genes and memes are replicators and their reproductive drive may be at odds with each other. For example, a sexually repressive meme cannot hope to replicate unless it replicates by infecting more and more brains as an infected person is less likely to reproduce biologically. One solution for such a meme may be to accept sexuality as a necessary sin, which persons are expected to commit, but can still be "saved" if the person "repents" by following the rituals and showing other signs of continuing dedication to the meme.

H. Leigh, *Genes, Memes, Culture, and Mental Illness,*
DOI 10.1007/978-1-4419-5671-2_25, © Hoyle Leigh, 2010

The ability to process incoming memes rationally is an important task of human education, and the more able a person is in this capacity, the less likely is the person to be a victim of later infection by an epidemic meme. Nevertheless, as in viral epidemics, there may be highly infectious memes that will infect even the most immunologically competent individuals. And some such memes may be quite innocuous despite their contagiousness, as in fashion or fads (like the hoola-hoop of the 1950s). Yet, at times they may be quite detrimental to health, such as certain dietary fads and drug use.

Endemic culture of violence in the ghettos is an example of an abundance of toxic memes in geographically segregated areas.

25.1.1 Eating Disorders

Some conditions, such as eating disorders, may start as a mild meme infection, i.e., imitating others, but then may become a final common pathway syndrome in interaction with existing dormant memes (e.g., disparaging selfplex, low self-esteem) and early gene × meme interaction (e.g., 5-HTTLPR *s/s* influenced by childhood abuse – Chapter 14). Once the syndrome develops, the physiologic effects such as of starvation may create or enhance psychiatric symptoms (Zandian et al., 2007).

In the case of anorexia nervosa, a strong distortion in body image coupled with a relentless pursuit of thinness in turn causes metabolic and endocrine changes that may result in further reduction in rational meme processing and perpetuation of the self-destructive behavior. Single nucleotide polymorphisms (SNP) of the brain-derived neurotrophic factor (BDNF) gene have been described in both anorexia nervosa and bulimia nervosa (Dmitrzak-Weglarz et al., 2007; Rybakowski et al., 2007; Sulek et al., 2007). The genetic polymorphism may be associated with personality traits such as persistence and harm avoidance that may predispose the individual to the meme takeover.

Altered pleasure mechanisms in the nucleus accumbens may also underlie eating disorders. After all, eating should be pleasurable for all organisms, so eating disorders may well be classified under pleasure spectrum disorders. The main reason I am discussing them here is that they have an overwhelming memetic component – deliberate pursuit of a distorted body image.

Direct stimulation of the serotonin receptor, 5-HT 4 in nucleus accumbens reduced the physiological drive to eat and increased CART (cocaine- and amphetamine-regulated transcript) mRNA levels in mice. MDMA (ecstasy) seems to stimulate the 5-HT 4 receptors in nucleus accumbens and release CART which results in its appetite suppressant effect (Jean et al., 2007). Memes may also act like MDMA, directly stimulating the serotonin receptors in nucleus accumbens causing appetite suppression.

What is the evolutionary significance of eating disorders? Some have argued that foregoing food and not feeling hungry (and even feeling pleasure without food), coupled with hyperactivity, might have adaptive value at times of scarcity as well as potential competition for mate (Faer et al., 2005; Gatward, 2007; Guisinger, 2003). Meme-induced pursuit of ideal body weight may trigger off an ancient adaptive gene-derived neurobiologic mechanism to deal with food scarcity.

There may be differential genetic polymorphisms between restrictive type of eating disorders and bulimia nervosa. The behaviors of bingeing and purging are strongly memetic as are the perfectionism and body image distortions in anorexia nervosa.

25.1.2 Destructive Meme Infections and Epidemics: Mass Hysteria, Factitious Illness, Suicide, Suicide Bombing, Aggression

We already discussed in Chapter 24 how memes may attach themselves to the brain's pleasure mechanism in the service of their own replication and perpetuation. Memes in the environment may at times acquire overwhelming power and infect the brain massively and take over the meme-processing apparatus and co-opt it for their own replication. Such memes may sweep through a whole population in a frenzy, as in mobilizing for war, religious fanaticism, and mass hysteria. In less virulent form, the memes may simply gain epidemic proportions as fads.

At the individual level, at times of stress, susceptible individuals may unconsciously adopt behaviors, emotions, or symptoms of others to whom they were exposed in earlier life. These may result in factitious symptoms or malingering (Palmer, 2007).

In the case of suicide, there is clear evidence of an infectious nature of the behavior on top of the often coexisting serious pathology such as depression and psychosis. Suicide can thus be considered to be a final common behavior pathway for various mental conditions, including depression, psychosis, neurotic distress, and situational distress. Epidemics and clusters of suicides have been reported, particularly among adolescents. Imitation of suicide depicted in media has also been reported (Gould, 1999, 2001; Gould and Shaffer, 1986; Gould et al., 1988; Phillips and Paight, 1987). In a vulnerable individual, or at times of stress-induced vulnerability, suicide memes may take hold and proliferate, leading to the suicidal behavior.

Suicide bombing is another example of memetic contagion. An upsurge of such terrorist acts often follows another. A recent survey of general population concerning suicide bombing revealed that Suni fundamentalism was associated with increased support for suicide bombing (Kazim et al., 2008). Terrorist groups may serve the function of a "family" for members of the society who lack a sense of belonging. Acts of terrorism may be seen as "propaganda by deed" to recruit members to the family and its beliefs. Terrorism is also instrumental in building a counterterror industry that may have its own culture and pathology (Palmer, 2007).

Aggression is another evolutionarily adaptive neurophysiologic entity common to all animals. Instrumental or purposeful aggression as in attacking a prey or in combat is different from affective or angry aggression in both behavior and physiology.

Conspecific aggression is usually related to establishment of sexual and social dominance and mostly exhibited by males. While physical aggression may have been adaptive in the stone age in achieving social and sexual dominance, physical aggression is memetically suppressed in modern societies which value memetic dominance over physical force. It should be noted, however, that such "civilized" behavior of gentlemen is a recent memetic acquisition in Western societies, and that there are still areas on the globe where physical violence and aggression are widely accepted.

In memetically civilized societies, however, physical violence is often a manifestation of mental retardation, low intelligence, brain damage, or other physical conditions that reduce the effectiveness of the frontal lobes concerned with memetic control of behavior. Certain memetic subcultures and meme infections, as with media violence, may provide a more permissive state for physical violence in susceptible individuals (Cantor, 2000; Mitrofan et al., 2008; Villani, 2001).

25.1.3 Irrational Beliefs and Delusions

Irrational beliefs and delusions may be shared memes within a subculture (e.g., religions, cults). Individuals with inadequate meme-processing abilities are likely to accept irrational and often anti-gene memes (e.g., sexual repression, denial of some forms of pleasure). Some, even though infected with such memes, may be able to set aside the irrational memes, and recognize their irrationality and not allow them to dominate their emotions and behavior. These are normal individuals who recognize that some of their beliefs are irrational, but temporarily and sporadically express allegiance to them for the sake of belonging to the communal activities that are pleasurable. On the other hand, some of the infected individuals may be able to derive pleasure only through means acceptable to the irrational memes, i.e., through loyalty and blind obedience to the group that shares the memes whose only concern is the propagation of the memes (religion, cult, -ism, etc.) themselves. This may lead fanaticism, suicide bombing, etc., as discussed in Chapter 24.

25.2 Treatment

As we discussed earlier, meme infection is a normal and necessary part of human development and acculturation. Only when there is conflict between gene-driven needs and meme-driven needs, and/or when there is conflict among the memes within the brain, including newly arrived ones, will there be symptoms and need for intervention.

As discussed in the previous section, education geared to evaluate and process memes rationally, i.e., in a way compatible with the adaptive gene-driven
requirements, is essential for primary prevention.

Encouraging individuals to utilize critical thinking as opposed to blindly following what is fashionable or "group-think" may be sufficient in dealing with
fads – in fashion, food, religion, or ideology. Insofar as the fad is innocuous, normal individuals may decide that the pleasure it affords outweighs any potential
detriment.

For more chronic syndromes, such as epidemics of fibromyalgia, chemical
sensitivity, and hypoglycemia, the memetic diagnosis connects an internal sense
of distress to an explanatory concept (misattribution). For treatment of these
conditions, see Section 23.1.4.

Eating disorders are memetically driven physiologic aberrations primed by
gene × meme interaction in early life. The first order of business in symptomatic
anorexia nervosa and bulimia is restoration of normal weight and physiology
through tube feeding and medications. Genotyping may be useful as 5-HTTLPR
s/s may be at a higher risk for anorexia nervosa rather than bingeing. In those
with s/s, serotonin reuptake blockers, the usual treatment for anorexia nervosa (and
obsessive–compulsive syndrome), may not be effective (Gorwood, 2004; Murphy
et al., 2004). Olanzapine might be effective in such patients (Dunican and DelDotto,
2007). Bulimia nervosa tends to respond to antidepressants and mood stabilizers
(Berkman et al., 2006; Couturier and Lock, 2007; Ramoz et al., 2007; Reinblatt
et al., 2008; Stefano et al., 2008).

Meme-oriented therapies include various individual psychotherapies, group
therapy, family therapy, and milieu therapy, which have varying degrees of efficacy (Guarda, 2008; Herpertz-Dahlmann, 2009; Herpertz-Dahlmann and Salbach-
Andrae, 2009; Keel and Haedt, 2008). Problems of mentalization, otherwise known
as theory of mind (see Chapters 8 and 11), have been postulated in anorexia nervosa and treatment geared to an understanding of how the body or body image is
representing mental distress has been proposed (Skarderud, 2007a, b, c).

There is clearly a need for a more specific meme-oriented therapy in eating
disorders. Such therapy should first recognize the memetic content of the eating disorder – how the patient perceives herself physically and as a person. Her strivings
should be taken at face value and as belonging to a selfplex. Then, collaboratively
with the therapist, the patient should delineate other selfplexes that may exist, e.g.,
when she was younger, how she imagined herself to be when age X. Then a rational
strategy may be developed to attain the shape and character the patient would like
to be, i.e., a new memetic ego ideal. An avatar utilizing virtual reality may be particularly useful. An avatar is an image of oneself shaped like the person she wants
to be, and seeing herself eat, exercise, and socialize may be an excellent self-model
to imitate.

Malignant meme infections, such as fanaticism, religious or otherwise, are potentially both self-destructive and other destructive, but as the affected are unwilling to
seek help, there is little psychiatry can do for them. Only when they are actually
attempting a criminal act, such as homicide or suicide bombing, could treatment

be attempted. For such criminal acts, the first order of business would be to isolate the fanatic memes from contaminating others, especially those who have not been immunized. Then, isolating them from sources of supportive and sustaining memes, i e , the pleasure connection, should reduce the reproductive power of the malignant memes. Then the educational process of identifying resident memes, and sorting them to constructive and destructive memes could begin. When irrational memes are deprived of their pleasure (dopamine) connection, they are likely to be discarded or replaced with more constructive memes.

Adjunctive general and specific meme-oriented therapies discussed in Chapters 17 and 18 can be used in conjunction with any of the therapies discussed in this chapter.

References

Berkman, N. D., Bulik, C. M., Brownley, K. A., et al. (2006) Management of eating disorders. *Evid Rep Technol Assess (Full Rep)*, **135**, 1–166.

Cantor, J. (2000) Media violence. *J Adolesc Health*, **27**, 30–34.

Couturier, J., Lock, J. (2007) A review of medication use for children and adolescents with eating disorders. *J Can Acad Child Adolesc Psychiatry*, **16**, 173–176.

Dmitrzak-Weglarz, M., Skibinska, M., Slopien, A., et al. (2007) BDNF Met66 allele is associated with anorexia nervosa in the Polish population. *Psychiatr Genet*, **17**, 245–246.

Dunican, K. C., DelDotto, D. (2007) The role of olanzapine in the treatment of anorexia nervosa. *Ann Pharmacother*, **41**, 111–115.

Faer, L. M., Hendriks, A., Abed, R. T., et al. (2005) The evolutionary psychology of eating disorders: Female competition for mates or for status? *Psychol Psychother*, **78**, 397–417.

Gatward, N. (2007) Anorexia nervosa: An evolutionary puzzle. *Eur Eat Disord Rev*, **15**, 1–12.

Gorwood, P. (2004) Eating disorders, serotonin transporter polymorphisms and potential treatment response. *Am J Pharmacogenomics*, **4**, 9–17.

Gould, M. S. (1999) Suicide clusters and media exposure. In *Suicide Over the Life Cycle* (S. Blumenthal and D. Kupfer eds.), pp. 517–532. American Psychiatric Publishing, Inc., Washington, DC.

Gould, M. S. (2001) Suicide and the media. *Ann N Y Acad Sci*, **932**, 200–221, discussion 221–204.

Gould, M. S., Shaffer, D. (1986) The impact of suicide in television movies. Evidence of imitation. *N Engl J Med*, **315**, 690–694.

Gould, M. S., Shaffer, D., Kleinman, M. (1988) The impact of suicide in television movies: Replication and commentary. *Suicide Life Threat Behav*, **18**, 90–99.

Guarda, A. S. (2008) Treatment of anorexia nervosa: Insights and obstacles. *Physiol Behav*, **94**, 113–120.

Guisinger, S. (2003) Adapted to flee famine: Adding an evolutionary perspective on anorexia nervosa. *Psychol Rev*, **110**, 745–761.

Herpertz-Dahlmann, B. (2009) Adolescent eating disorders: Definitions, symptomatology, epidemiology and comorbidity. *Child Adolesc Psychiatr Clin N Am*, **18**, 31–47.

Herpertz-Dahlmann, B., Salbach-Andrae, H. (2009) Overview of treatment modalities in adolescent anorexia nervosa. *Child Adolesc Psychiatr Clin N Am*, **18**, 131–145.

Jean, A., Conductier, G., Manrique, C., et al. (2007) Anorexia induced by activation of serotonin 5-HT4 receptors is mediated by increases in CART in the nucleus accumbens. *Proc Natl Acad Sci U S A*, **104**, 16335–16340.

Kazim, S. F., Aly, Z., Bangash, H. K., et al. (2008) Attitudes toward suicide bombing in Pakistan. *Crisis*, **29**, 81–85.

Keel, P. K., Haedt, A. (2008) Evidence-based psychosocial treatments for eating problems and eating disorders. *J Clin Child Adolesc Psychol*, **37**, 39–61.

Mitrofan, O., Paul, M., Spencer, N. (2008) Is aggression in children with behavioural and emotional difficulties associated with television viewing and video game playing? A systematic review. *Child Care Health Dev*, **35**, 5–15.

Murphy, G. M., Jr., Hollander, S. B., Rodrigues, H. E., et al. (2004) Effects of the serotonin transporter gene promoter polymorphism on mirtazapine and paroxetine efficacy and adverse events in geriatric major depression. *Arch Gen Psychiatry*, **61**, 1163–1169.

Palmer, I. (2007) Terrorism, suicide bombing, fear and mental health. *Int Rev Psychiatry*, **19**, 289–296.

Phillips, D. P., Paight, D. J. (1987) The impact of televised movies about suicide. A replicative study. *N Engl J Med*, **317**, 809–811.

Ramoz, N., Versini, A., Gorwood, P. (2007) Eating disorders: An overview of treatment responses and the potential impact of vulnerability genes and endophenotypes. *Expert Opin Pharmacother*, **8**, 2029–2044.

Reinblatt, S. P., Redgrave, G. W., Guarda, A. S. (2008) Medication management of pediatric eating disorders. *Int Rev Psychiatry*, **20**, 183–188.

Rybakowski, F., Dmitrzak-Weglarz, M., Szczepankiewicz, A., et al. (2007) Brain derived neurotrophic factor gene Val66Met and -270C/T polymorphisms and personality traits predisposing to anorexia nervosa. *Neuro Endocrinol Lett*, **28**, 153–158.

Skarderud, F. (2007a) Eating one's words, part I: 'Concretised metaphors' and reflective function in anorexia nervosa–an interview study. *Eur Eat Disord Rev*, **15**, 163–174.

Skarderud, F. (2007b) Eating one's words, part II: The embodied mind and reflective function in anorexia nervosa–theory. *Eur Eat Disord Rev*, **15**, 243–252.

Skarderud, F. (2007c) Eating one's words: Part III. Mentalisation-based psychotherapy for anorexia nervosa–an outline for a treatment and training manual. *Eur Eat Disord Rev*, **15**, 323–339.

Stefano, S. C., Bacaltchuk, J., Blay, S. L., et al. (2008) Antidepressants in short-term treatment of binge eating disorder: Systematic review and meta-analysis. *Eat Behav*, **9**, 129–136.

Sulek, S., Lacinova, Z., Dolinkova, M., et al. (2007) Genetic polymorphisms as a risk factor for anorexia nervosa. *Prague Med Rep*, **108**, 215–225.

Villani, S. (2001) Impact of media on children and adolescents: A 10-year review of the research. *J Am Acad Child Adolesc Psychiatry*, **40**, 392–401.

Zandian, M., Ioakimidis, I., Bergh, C., et al. (2007) Cause and treatment of anorexia nervosa. *Physiol Behav*, **92**, 283–290.

Chapter 26
Challenges for the Future

Contents

26.1 Genes and Memes – How to Achieve a Peaceful Coexistence

Memes were created by genes in the service of better survival and replication of the organism, i.e., genes. Once memes achieved widespread portability and replicability, however, some memes evolved in a deviant path to come in conflict with the survival and welfare interests of the individual genetic organism, i.e., irrational memes, self-destructive memes.

Mental health may be achieved in a democracy of various memes in the brain which is possible only if the brain possesses the capability to process and manipulate memes in the service of the genetic organism (see Chapter 12). Education is the means through which meme-processing ability is learned and strengthened. An important challenge for the human race is then how to consciously design and implement educational methods specifically designed to enhance the meme-processing ability. This involves exposure to a variety of both salutary and harmful memes and teaching how to evaluate such memes and how to sort and filter incoming memes. Specific techniques of dealing with environments that are flooded with memes detrimental to the interests of the organism must be developed and taught, which may include both broad-spectrum anti-meme procedures such as relaxation and meditation techniques as well as specific anti-meme procedures yet to be developed (see Chapters 17 and 18).

H. Leigh, *Genes, Memes, Culture, and Mental Illness,*
DOI 10.1007/978-1-4419-5671-2_26, © Hoyle Leigh, 2010

Identifying individuals who are vulnerable to infection by detrimental memes through genetic testing and environmental evaluation is another important challenge. Once such individuals are identified in childhood, specific nurturing memetic environments could be provided for them that would mitigate the vulnerability (see Chapter 19).

Models of mental health that show how to deal with conflicting memes and achieve a memetic democracy in the brain should be developed and made available. This could include actual scenarios of conflict resolution, both interpersonal and intrapsychic. The use of avatars in virtual reality might be particularly useful in this regard.

26.2 Need for New Diagnostic and Therapeutic Approaches and Tools

It should be clear that new diagnostic and therapeutic approaches and tools must be developed specifically designed for gene × meme interaction. For example, an inventory of existing memes in the brain and their configuration, i.e., which memeplexes are dominant, and which are dormant, and which are in rebellion with the dominant ones, would be a particularly useful diagnostic tool. For this purpose, computerized meme scans might be developed utilizing such techniques as time-limited free association and word association test. Existing projective tests, such as the Rorschach might be reinterpreted in terms of memetic content and conflicts.

A reclassification of mental illness taking into account the gene × meme interactions, as I have attempted to do in this book, would naturally lead to rational treatment approaches that are both gene- and meme-oriented.

Broad-spectrum anti-meme therapies such as relaxation, massage, music therapy, etc., should be emphasized and practiced more widely in psychiatric treatment settings, not just as an adjunct but as a main procedure in combating noxious meme infections just like broad-spectrum antibiotics in bacterial infections.

Specific meme-oriented therapies geared to neutralizing specific toxic memes must be developed. Such therapies would include infusions of specific neutralizing memes in the form of words, and/or sounds, and/or visual imagery, or combinations thereof. Virtual reality and avatars may be of particular importance in specific memetic therapies. For example, seeing oneself as an avatar with the ability to solve specific memetic and/or meme × gene conflicts would empower the patient to identify with the avatar and imitate it, resulting in the incorporation of the ability meme.

26.3 Testable Hypotheses of Gene × Meme × Environment Interaction

The essence of our model of mental health and illness is that genes do not interact with environment directly, but through memes that enter the brain and are processed by the brain in interaction with and filtered by existing resident memes. The nature and strength of the already existing memes, therefore, modify whether and how environmental stresses are perceived and thus interact with the genes. Some testable hypotheses that arise from this model would include:

1. Documentation of resident memes through meme scan or other means should predict how a specific stressor such as childhood abuse may have resulted in genetic change, i.e., which genes are turned on and off (*epigenesis*). This should be testable through DNA analysis. For example, what specific memes are associated with methylation or acetylation of the serotonin transporter promoter gene (SERT, 5-HTTLPR)? With MAOA? Does the proliferation of specific memes, e.g., suicidal ideation, occur in the presence of specific gene configurations, such as the activation of the 5-HTTLPR *s*?
2. The status of such genetic changes will be accompanied with differential brain and physiologic *arousal patterns to specific meme infusion*. The brain function should be measurable through imaging techniques such as PET and fMRI.
3. Evaluation of *current status of memes* in the brain, i.e., what the dominant memeplexes are, how much conflict or harmony there is between the dominant memeplexes and the nondominant ones, will predict the degree of mental health or illness of the individual.
4. Meme-oriented therapies will result in *changes in brain function*. Broad-spectrum anti-meme therapies should show a generalized change in the meme-processing activity of the brain, while specific meme-oriented therapies will show more specific and subtle changes. These should be demonstrable with imaging techniques.
5. *Immunization* against toxic memes will result in measurable differences in the susceptibility to later infusion of toxic memes.
6. There will be measurable differences in the state of mental health between those with high levels of *education* and thus high levels of meme-processing ability and those with low levels.

26.4   Memes, Social Sciences, and Neuroscience

The concept of memes received mixed, and often hostile, response from experts in such social science disciplines such as anthropology, sociology, and psychology. They claim, often rightly, that existing concepts in their disciplines are adequate in explaining the phenomena at hand without invoking memes.

The hostile attitudes seem to be mostly determined by a sense of stepping on the toes of the social scientists by biology as memes are ultimately based on biological replicators. The contribution of memetics to social sciences is not to usurp existing concepts but to provide an underlying mechanism for them. Just as the laws of physics are not nullified by the discovery of atoms or quantum mechanics, existing concepts in social sciences are not damaged by the concept of memes.

Rather, memes provide the basic mechanism of the interaction between culture and human brains, i.e., how social milieu may affect brains and how brains may affect social milieu.

It is in neuroscience that, I believe, the concept of memes can be most useful as it provides a bridge that connects the perceived environment, memory, and genes. As the quantum theory is most applicable and manifest in the microuniverse of subatomic particles, memes as memory and brain code provide a powerful model of gene × meme × environment interaction in the microcosm of the brain that results in mental health and illness.

26.5 Ethical Considerations

Ethical considerations may arise concerning some of the diagnostic and therapeutic techniques that are directed toward memes and memeplexes. For example, certain specific and general anti-meme therapies might incorporate "brainwashing" techniques. Development of *meme scans* may be seen to be intrusions of privacy.

Just as cutting and excising tissue are intrusive but necessary parts of surgery, some meme-oriented intrusive techniques may be useful provided informed consent is obtained. An ethical dilemma may exist, however, when we posit competing selfplexes, and some of the selfplexes (i.e., parts of the mind) may object to the procedure while others consent. This would be particularly problematic in brains in which memetic democracy, and thus mental health, has not been attained (see Chapters 11 and 12). The solution to this problem may be found in the memetic collaboration between the therapist and the patient that will enhance the selfplex(es) geared toward the needs of the *organism* that is the individual patient.

Our model of the individual as a government of selfplexes is a deterministic model with a large degree of freedom (see Chapter 11). Free will, to the extent that it is the processing of memes representing choices important enough to reach consciousness, is subject to how the selfplexes are configured. In a memetic democracy, its exercise will be the result of a debate of conflicting sides. In an autocracy, free will may not exist as choices may be automatic based on irrational dogmas.

Ethics is itself composed of memeplexes, derived from both genetic evolution and memetic evolution. Unlike certain religious and cultural prescriptions and proscriptions that are runaway proliferations of toxic memes, ethics is universally accepted as serving the interests and needs of both genes and memes.

26.6 Post-human Evolution of Memes

It is with some wistfulness that we see memes, the offspring of our genes, have achieved an evolutionary life of their own in artifacts and cyberspace. Indeed, memes have flown away from the confines of the planet earth as in the voyager interstellar record (see Chapters 8 and 10).

Memes may have achieved, or will shortly achieve, the ability to replicate themselves and evolve independently of humans in both space and cyberspace. Memes may be seen to be a paradigm-shifting evolution of the human race in which genetic evolution, having reached a level of impasse (e.g., the birth canal is too narrow for the increasing size of the head), yields to an alternative mode of evolution in the form of memes. There is, after all, continuity in this as genes and memes are both packets of information, and in a broader sense, genes may be seen to be a subset of memes that are encoded in DNA.

Regardless of the evolutionary future of memes, they are currently mostly in a symbiotic relationship with our genes, and our mental health depends on the successful maintenance of the symbiosis through judicious processing of memes in the interest of ourselves, the result of our individual gene $\times$ meme $\times$ environment interaction.

Index

A

Abuse, 7, 158, 160, 170–171, 174–178, 204, 213, 215, 224, 231, 234, 238, 244, 257, 261–265, 268, 277
Acculturation, 270
Acetylation, 16, 18–19, 213, 277
Acrophobia, 239
ACTH, 14, 145
Active passivity, 204
Acute stress, 12–13, 21, 240, 245, 250
Acute stress disorder (ASD), 12, 160, 171, 223, 224, 237–247
Addiction, 25, 146, 171, 198, 200, 224, 261–265
Adenine, 41, 52–53, 61
Adjustment reaction, 245
Advertising, 20, 39, 209
Aggression, 14, 231–232, 234, 269–270
Ailurophobia, 239
Alcohol, 37, 143–144, 158, 167, 174, 177, 232, 262–265
al-Farabi, 198
Algorithm, 54, 95
Alienist, 3
Allostasis, 11, 20
Allostatic load, 11
Altered state, 135–136
Altruism, 55, 115, 148, 218
Ammonia, 52
Amnesia, 251
Amygdala, 5–6, 12–15, 21, 89, 100–102, 127–128, 131, 144–147, 173, 176, 209, 214, 232, 237–238, 243
Amyotrophic lateral sclerosis, 43
Ancestors, 30, 37–39, 58, 64, 158
Anesthesia, 252
Aneuploid, 63
Anhedonia, 226, 243, 263
Anorexia nervosa, 160, 224, 268–269, 271

Anterior cingulate, 6, 12, 127, 134, 147, 173, 214, 229, 232, 250
Anterior cingulate gyrus, 12–13, 147, 229
Anthropology, 120–122, 277
Antianxiety agent, 245–246
Antidepressant, 6–7, 13, 103, 177–178, 196, 245–246, 271
Antileptons, 51
Antimatter, 51
Antiparticle, 51
Antipsychotic, 4, 196, 235, 246
Antiquarks, 51
Antisocial, 7, 32, 129, 160, 169, 171, 213, 223, 226, 229–235, 262
Antisociali, 169, 226
Antisocial personality, 7, 160, 171, 213, 223, 231–232, 234
Anxiety, 4–8, 12, 14, 26, 32, 128–129, 135, 142, 147, 151, 157, 159–160, 168–173, 181–183, 198, 200, 209, 215, 223, 225–226, 233, 237–247, 253, 256–257, 262–263
Anxiety-mood spectrum syndrome, 237–247
Arachnophobia, 239
Archaea, 55–56, 79
Archean, 52, 56, 79–80
Archean period, 52
Artificial selection, 59
Asset, 168, 170–171, 173–174, 176
Ataques de nervios, 26–27
Ataxia, 252
Atheoretical, 166
Attention, 7, 14, 100, 102–103, 113, 131–133, 169, 181, 188, 196–200, 205, 215, 229–234, 237–239, 243, 250, 253, 263
Attention-cognition, 160, 171, 223, 226, 229–235, 263

H. Leigh, *Genes, Memes, Culture, and Mental Illness*,
DOI 10.1007/978-1-4419-5671-2, © Hoyle Leigh, 2010

Lightning Source UK Ltd.
Milton Keynes UK
UKOW020216081111

181640UK00004B/62/P